DIAGNOSTIC AND OPERATIVE HYSTEROSCOPY: A TEXT AND ATLAS

Diagnostic and Operative Hysteroscopy: A Text and Atlas

MICHAEL S. BAGGISH, M.D.
Professor and Chairman
Department of Obstetrics and Gynecology
State University of New York
  Health Science Center
Chief, Obstetrics and Gynecology
Crouse-Irving Memorial Hospital
Syracuse, New York

JACQUES BARBOT, M.D.
University Paris V and VI
Ancien Interne des Hopitaux de Paris
Chef de Service Adjoint Hopital de Courbevoie
Hopital Marcelin-Berthelot-Courbevoie
Hopital St. Jacques
Paris, France

RAFAEL F. VALLE, M.D.
Associate Professor of Obstetrics and Gynecology
Northwestern University Medical School
Attending Physician
Prentice Women's Hospital and Maternity Center
Northwestern Memorial Hospital
Chicago, Illinois

YEAR BOOK MEDICAL PUBLISHERS, INC.
CHICAGO • LONDON • BOCA RATON

3 4 5 6 7 8 9 0 93 92 91 90 89

Library of Congress Cataloging-in-Publication Data

Baggish, Michael S.
    Diagnostic and operative hysteroscopy: a text and atlas / Michael S. Baggish, Rafael F. Valle, Jacques Barbot.
        p.   cm.
    Includes bibliographies and index.
    ISBN 0-8151-0460-X
    1. Hysteroscopy.   2. Hysteroscopy—Atlases.   I. Valle, Rafael F.   II. Barbot, Jacques.   III. Title.
    [DNLM: 1. Endoscopy—atlases.   2. Uterine Diseases—diagnosis—atlases.   3. Uterine Diseases—therapy—atlases.   4. Uterus—atlases.   WP 17 B144h]
RG304.5.H97B34   1989
618.1′407545—dc19
DNLM/DLC   88-27672
for Library of Congress   CIP

Sponsoring Editor: James Ryan
Associate Managing Editor, Manuscript Services: Deborah Thorp
Project Manager: Carol Reynolds
Proofroom Manager: Shirley E. Taylor

This book is dedicated with love and admiration to our mothers, who made this all possible:

Sylvia Zachariah Baggish
Yvonne Louise Barbot
Beatriz Valle Valle

CONTRIBUTORS

LESLIE AREY, PH.D, SC.D., L.L.D. (DECEASED)
Professor Emeritus of Cell Biology and Anatomy
Northwestern University Medical School
Chicago, Illinois

SHAWKY Z. A. BADAWY, M.D.
Professor, Department of Obstetrics and Gynecology
Director of Reproductive Endocrinology
State University of New York, Health Science Center
Crouse Irving Memorial Hospital
Syracuse, New York

MICHAEL S. BAGGISH, M.D.
Professor and Chairman
Department of Obstetrics and Gynecology
State University of New York
Health Science Center
Crouse-Irving Memorial Hospital
Syracuse, New York

JACQUES BARBOT, M.D.
University Paris V and VI
Ancien Interne des Hopitaux de Paris
Chef de Service Adjoint Hopital de Courbevoie
Hopital Marcelin-Berthelot-Courbevoie
Hopital St. Jacques
Paris, France

FRED M. GARDNER, PH.D.
Professor of Physics
University of Hartford
West Hartford, Conneticut

DORIS LAUREY, R.N.
Team Leader, Laser Service
Crouse Irving Memorial Hospital
Syracuse, New York

W. DWAYNE LAWRENCE, M.D.
Associate Professor of Pathology
Wayne State University School of Medicine
Chief of Anatomic Pathology
Hutzel Hospital
Detroit, Michigan

JACK M. LOMANO, M.D.
Clinical Assistant Professor
Ohio State University
Director of Education and Development
Grant Laser Center
Columbus, Ohio

JANICE E. LUKE, R.N., B.S.N.
Head Nurse, Urology/Gynecology
State University of New York
Health Science Center
Syracuse, New York

CHARLES M. MARCH, M.D.
Professor, Department of Obstetrics and Gynecology
University of Southern California School of Medicine
Los Angeles, California

JOHN L. MARLOW, M.D.
Director, Continuing Medical Education
Columbia Hospital for Women Medical Center
Assistant Professor
Department of Obstetrics and Gynecology
George Washington University School of Medicine
Assistant Clinical Professor
Department of Obstetrics and Gynecology
Georgetown University School of Medicine
Washington, D.C.

BEVERLY MAYETTE, R.N.
Team Leader, Gynecologic Operating Room
Crouse Irving Memorial Hospital
Syracuse, New York

LUCA MENCAGLIA, M.D.
Professor of Obstetrics and Gynecology
Institute of Obstetrics and Gynecology
University of Perugia
Perugia, Italy

ROBERT S. NEUWIRTH, M.D.
Professor of Obstetrics and Gynecology
College of Physicians and Surgeons
Columbia University
Director of Obstetrics and Gynecology
St. Luke's-Roosevelt Hospital Center
New York, New York

ANTONIO PERINO, M.D.
Associate Professor
Department of Obstetrics and Gynecology
University of Palermo
Palermo, Italy

THEODORE P. REED III, M.D.
Clinical Professor of Obstetrics and Gynecology
Thomas Jefferson University
Associate Director of Obstetrics and Gynecology and
  Residency Education
Union Memorial Hospital
Baltimore, Maryland

ROBERT E. SCULLY, M.D.
Professor of Pathology
Harvard Medical School
Pathologist, Massachusetts General Hospital
Boston, Massachusetts

MARGARET A. THOMPSON, Ph.D
Assistant Professor
Department of Obstetrics and Gynecology
State University of New York
Health Science Center
Syracuse, New York

RAFAEL F. VALLE, M.D.
Associate Professor of Obstetrics and Gynecology
Northwestern University Medical School
Attending Physician
Prentice Women's Hospital and Maternity Center
Northwestern Memorial Hospital
Chicago, Illinois

FOREWORD

Hysteroscopy has now become both an exciting and an indispensable part of modern gynecology. This is due in part to technical advances in endoscopy but is also due to the fact that the contemporary practitioner desires to obtain the most direct information on uterine pathology in the shortest possible time and with minimal risk and cost to the patient. Hysteroscopy thus provides accuracy for intrauterine diagnosis at a level unequaled by any other diagnostic procedure, and is certainly less traumatic than traditional methods of uterine sampling or radiological visualization. Evolving techniques of hysteroscopy also allow for the performance of both simple and advanced intrauterine surgery with impressive results, often avoiding the risk and expense of laparotomy. Diagnostic and operative hysteroscopy have added important new horizons for the diagnosis and treatment of intrauterine disease.

Hysteroscopy has intrigued gynecologists for over a century, but initial attempts to visualize the interior of the uterus either failed or were frequently inadequate because of primitive instruments and the inability to properly distend the muscular walls of the uterus. A particular problem facing the pioneers in this field was the fact that it was often difficult to traverse the internal os in an atraumatic fashion. Dilatation and manipulation often created stretching of the endocervical and endometrial tissues with associated bleeding and concomitant impairment of clear visualization, which is so essential in diagnostic procedures. With the advent of fiberoptic instrumentation with improved lens systems and telescopes, and the ability to traverse the endocervical canal atraumatically and to distend the uterine cavity using either viscous solutions or aqueous fluids administered under pressure, or with the use of carefully controlled carbon dioxide insufflation, the era of modern hysteroscopy evolved.

As interest developed in hysteroscopy as a useful tool in clinical practice, technical developments quickly followed. These included the development and introduction of contact hysteroscopy as well as the development and introduction of several microhysteroscopes that have made office hysteroscopy a truly practical, safe, and convenient technique, complementing the now traditional procedures for panoramic intrauterine visualization. Presently, we are seeing an expanded enthusiasm on the part of both clinicians and manufacturers for the development of new operative hysteroscopes with improved mechanical instrumentation, as well as with laser capability.

This volume fills an important void in the field of hysteroscopy. It is not only a thorough presentation of current techniques and a clear appraisal of the instrumentation available, but it is also a review of the embryology, anatomy, physiology, and pathology of the uterus, with particular emphasis on those items that relate directly to hysteroscopy. The technique of hysteroscopy is a skill-based technique and requires careful attention to detail as well as patience and practice. This volume provides the reader with all of the background information necessary to learn basic hysteroscopy and to prepare for operative procedures, and to be in a position to take advantage of new developments as they appear. There are many new techniques on the endoscopic horizon that will undoubtedly find a place in the hysteroscopic armamentarium of the future, and these techniques of embryoscopy, hysteroscopic sterilization, and laser hysteroscopy are not neglected in this volume. This volume, therefore, provides the reader with not only the fundamentals to learn hysteroscopy but with the background material to allow for growth and development as the field advances.

The editors of this textbook and atlas of hysteroscopy, along with the contributors, are all experts who have been personally involved in the development of hysteroscopic techniques. All are writing from personal experience with endoscopy and are presenting the state of the art of gynecologic endoscopy. It is my belief that this volume will be an important and a classic landmark in the history of uterine endoscopy.

Hysteroscopy has already assumed an important place in gynecologic practice. As stated earlier, as a diagnostic technique, hysteroscopy affords a high level of accuracy in detecting intrauterine conditions that may not be revealed by other methods. In modern gynecologic practice, hysteroscopy is indicated whenever intrauterine disease is suspected and whenever the clinician is considering intervention. With the expansion of the technique and the availability of sophisticated instruments for ambulatory hysteroscopy in the office setting and for specialized operative procedures, new high standards for gynecology have appeared. This volume presents those new areas to the reader in a most informative and comprehensive fashion.

This is the state of the art of modern hysteroscopy.

JOHN J. SCIARRA, M.D., Ph.D.
Professor and Chairman
Department of Obstetrics and Gynecology
Northwestern University
Chicago, Illinois

PREFACE

The idea for a book about hysteroscopy was conceived in 1981. At that time, substantial interest was evident relative to techniques of modern contact hysteroscopy and it was believed that a descriptive atlas dedicated to this subject would be most timely. Work on the atlas began in earnest during 1982 and an extensive number of slides and photographs were collected.

As the work proceeded it became obvious that the scope of the subject matter was too limited. Analysis of questions raised by participants at seminars and workshops indicated a definite need for a more thorough treatment of hysteroscopy. Therefore, the planned atlas was altered so as to cover panoramic as well as contact hysteroscopy. Year Book Medical Publishers contracted for the manuscript; additional pictures were steadily accumulated and a brief accompanying text was written.

By 1985, the gynecologic community recognized the real benefits of diagnostic and operative hysteroscopy and the number of teaching seminars burgeoned to meet the demand of those wishing to learn these endoscopic techniques. Perceptive individuals within the specialty had in fact predicted that hysteroscopy would become our major endoscopic focus during the 1980s. Once more the subject matter for the book was scrutinized to update and to satisfy the needs of those individuals wishing to learn and practice uterine endoscopy. On this occasion a decision was made to broaden the appeal of the book by combining the extensive photographs and illustrations with an equally comprehensive text. The number of chapters doubled as a result of this formulation. The format evolved to follow the pattern of an ideal instructional seminar which would have limitless time as well as exceptional faculty available to teach it.

We have endeavored in the following pages to present not only an expansive tour de force about hysteroscopy, but also an easily readable book encompassing detailed information about the uterus itself. To this end, the early chapters deal with gross anatomy, embryology, histology, physiology, and pathology of this organ.

Logically, the initial section of the book also includes important chapters dealing with the history of hysteroscopy and optical physics. The next section continues in a step-by-step fashion, building on the knowledge gained in previous chapters, and covers the basic rudiments of instrumentation, distending media, and maintenance of equipment. The third section opens with a chapter entitled "How to Learn Hysteroscopy" and continues with subgroupings of specific methodology. The fourth section considers hysteroscopic diagnosis and a comparison between hysteroscopy and hysterography. The fifth section is devoted to operative hysteroscopy and the sixth section to specialized operative techniques including hysteroscopy during pregnancy. Finally, the last three chapters consider photography, the future, and how to establish a hysteroscopy program.

As can be readily seen this book is a joint venture in every sense of the word. The editors have not compromised quality especially in the selection of contributory authors. Only the best and uniquely qualified experts were selected to participate. In several sections vital subjects were singled out for more complete coverage. These strategic chapters emphasize areas that we consider significantly important areas for future growth.

Pictures and illustrations comprise a substantial portion of this book. Whenever possible, color plates have been selected to detail hysteroscopic findings and to demonstrate operative manipulations. Halftone and line drawings are used to illustrate aspects that would otherwise not be possible to show in photographs or that could be more emphatically demonstrated by pen and ink.

We wish to recognize Mr. Jose Ruiz for his exceptional artistic talent as well as his calm countenance in the face of sometimes less-than-reasonable demands.

We express our gratitude to the secretarial staff for their industry and unending patience, but especially for their typing and transcribing skills. This untiring group includes: Emilie Welch, Jackie Kinney, Emily Stamm, Maria Burgess.

The administrative skills and editing expertise of Paula Belofsky deserve special thanks. Finally, we appreciate the contributions of those at Year Book: the continuous faith and encouragement of Jim Ryan, the sponsoring editor of this book, and the expert advice of Deborah Thorp and Carol Reynolds.

The following hysteroscopy instrument companies have closely cooperated with the editors by providing photographs of their equipment for inclusion in this volume: Bryan Corporation, Woburn, Mass.; Ciron ACMI, Santa Barbara, Calif.; Cabot Medical, Langhorne, Pa.; Weck Instrument Company, Chicago, Ill., Olympus, Lake Success, New York; Karl Storz, Culver City, Calif.; and Richard Wolf, Rosemont, Ill.

Michael S. Baggish, M.D.
Jacques Barbot, M.D.
Rafael F. Valle, M.D.

CONTENTS

COLOR PLATES

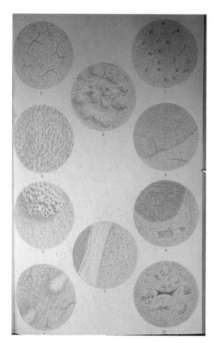

PLATE 1.—Drawings of Charles David illustrating lesions that he observed: normal uterine cavity; mucoid polyp; fibroma; cancer of corpus; uterus didelphis; uterus after normal delivery; placental retention; and uterine perforation.

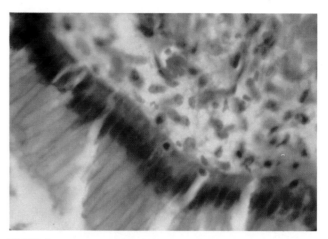

PLATE 3.—Detail of endocervical mucous epithelium.

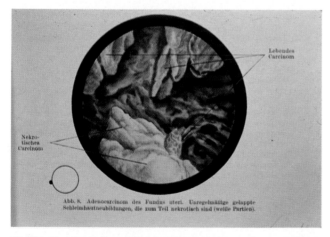

PLATE 2.—Adenocarcinoma of the uterus as seen by Gauss and painted by Heinrich Hoheiser-Neisse.

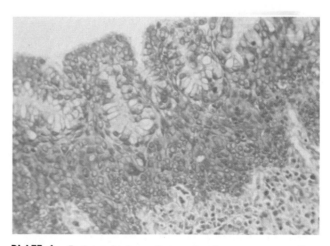

PLATE 4.—Endocervical papillae and surface mucus-secreting epithelium with extensive squamous metaplasia.

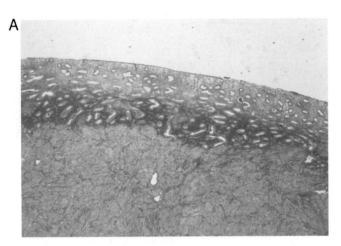

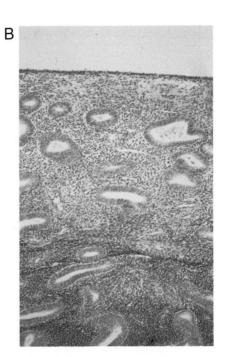

PLATE 5.—**A** and **B,** resurfacing stage (days 6 to 8) of the menstrual cycle.

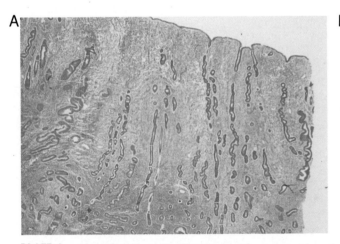

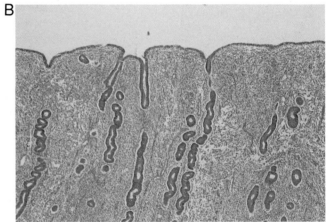

PLATE 6.—**A** and **B,** late proliferative stage of the menstrual cycle (days 12 through 14).

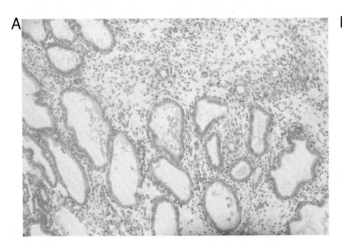

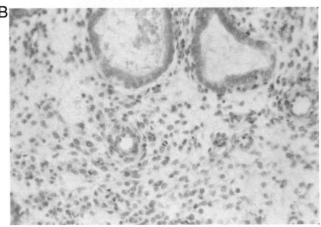

PLATE 7.—**A** and **B,** secretory stage of the cycle (day 23).

A

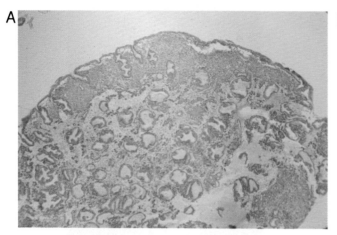

B

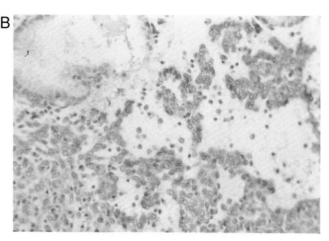

PLATE 8.—A, photomicrograph (early stage) showing initial breakup of the endometrium. **B,** detail of clumped stroma, in-flammatory cells, and disintegrating glands typical of endometrium during menstruation.

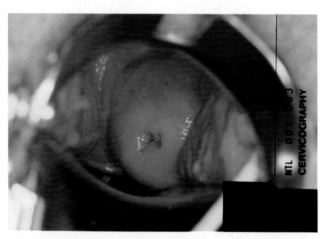

PLATE 9.—The cervix projects into the vagina in a slightly posterior direction. The external os is evident. The upper extent of the vagina is divided into four fornices.

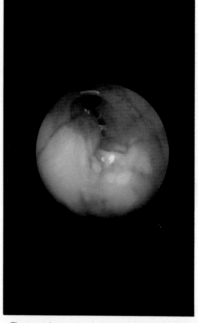

PLATE 10.—The endocervical mucosa as seen in panoramic hysteroscopy shows numerous folds and clefts. The mucosa is light pink and usually fills the area around the internal os.

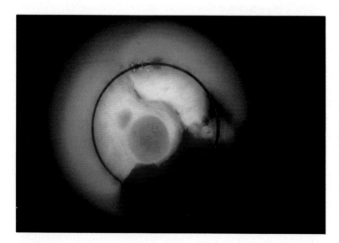

PLATE 11.—Small retention cysts may also be seen in the normal endocervical canal.

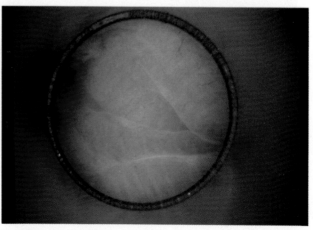

PLATE 12.—The uterine walls are closely applied, and the cavity is more potential than real. Proliferative endometrium, as seen on contact hysteroscopy, is almost translucent with fine vessels.

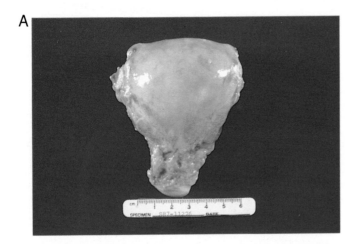

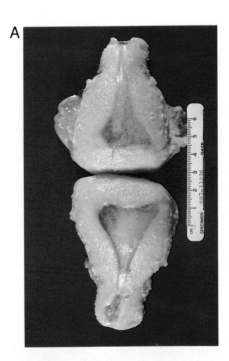

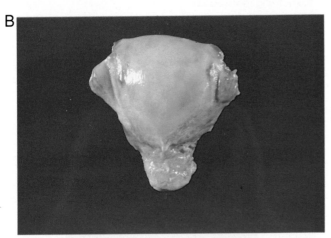

PLATE 13.—**A,** the convex posterior wall of the uterus is covered with peritoneum. **B,** the anterior aspect of the uterus is flattened. Two thirds of its surface is covered with peritoneum which reflects from the upper portion of the urinary bladder.

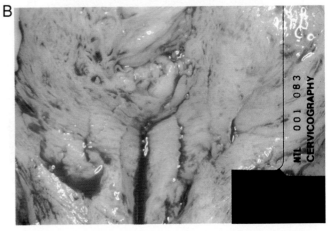

PLATE 14.—**A,** the endometrium appears orange-tan and varies in thickness depending on the phase of the menstrual cycle. The myometrium is four to five times thicker than the endometrium. **B,** magnified view of the opened uterus. The large and numerous myometrial vessels are apparent.

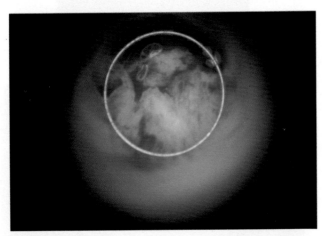

PLATE 15.—Secretory endometrium as viewed by contact hysteroscopy. The mucosa has a reddish hue and is polypoid.

A

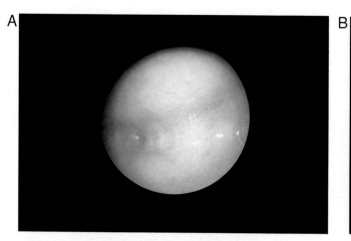

B

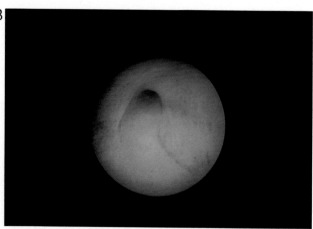

PLATE 16.—A, the tubal ostium is recessed and appears as a small, round opening at the terminal extremity of the cornu. **B,**

magnified detail of tubal ostium.

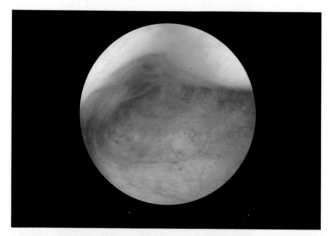

PLATE 17.—Submucosal endometrial capillaries form a netlike pattern. The endometrium has a rich vascular supply and bleeds with the slightest trauma.

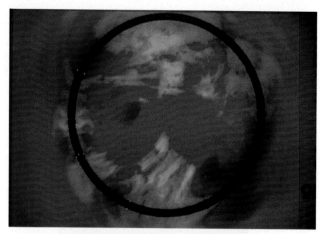

PLATE 18.—Contact hysteroscopy may reveal small holes or diverticula in the otherwise intact endometrium.

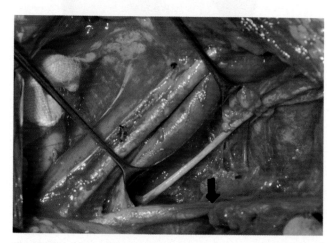

PLATE 19.—The uterine artery arises from the hypogastric artery (seen lateral to the ureter) *(arrow).*

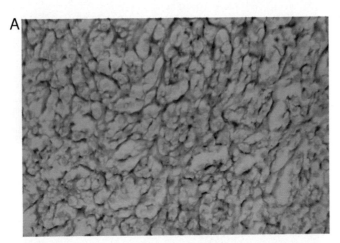

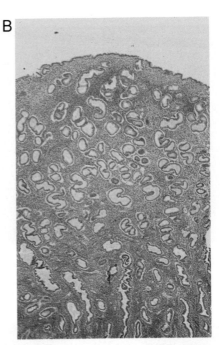

PLATE 20.—**A,** the endometrial glands and stroma are surrounded by a structural reticulum network. This section (reticulum stain) illustrates the basket weave pattern of these fibers. **B,** the endometrium is divided into a static portion, the basalis, and a functioning portion. The latter varies in thickness during the proliferative and secretory phases of the menstrual cycle.

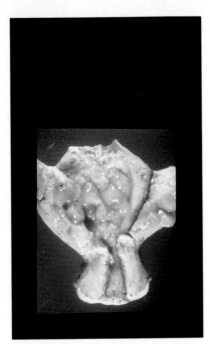

PLATE 21.—Secretory phase. The endometrium is yellow-white, glistening, and polypoid. Microscopic examination revealed this endometrium to be at day 19 of the cycle.

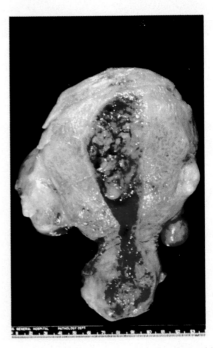

PLATE 22.—Endometrial hyperplasia. The endometrial cavity is occupied by thickened, irregularly polypoid, yellow-tan tissue without evidence of necrosis.

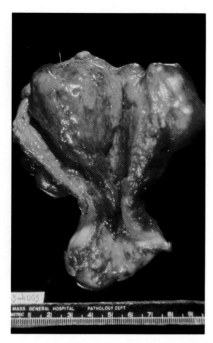

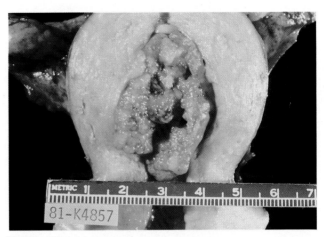

PLATE 25.—Endometrial adenocarcinoma. The endometrial cavity is occupied by a bulging, irregularly polypoid tumor with a pebbly surface. Opaque yellow foci are visible.

PLATE 23.—Endometrial polyp. Virtually the entire endometrial cavity is occupied by a large, broad-based, sessile polyp; ×13.

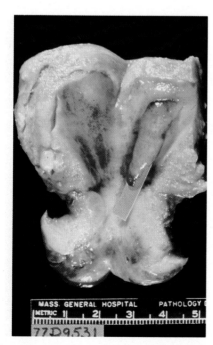

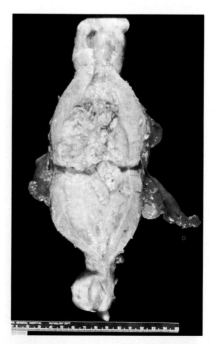

PLATE 26.—Endometrial adenocarcinoma. The anterior and posterior endometrial surfaces are occupied by yellow-tan, irregularly piled-up tumor, which terminates abruptly at the internal cervical os.

PLATE 24.—Endometrial polyp. An elongated slender polyp is attached to the fundus and extends to the internal cervical os. The surrounding endometrium appears flattened and atrophic.

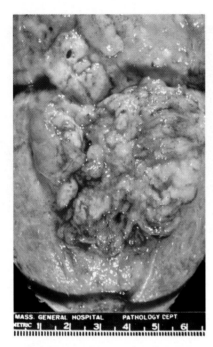

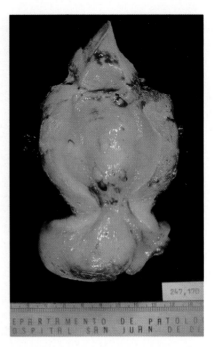

PLATE 27.—Higher magnification of tumor in Plate 26 shows the opaque, pale-yellow, irregularly polypoid surface of the tumor.

PLATE 29.—Low-grade stromal sarcoma (endolymphatic stromal myosis). Tumor bulges into the endometrial cavity and may be seen as worm-like extensions protruding from the vessels within the myometrium.

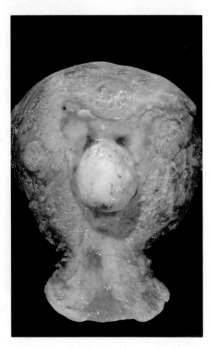

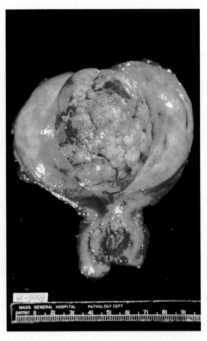

PLATE 28.—Submucosal leiomyoma. The tumor forms a pedunculated rounded mass attached to the endometrium by a short broad pedicle.

PLATE 30.—Malignant müllerian mixed tumor; homologous (carcinosarcoma). A large polypoid mass distends the edometrial cavity.

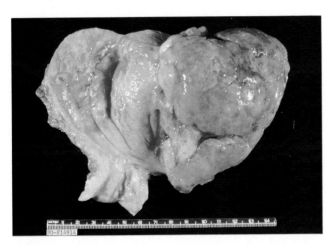

PLATE 31.—Malignant müllerian mixed tumor; heterologous. The large polypoid tumor exhibits extensive areas of yellow to green necrotic tissue.

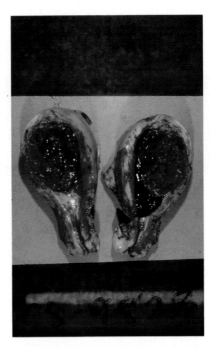

PLATE 32.—Choriocarcinoma. The endometrial cavity is filled with soft, markedly hemorrhagic tumor.

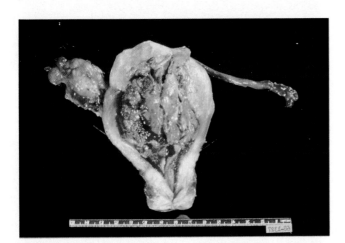

PLATE 33.—Placental polyp. The endometrial cavity contains soft, polypoid, yellow-red tissue.

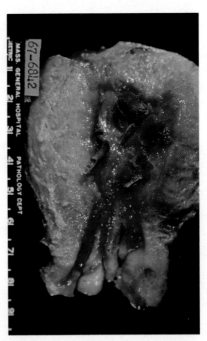

PLATE 34.—Irregular yellow-brown fragments of bone are embedded within the endometrium. A fragment protruding from the endometrium in the left portion of the photograph has a tubular configuration.

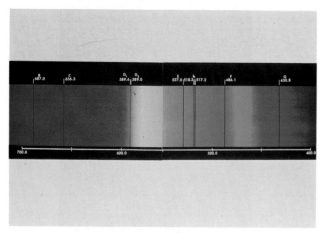

PLATE 35.—The white light visible spectrum, extending from wave lengths of approximately 400 to 750 μm.

A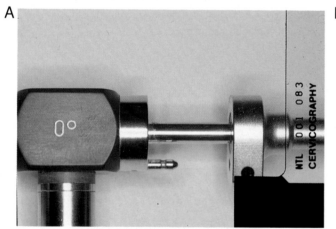

B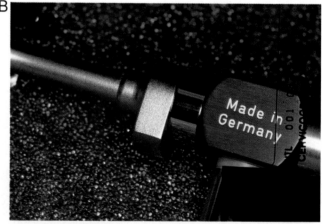

PLATE 36.—**A,** the interlock between the telescope and sheath should engage quickly and smoothly. **B,** when completely en-gaged the telescope/sheath interface should not leak.

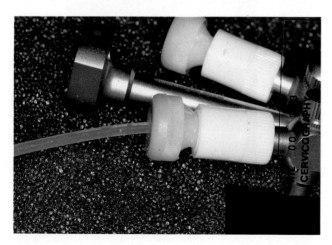

PLATE 37.—Leaf gaskets cannot slip off or leak. They have Luer-lock type of attachment to the operating channels.

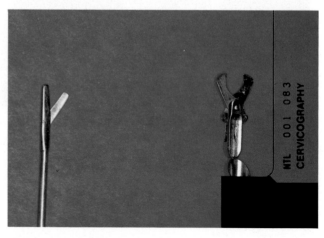

PLATE 38.—Close-up comparison between semirigid and heavier rigid scissors.

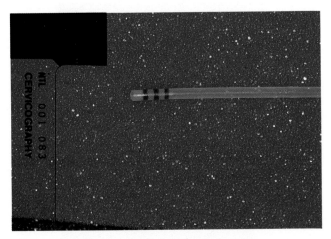

PLATE 39.—Terminus of aspirating cannula. Bands at the end of the cannula are 1 mm apart and may also serve as a measuring device.

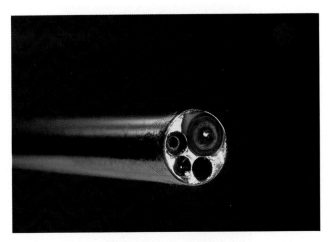

PLATE 40.—Baggish dual operating sheath.

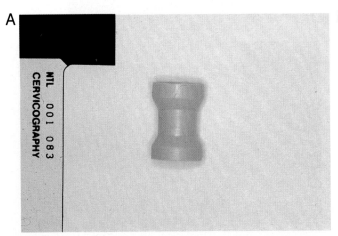

A

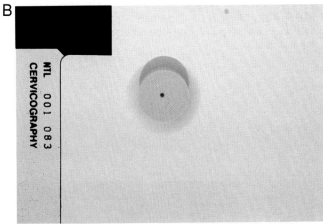

B

PLATE 41.—**A,** standard urologic-type nipple which slips over the operating channel stopcock valve. **B,** the appropriate nipple has a pinpoint opening.

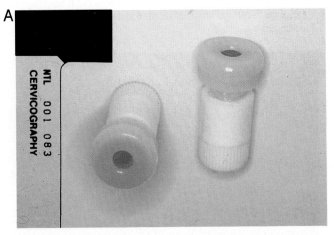

A

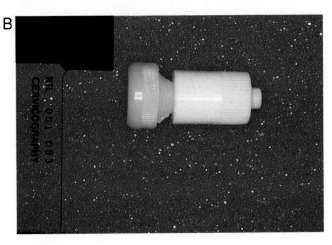

B

PLATE 42.—**A,** new leaf-type plug attaches directly to operating channel(s). **B,** the Luer-type fitting precludes slipping and/or leakage.

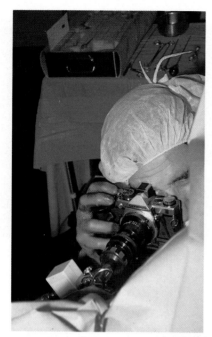

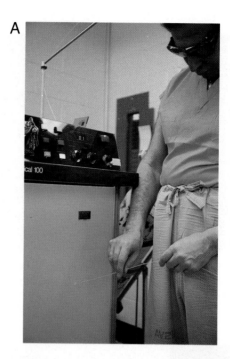

PLATE 43.—Olympus OM-2 camera with special adaptor is attached to the hysteroscope. A flash cube is seen to the left of the camera.

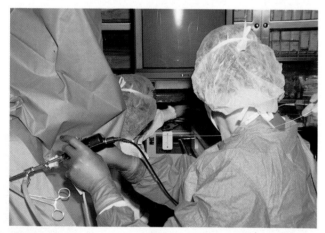

PLATE 44.—Operative hysteroscopy is performed indirectly by viewing the video monitor. Note the operator sits upright rather than crouched.

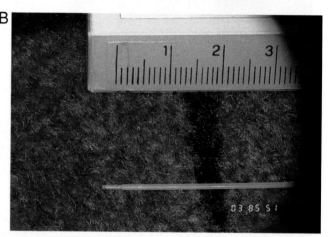

PLATE 45.—**A,** laser light is conducted by means of a fiber which can be introduced through the operating channel of the hysteroscope. The Nd-YAG beam is not visible but is targeted by the orange-red helium neon beam. **B,** closeup of 600-μm quartz fiber for Nd-YAG laser.

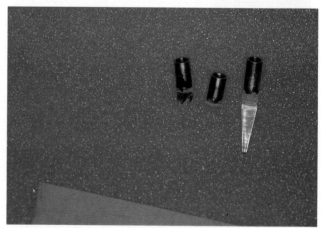

PLATE 46.—Sapphire lenses focus the Nd-YAG laser beam to a fine point but must maintain contact with the tissue.

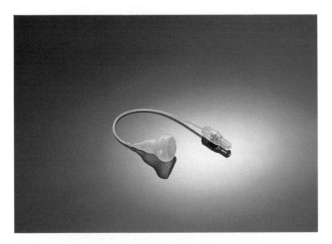

PLATE 47.—A specially designed intrauterine balloon may be inflated to control bleeding after operative hysteroscopy.

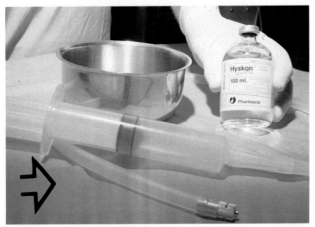

PLATE 48.—A large-bore connecting tube *(arrow)* is interposed between the fluid-filled syringe and the hysteroscope sheath.

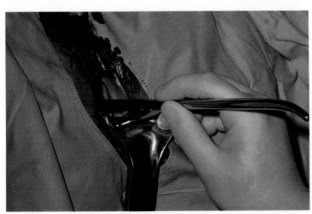

PLATE 49.—Dilatation of the cervix may be necessary. Pratt dilators lubricated with Hyskon are the least traumatic instruments with which to accomplish this maneuver.

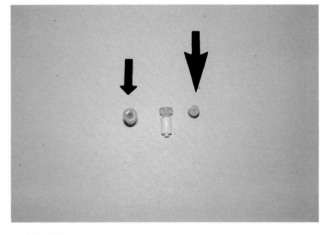

PLATE 50.—A nipple *(large arrow)* or Luer-lock leaf gasket *(small arrow)* should be placed over the operative channel port to prevent leakage.

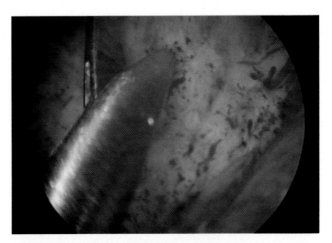

PLATE 51.—A semirigid scissors has been inserted through the operating channel and is seen within the uterine cavity. The scissor blade is opened on the left. The shaft of the scissors appears larger because it is closer to the lens of the telescope.

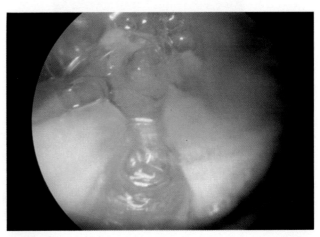

PLATE 52.—A groove has been placed in the endometrium (posterior wall) by the pressure of the hysteroscope.

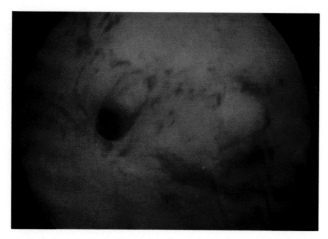

PLATE 53.—The hysteroscope has been brought close to the tubal ostium. Particles of blood are flowing toward the opening.

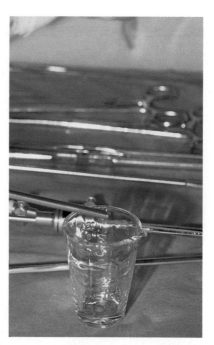

PLATE 55.—Prior to inserting the endoscope into the uterus, the Hyskon is flushed through the system to eliminate air bubbles.

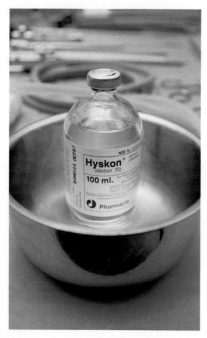

PLATE 54.—Hyskon or 32% dextran is a crystal-clear fluid with the consistency of honey. As illustrated here, it is packaged in 100-cc vials.

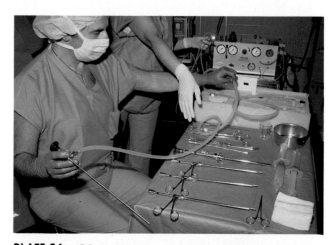

PLATE 56.—CO_2 medium is clearly advantageous for diagnostic hysteroscopy using the 5-mm diagnostic sheath.

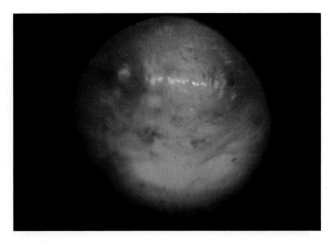

PLATE 59.—Atrophic endometrium in a postmenopausal woman.

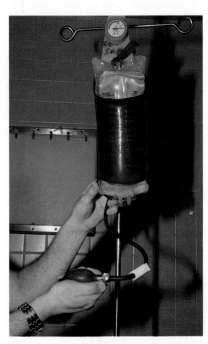

PLATE 57.—Sterile water or saline is available in any operating suite in 500-, 1,000-, and 3,000-cc bags.

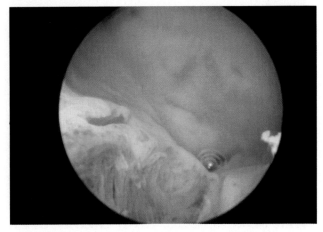

PLATE 60.—Close-up view of a secretory endometrium.

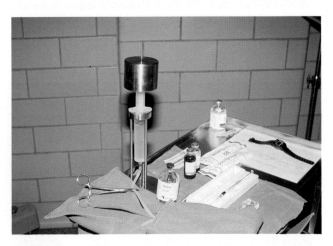

PLATE 58.—A rather simple Hyskon pump consisting of a weight engaged onto the plunger of a plastic syringe.

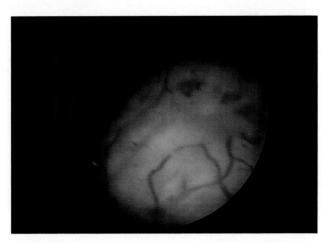

PLATE 61.—Submucous myoma. Note the surface vessels and its projection into the uterine cavity.

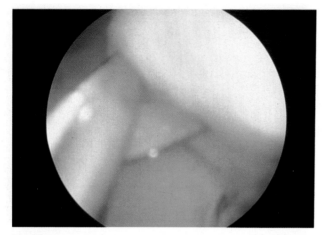

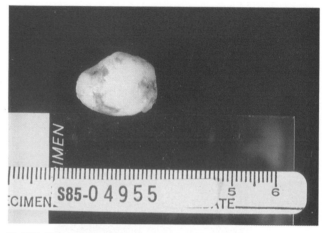

PLATE 62.—The scissors pushes the myoma upward to gain access to the pedicle.

PLATE 63.—The specimen shown in Plates 61 and 62, after excision and removal.

A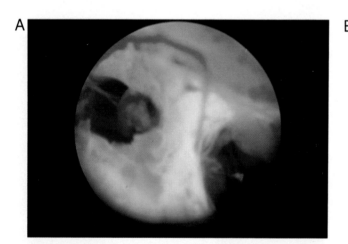

B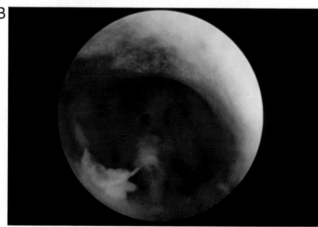

PLATE 64.—**A,** hysteroscopy showing "curtain-like" adhesions connecting the anterior and posterior uterine walls. **B,** uterine

cavity dissected free of adhesions.

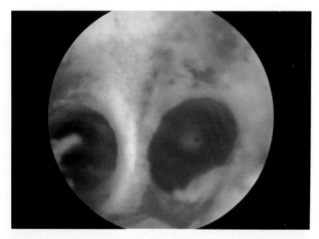

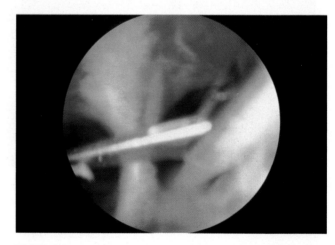

PLATE 65.—Complete uterine septum as viewed from the internal os of the cervix.

PLATE 66.—Panoramic view of hysteroscopically guided division of the septum (see Plate 65).

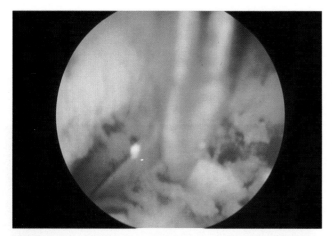

PLATE 67.—Completion of septum incision. The fundus has been reached and the procedure is terminated (see Plates 65 and 66).

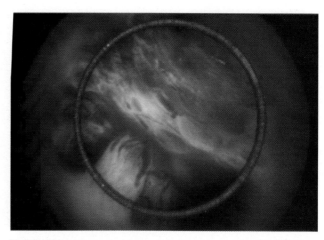

PLATE 70.—Because the endoscope views within the tissue itself, such details as the cysts of benign hyperplasia are easy to see.

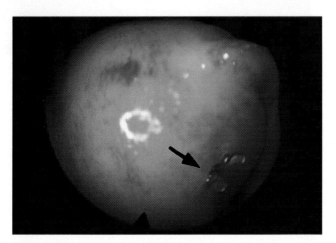

PLATE 68.—Uterine perforation *(arrow)* may occur during sounding, dilation, or operative manipulations. A simultaneous laparoscopy during certain operations is a worthwhile safeguard.

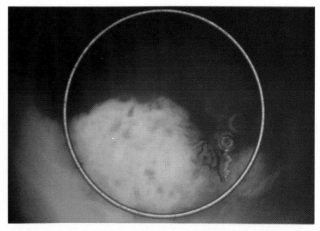

PLATE 71.—Accurate measurement of lesions observed by contact hysteroscopy is possible because the diameter of the viewing circle is known, (e.g., 6 mm). The myoma seen in this slide measures approximately 3 to 4 mm.

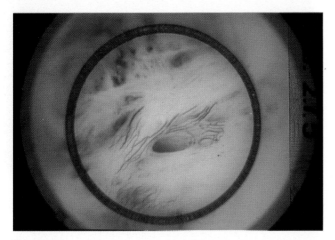

PLATE 69.—Contact hysteroscopic photograph of the endocervical canal showing vascular pattern and vessels 20 μm apart. Small "gland" openings may be seen.

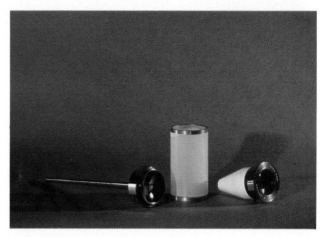

PLATE 72.—The contact hysteroscope consists of an optical guide *(left),* a light collecting chamber *(center),* and a magnifying eyepiece *(right).*

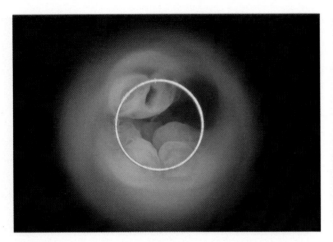

PLATE 73.—Details of the endocervical mucosa are observed. Mucosal (pink) papillae are separated by clefts or tunnels.

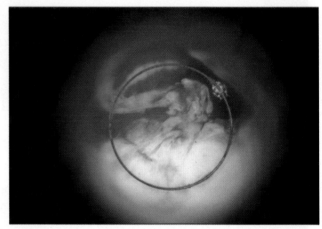

PLATE 75.—Secretory endometrium is reddish in color, has a polypoid pattern, and adheres firmly to the base.

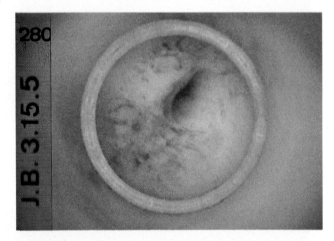

PLATE 74.—The tubal ostium is seen within the focusing circle. The area outside the circle represents reflected light.

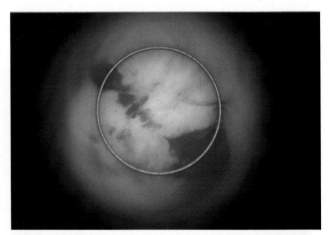

PLATE 76.—Atrophic endometrium is thin, white, and flat. It is generally devoid of vessels.

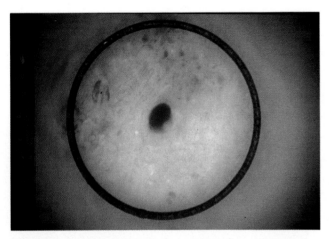

PLATE 77.—Tubal ostium as seen by contact hysteroscopy during early proliferative phase.

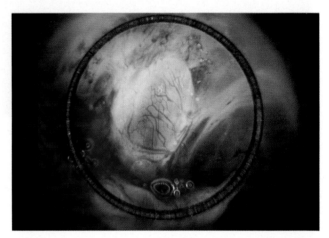

PLATE 79.—There is a small inclusion cyst in the upper endocervical canal. A normal, branching vascular pattern is evident.

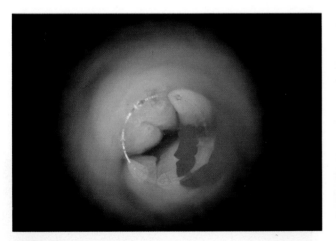

PLATE 78.—Detailed view of the endocervical canal; the crypts are frequently called glands. The cervical mucosa is pink-white and generally is thrown up into folds.

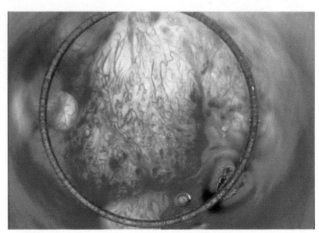

PLATE 80.—This endocervical polyp appears orange-red. The shaggy vascular network is characteristic of these lesions.

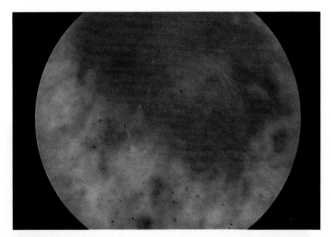

PLATE 81.—Cervical endometriosis appears as blue-black implants.

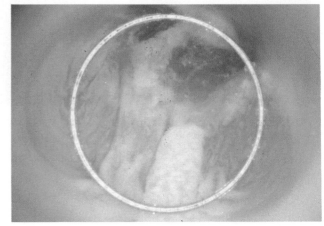

PLATE 83.—The lesion can be seen to extend less than 6 mm into the canal. The atypical epithelium is tongue-shaped, white, and shows a punctate vascular pattern.

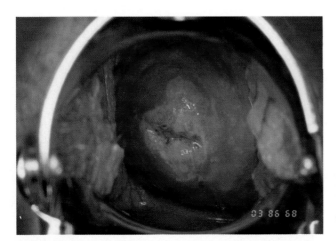

PLATE 82.—Colpophotograph showing an extensive abnormal transformation zone and CIN extending into the cervical canal.

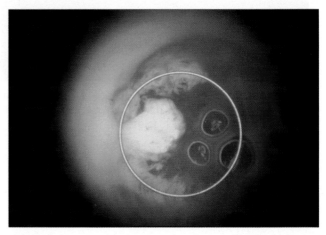

PLATE 84.—A small, stark white atypical focal lesion protrudes into the endocervical canal. The appearance suggests adenocarcinoma.

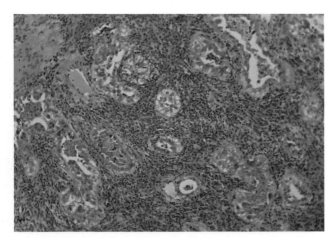

PLATE 85.—Histologic section confirms the diagnosis of primary adenocarcinoma of the endocervix (×100).

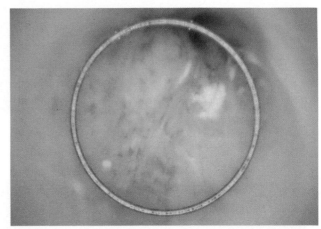

PLATE 87.—Contact endoscopy shows grayish neoplastic epithelium and luminescent particles, characteristic of invasive cancers elsewhere in the uterus.

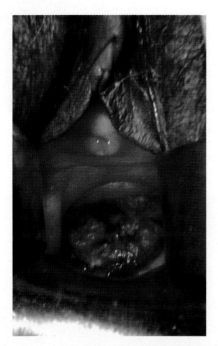

PLATE 86.—An exophytic invasive epidermoid carcinoma of the cervix.

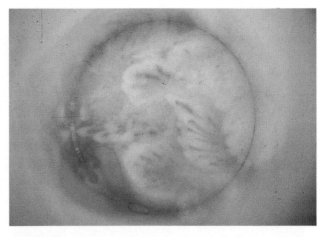

PLATE 88.—View of lower urethra showing condylomata acuminata filling the canal.

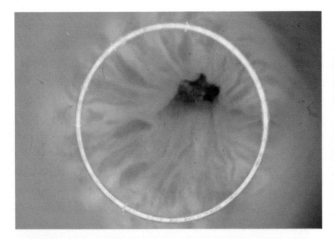

PLATE 89.—Contact urethroscopy provides an excellent view of the entire urethral canal.

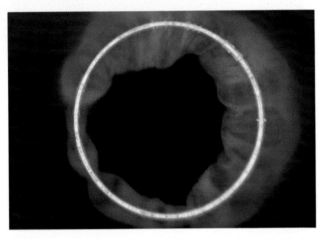

PLATE 90.—The urethral sphincter viewed from the urethral side. The sphincter is normal.

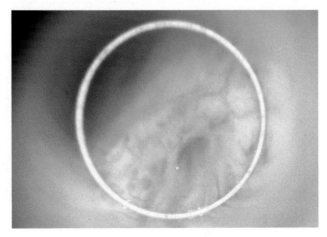

PLATE 91.—The left ureteral orifice and a portion of the ureteric ridge is seen.

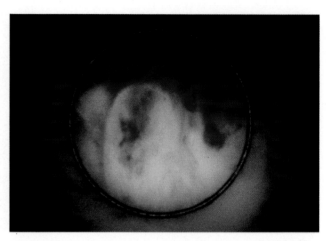

PLATE 92.—Nonfunctioning endometrial polyps (polypoid endometrium). These lesions are white with large, central vascular channels.

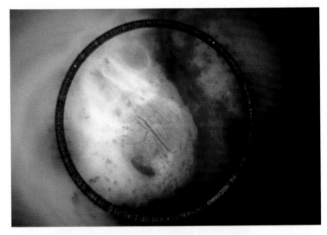

PLATE 93.—This polyp shows evidence of retrogressive hyperplasia. This results from estrogen stimulation in the perimenopausal period followed by cessation of ovarian function and atrophy.

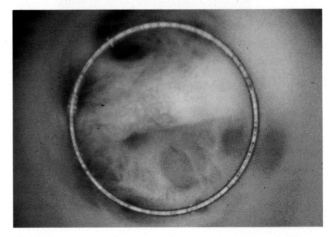

PLATE 94.—Uterine walls show cystic glands and open craters. These findings are appreciated by contact hysteroscope, which lies somewhere between panoramic hysteroscopy and light microscopy.

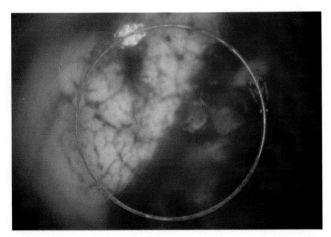

PLATE 95.—Atypical endometrial hyperplasia is characterized by greater glandular proliferation and is frequently associated with abnormal vessels.

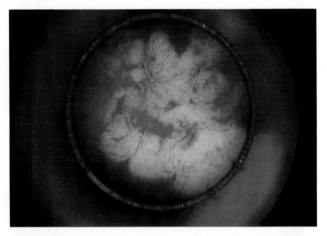

PLATE 97.—The cerebral pattern of adenocarcinoma is brain-like, with vessels outlining a gyri appearance. Note the small villi at the periphery of the lesion.

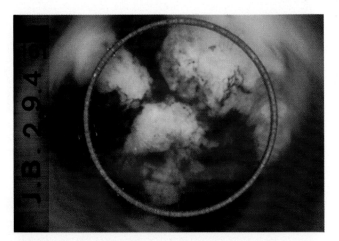

PLATE 96.—This is a typical vegetating pattern. The mucosa has a fluffy appearance and bears a resemblance to gray-white cumulus clouds.

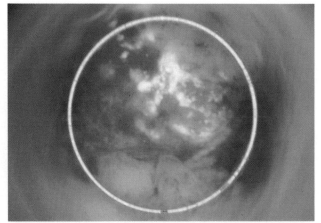

PLATE 98.—Luminescent or fluorescent pattern has been observed in many carcinomas of the endometrium and is a characteristic contact endoscopic finding associated with invasive tumors.

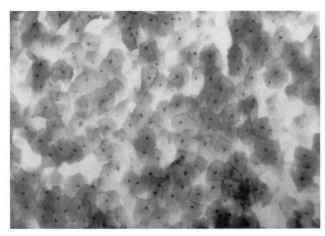

PLATE 99.—Atypical vessels such as those seen with invasive carcinoma of the cervix (by colposcopy) have been observed with poorly differentiated adenocarcinoma of the endometrium.

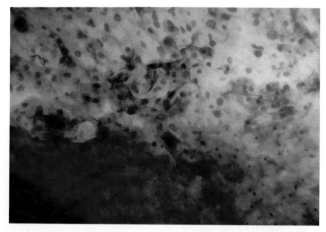

PLATE 102.—MCH contact vision (×150). Squamous cell epithelium with large cytoplasm and picnotic nuclei.

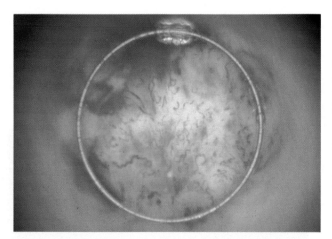

PLATE 100.—Endoscopic investigation of the vagina in a pre-pubertal girl suspected of having a congenital abnormality.

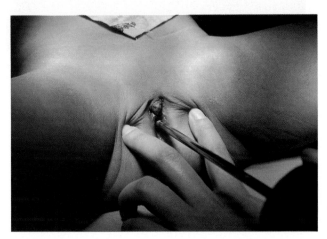

PLATE 103.—MCH contact vision (×150). There is marked contrast between CIN II immature cells and mature iodine-positive squamous cell epithelium. Lower limit of the lesion is shown. (CIN = cervical intraepithelial neoplasia; see later text).

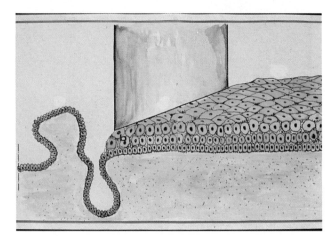

PLATE 101.—Contact vision allows one to observe the superficial cell layers of the epithelium lining the female genital tract (shown here in artist's rendering).

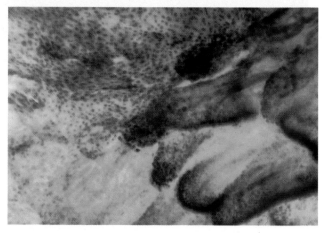

PLATE 104.—MCH contact vision (×150). SCJ with squamous normal immature cells and finger-in-glove pattern of cylindric cells is seen at the right side.

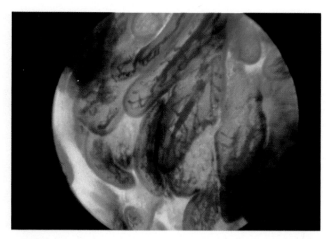

PLATE 105.—MCH contact vision (×150). Note typical papillary aspect of cylindrical epithelium behind the SCJ.

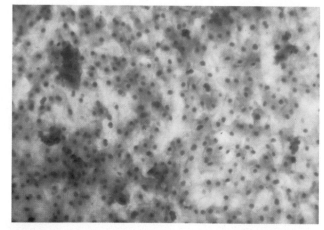

PLATE 107.—MCH contact vision (×150). Slight cellular abnormalities in immature metaplasia.

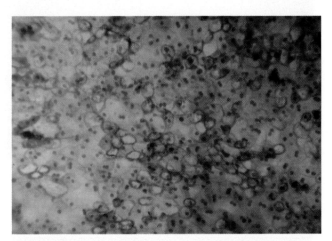

PLATE 106.—MCH contact vision (×150). Presence of viral cytopathic effect (koilocitosis) is seen on the cervical squamous epithelium.

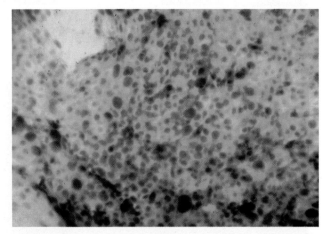

PLATE 108.—MCH contact vision (×150). Severe nuclear abnormalities in CIN III. (Contrast with Plate 118.)

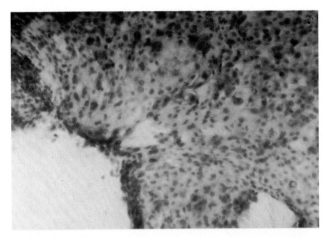

PLATE 109.—MCH contact vision (× 150). Upper endocervical limit of CIN III lesion. This is also the epicenter of the lesion.

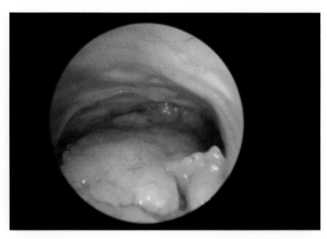

PLATE 112.—Polypoid hyperplasia located on the posterior wall; the rest of the endometrial mucosa is atrophic. In this case it is very easy to miss the lesion with a blind sampling technique.

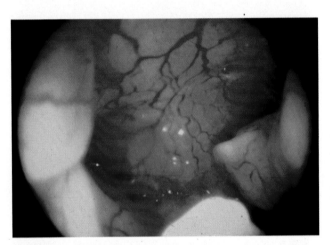

PLATE 110.—Hysteroscopic panoramic observation of an endometrial polypoid hyperplasia.

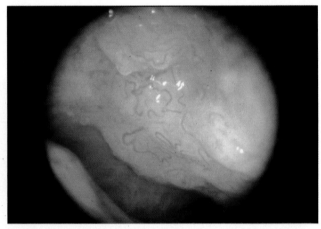

PLATE 113.—Close-up hysteroscopic observation showing atypical vascularization associated with adenomatous hyerplasia.

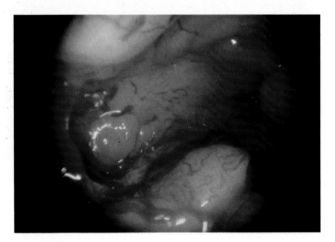

PLATE 111.—Panoramic vision of simple hyperplasia; note the irregular surface of the endometrial mucosa and the abnormal vascularization.

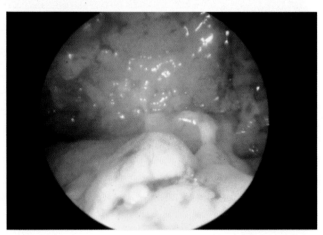

PLATE 114.—Panoramic picture of a well-differentiated adenocarcinoma of the endometrium; note the cerebroid pattern typical of this lesion.

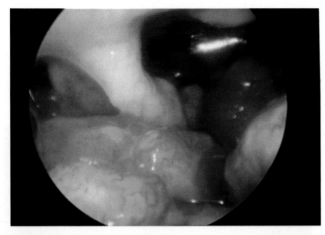

PLATE 115.—Panoramic vision of a completely altered uterine architecture in a patient with undifferentiated adenocarcinoma of the endometrium.

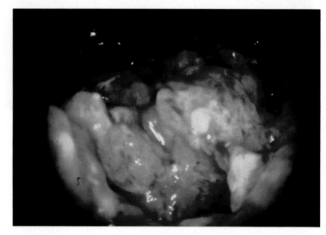

PLATE 117.—Overall hysteroscopic observation of a moderately differentiated endometrial carcinoma.

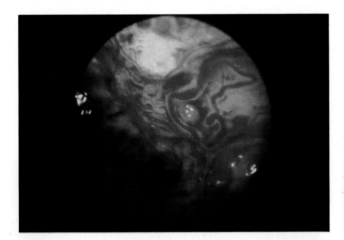

PLATE 116.—Impressive atypical vessels in a case of undifferentiated endometrial cancer.

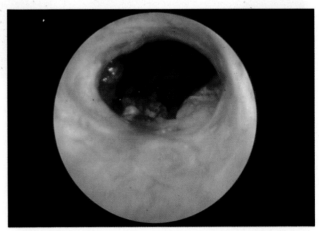

PLATE 118.—Same patient as Plate 108. Overall hysteroscopic observation showing the internal orifice and the upper portion of the cervical canal without spreading of the neoplasia.

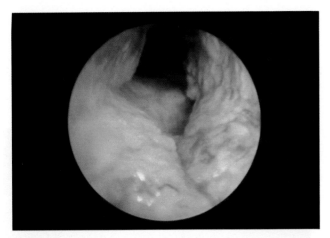

PLATE 119.—The cervical canal in this case is involved by the neoplastic spreading.

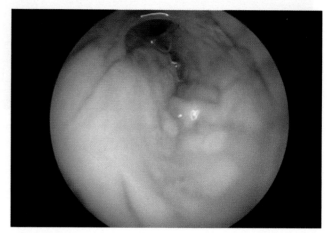

PLATE 121.—Detail of the endocervical canal showing longitudinal and oblique folds.

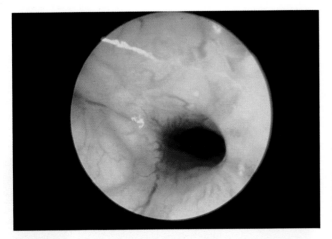

PLATE 120.—Normal hysteroscopic appearance of the endocervical canal. The internal os is opened by the pressure of the gas.

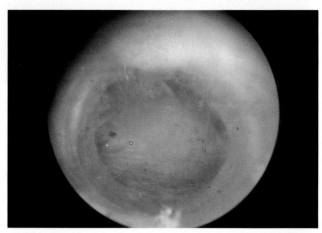

PLATE 122.—Hysteroscopic view of the normal endometrial cavity just after passing the internal os demonstrates the opening dividing the cavity into two chambers. The upper chamber, which is the largest, appears narrow because of the visual distortion.

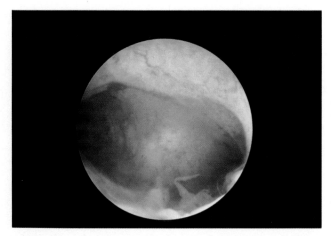

PLATE 123.—Normal hysteroscopic appearance of the endometrial cavity just before passing the oval, sharp-edged opening separating the cylindrical-looking lower chamber from the upper chamber, including the fundus and two horns.

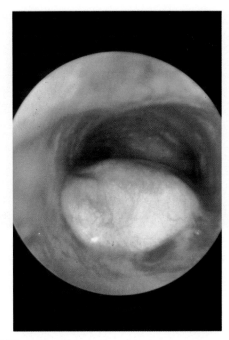

PLATE 125.—CO_2 panoramic hysteroscopy showing the polyp seen in Figure 16–4.

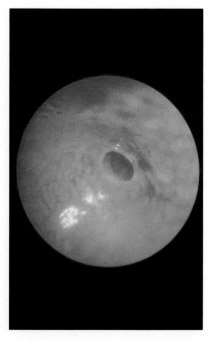

PLATE 124.—Hysteroscopic view of the tubal ostium showing the mucosal fold which circumscribes it and causes the misleading sphincter-like aspect on the hysterogram.

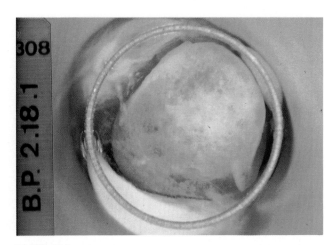

PLATE 126.—Contact hysteroscopy of the same polyp seen in Plate 125.

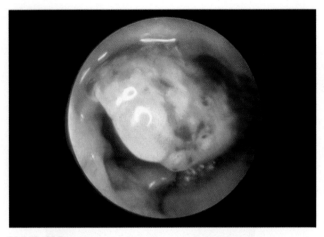

PLATE 127.—The corresponding (see Fig 16–6) hysteroscopic study confirms the presence of a submucous myoma.

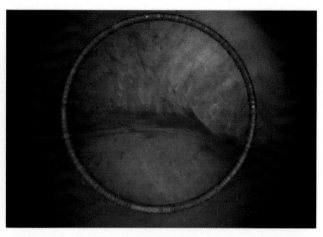

PLATE 129.—Diffuse hyperplasia as seen by contact hysteroscopy. The thickened walls of the uterus are closely opposed.

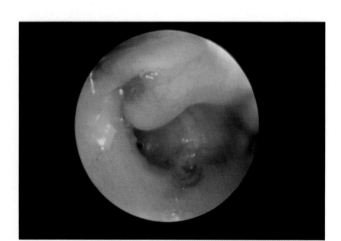

PLATE 128.—Hysteroscopy finding (See Fig 16–7) is suggestive of hyperplasia mucosa. The protrusions are responsible for the filling defects on the hysterogram.

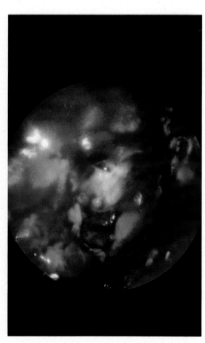

PLATE 130.—Hysteroscopy confirmed the invasive carcinoma having the gross appearance of the vegetating type.

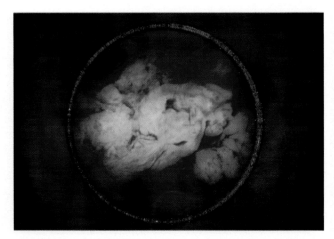

PLATE 131.—Contact hysteroscopy shows a pattern consistent with the vegetative type of adenocarcinoma.

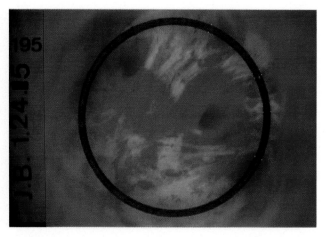

PLATE 133.—Contact hysteroscopy view of adenomyosis. The openings of the diverticula are visible and vary in size.

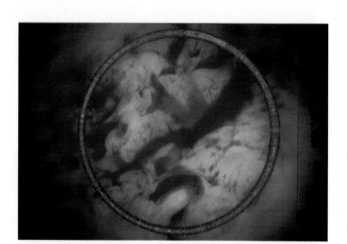

PLATE 132.—Thin atrophic endometrium. The large basilar vessels are seen through the thin mucosa.

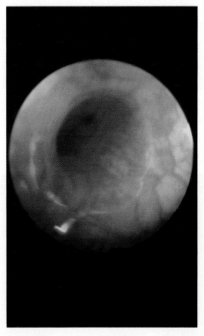

PLATE 134.—Adenomyosis just above the tubal ostium. Numerous thin vessels around the uterine cornu are seen.

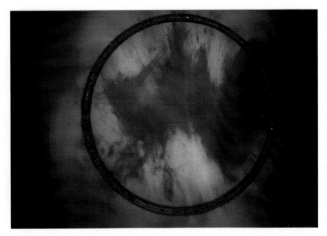

PLATE 135.—Hysteroscopic view taken while extensive adhesions are broken up.

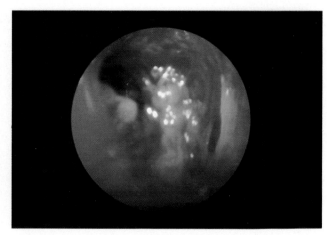

PLATE 138.—Hysteroscopy reveals placental retention.

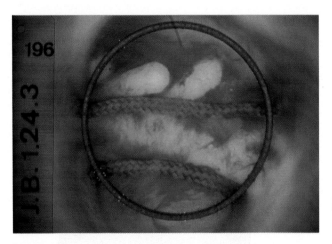

PLATE 136.—Contact hysteroscopy identifies a Dalkon Shield and multifilament strings coiled in the uterine cavity.

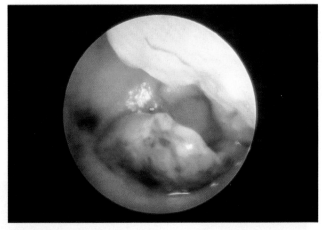

PLATE 139.—Hysteroscopy (compare with Fig 16–21) reveals one filling defect due to a submucous myoma and the other related to a large area of focal hyperplasia.

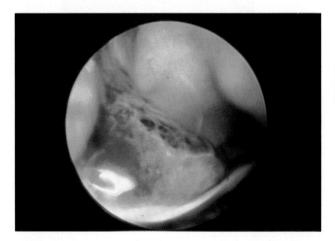

PLATE 137.—Hysteroscopy shows that the filling defect (see Fig 16–18) is in fact due to a large blood clot occupying the right horn.

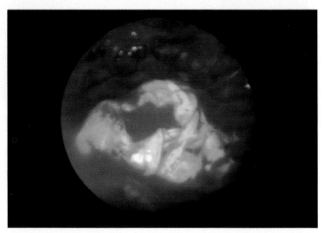

PLATE 140.—Placental retention showing whitish coloration and producing hemorrhage two months following abortion.

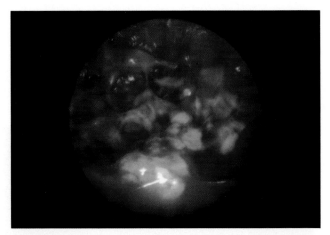

PLATE 141.—Retained placental fragments associated with persistent bleeding.

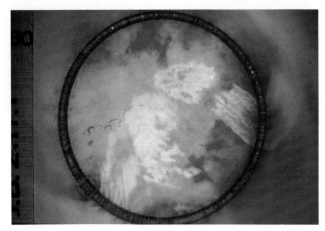

PLATE 143.—Hysteroscopic study of the patient in Figure 16–22 reveals a severe case of endometrial ossification with multiple calcified structures filling the endometrial cavity. This diagnosis is impossible by hysterography.

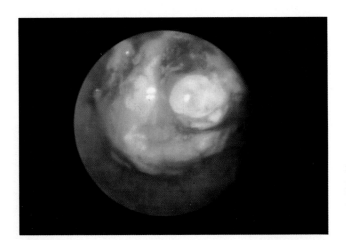

PLATE 142.—Old placental polyp found 3 months after an abortion.

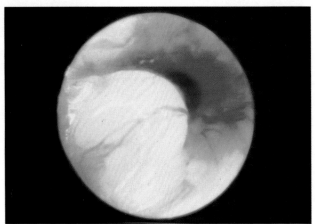

PLATE 144.—Myoma located within the endocervical canal. This abnormality is difficult to diagnose by hysterography.

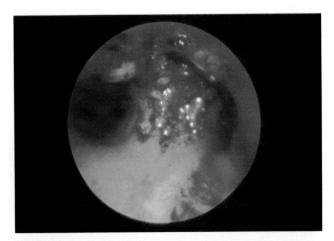

PLATE 145.—Hysteroscopy reveals the presence of a septum. However, it is difficult to infer from this view any perspective about the configuration of the endometrial cavity.

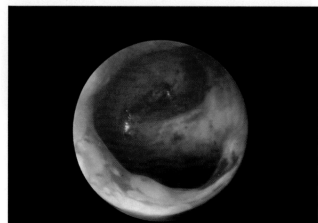

PLATE 147.—Hysteroscopic view of an intrauterine adhesion.

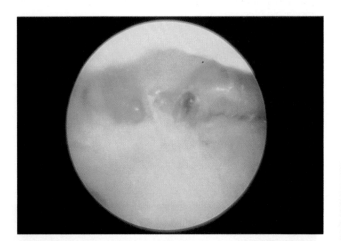

PLATE 146.—Hysteroscopy shows an important uterine adhesion. The upper part of the cavity appears completely obliterated, and only a small opening is visible on the fibrous wall.

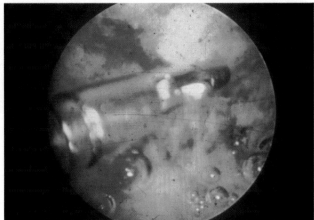

PLATE 148.—View of flexible hysteroscopic scissors dividing the adhesions pictured in Plate 147.

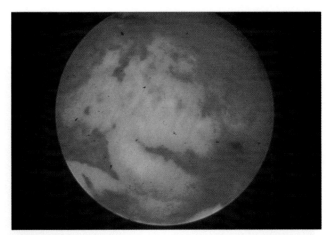

PLATE 149.—View of uterine cavity immediately after lysis of the adhesions in Plate 147. The left tubal ostium is now visible.

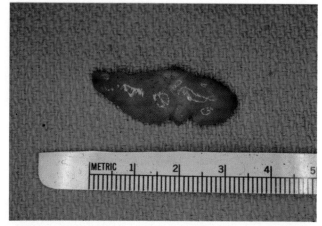

PLATE 151.—Endometrial polyp that had been located just above the internal os in a patient with abnormal bleeding who had undergone curretage six times.

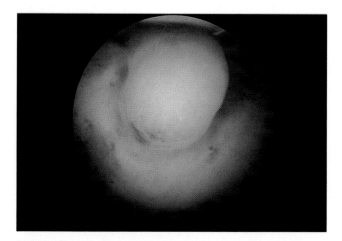

PLATE 150.—Hysteroscopic view of an endometrial polyp.

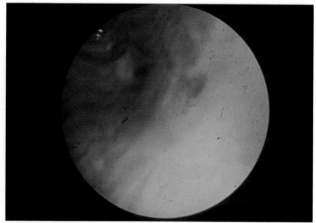

PLATE 152.—Hysteroscopic view of tubal ostium.

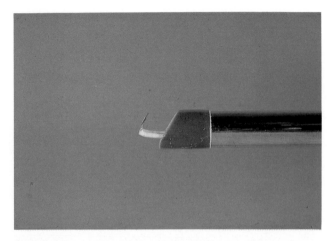

PLATE 153.—Cutting loop of resectoscope used to resect myoma.

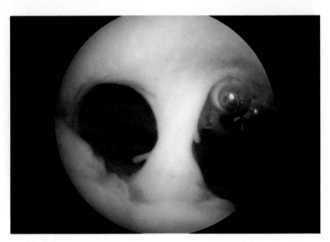

PLATE 156.—Hysteroscopic view of uterine septum.

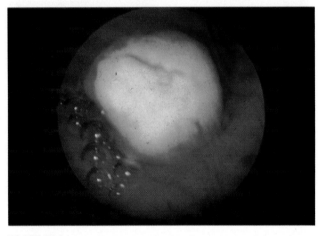

PLATE 154.—Pedunculated myoma viewed by hysteroscopy.

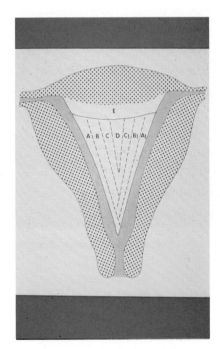

PLATE 157.—Diagram of surgical approach to wide uterine septum. Sequential incisions are made through all of area *A,* then *A,* *B,* *B,* *C,* *C,* and *D.* Finally the residual notch *E* is incised.

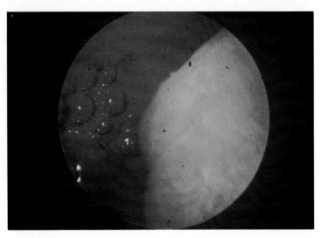

PLATE 155.—Broad-based, sessile myoma resected by hysteroscopy.

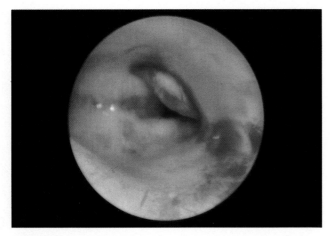

PLATE 158.—Small endometrial polyp located near the tubal ostium. Normal endometrium surrounds it.

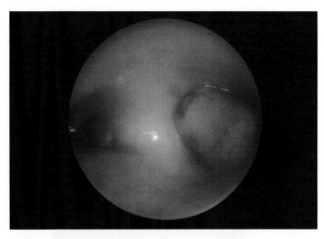

PLATE 160.—Polyp located within the cornu and completely blocking the left ostium.

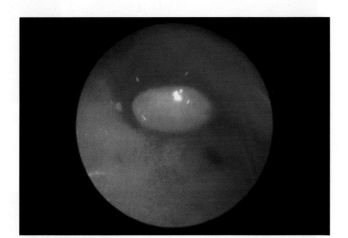

PLATE 159.—Another small functioning polyp. Note the tubal ostium just below the polyp.

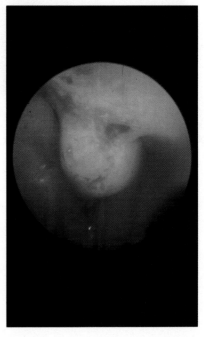

PLATE 161.—Broad-based pedicle of polyp arising from the anterior uterine wall.

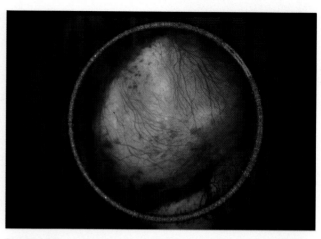

PLATE 162.—A polyp viewed by the contact hysteroscope. The polyp may be accurately measured because it can be related to the focal circle of the endoscope.

A

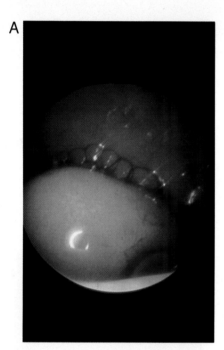

B

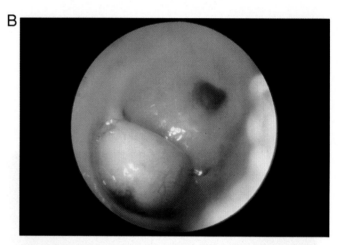

PLATE 163.—**A,** a large functional polyp covered with normal endometrium spread over the posterior wall of the uterine cavity. CO$_2$ bubbles are seen above the polyp. **B,** an endometrial polyp with a thin pedicle tending to take the appearance of a nonfunctional lesion as it grows bigger.

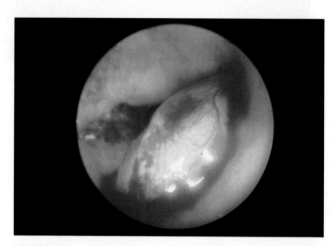

PLATE 164.—Nonfunctional endometrial polyp. It is whitish and flat, with a thin pedicle.

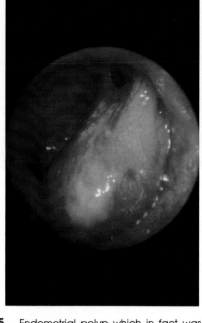

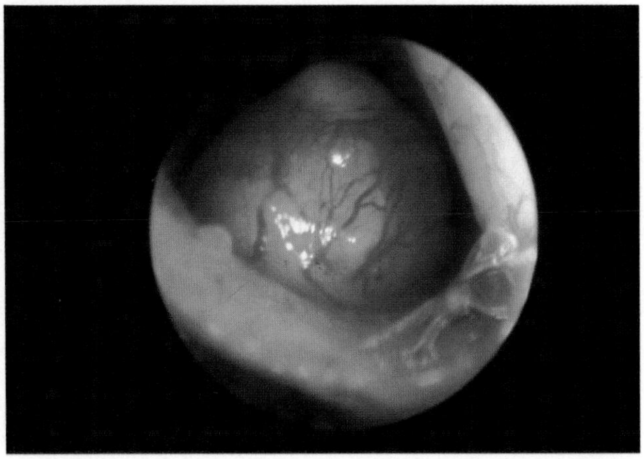

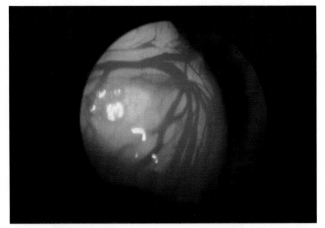

PLATE 167.—A submucous myoma bulging into the uterine cavity.

PLATE 165.—Endometrial polyp which in fact was diagnosed as adenomyosis on histologic examination.

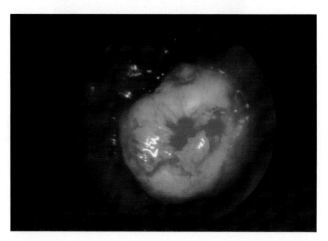

PLATE 168.—A network of dilated vessels can be seen on the surface of the myoma.

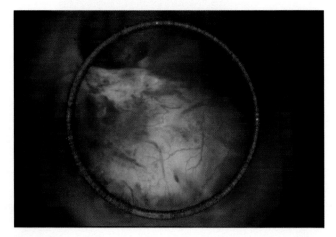

PLATE 166.—Thin, atrophic endometrium covers this polyp. The vascular pattern is detailed by contact hysteroscopy.

PLATE 169.—Submucous myoma during an episode of bleeding. Blood oozes from the network of dilated vessels.

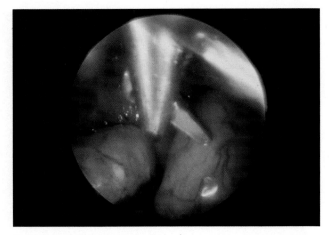

PLATE 170.—Two large pedunculated myomas before division of the pedicles by the scissors.

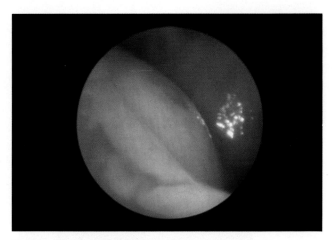

PLATE 171.—Slight protrusion (lower) created by intramural myoma, which is covered with normal endometrium.

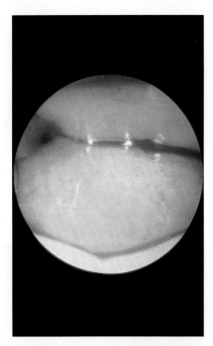

PLATE 172.—Simple endometrial hyperplasia. The mucosa is *not* polypoid. The diagnosis is confirmed with histologic evaluation of a sample of endometrium.

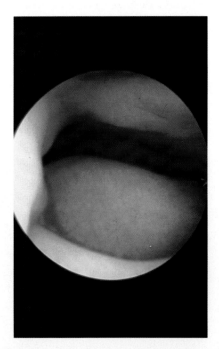

PLATE 173.—The endometrium (posterior wall) is thick and wavelike. The pattern is consistent with early polypoid hyperplasia.

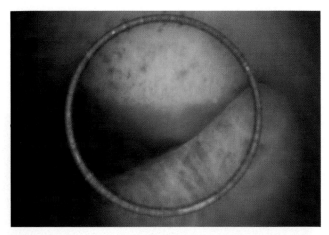

PLATE 174.—Contact hysteroscopy shows thick, plush uterine walls associated with endometrial hyperplasia.

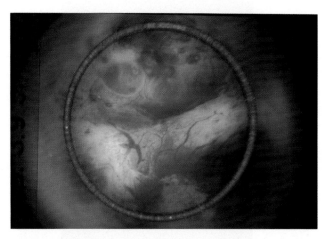

PLATE 177.—Hyperplastic epithelium is fragile and tears off easily during manipulation with the hysteroscope.

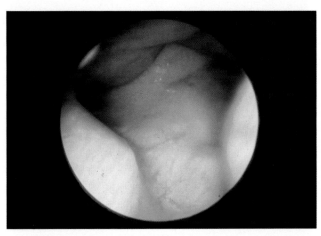

PLATE 175.—Diffuse polypoid hyperplasia of the endometrium. The hysteroscope has "grooved" the posterior wall.

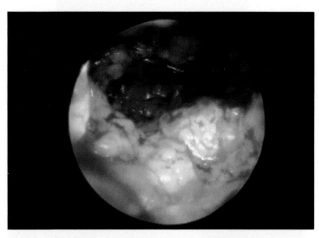

PLATE 178.—Endometrial carcinoma exhibiting its most common appearance (i.e., the vegetating pattern).

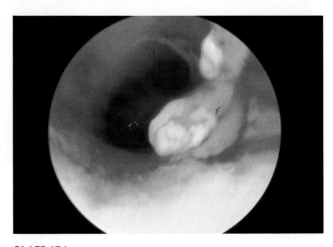

PLATE 176.—Panoramic hysteroscopy of focal polypoid hyperplasia.

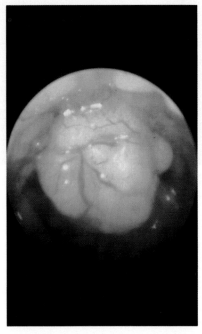

PLATE 179.—The polypoid type of endometrial carcinoma.

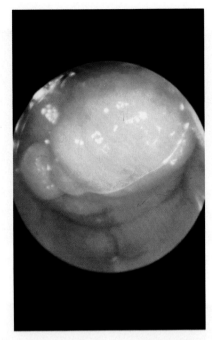

PLATE 180.—The nodular pattern of endometrial carcinoma implanted on the uterine fundus and growing toward the internal os.

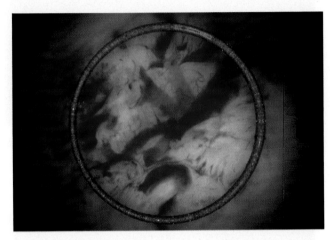

PLATE 182.—Contact hysteroscopic view showing gray-white coloration with irregular vegetations.

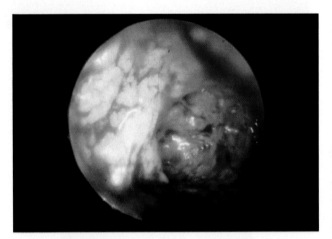

PLATE 181.—The cerebroid pattern of endometrial carcinoma has a brainlike appearance.

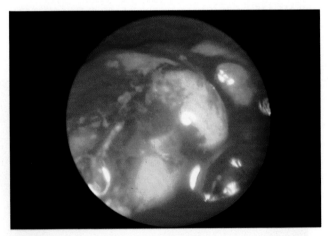

PLATE 183.—Extensive ulcerative type of endometrial carcinoma causing profuse bleeding.

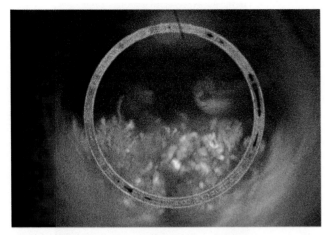

PLATE 184.—Contact hysteroscopy of adenocarcinoma involving the internal os of the cervix.

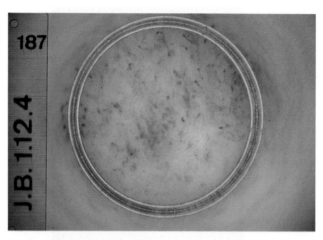

PLATE 187.—Contact hysteroscopy shows small diverticulae of the uterine fundus.

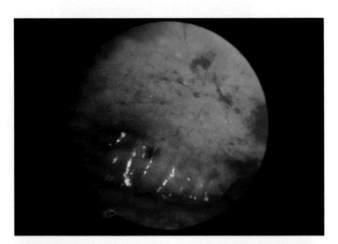

PLATE 185.—Endometrial atrophy associated with bleeding in a postmenopausal woman. Note filmy petechial mucosa with relief of the underlying myometrium.

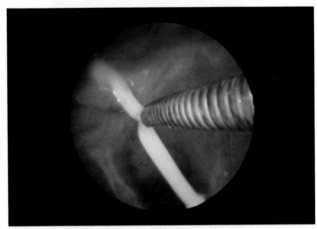

PLATE 188.—The arms of the "T" of the IUD are oblique, and the lower arm is embedded.

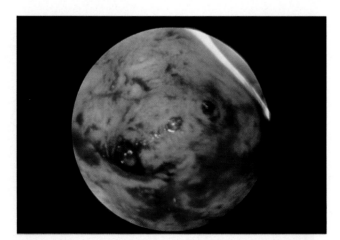

PLATE 186.—Adenomyosis showing diverticula of the uterine fundus.

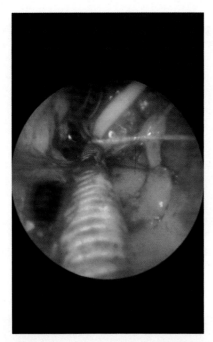

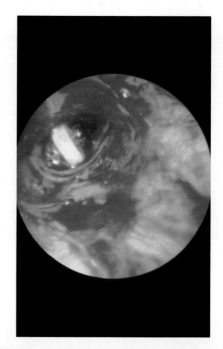

PLATE 189.—The IUD string is ascended and the device is displaced, with one arm embedded in the myometrium and the stem covered with blood and ragged mucosa.

PLATE 190.—The IUD has perforated the uterine fundus.

A

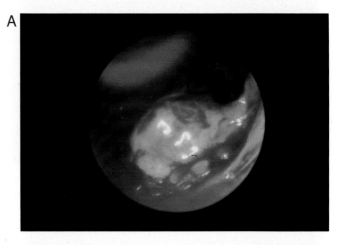

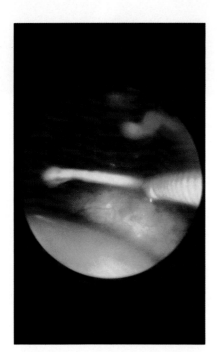

B

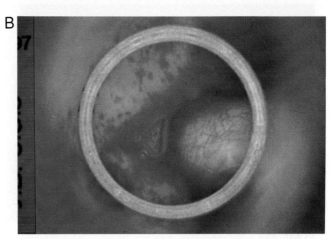

PLATE 191.—Pregnancy associated with an "in situ" IUD. The device lies on top of the gestational sac.

PLATE 192.—**A,** panoramic view of a uterine polyp. **B,** close-up (contact) view of a functioning polyp (left).

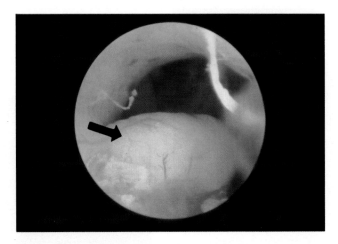

PLATE 193.—Submucous myoma *(arrow)* in the lower corpus.

A

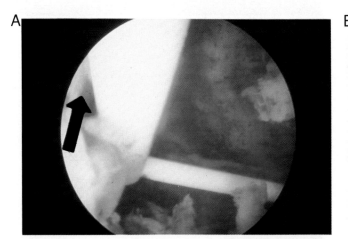

B

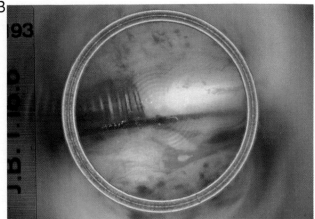

PLATE 194.—**A,** hysteroscopic view of Progestasert device. The arm is seen in the background; the stem is close to the objective

lens *(arrow)*. **B,** close-up view of the stem of a copper T IUD.

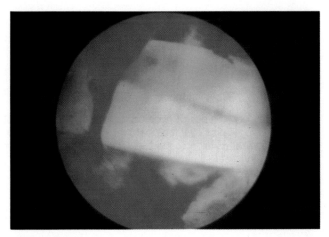

PLATE 195.—Broken terminal portion of a plastic curette found during hysteroscopy for abnormal bleeding.

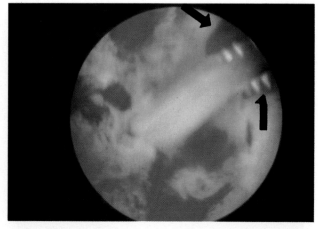

PLATE 196.—Jaws of grasping forceps *(arrows)* removing the foreign body shown in Plate 195.

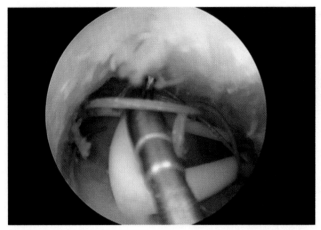

PLATE 197.—Hysteroscopic removal of an embedded Progestasert T IUD in the uterine cavity.

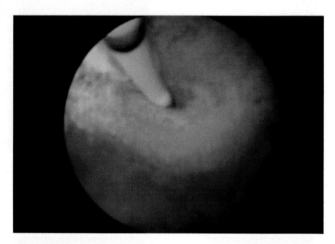

PLATE 200.—Tubal cannulation.

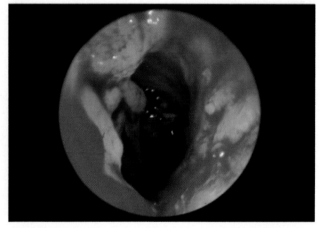

PLATE 198.—Panoramic hysteroscopy showing metastatic adenocarcinoma (primary) metastatic to the upper endocervix.

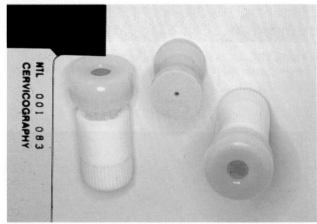

PLATE 201.—Two types of hysteroscopy plugs. The older urologic-type nipple slips over the operative channel. The leaf-type plug actually attaches onto the Luer-lock fitting and will not slip off.

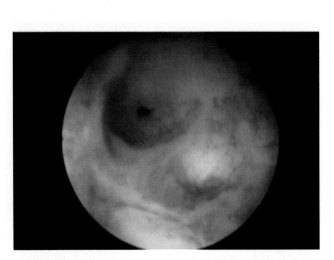

PLATE 199.—Hysteroscopic view of tubal opening.

A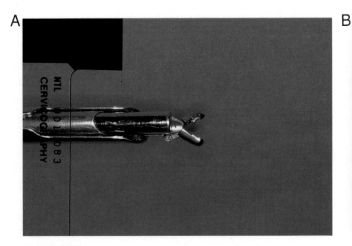

B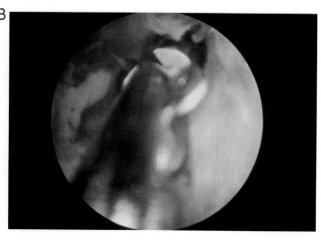

PLATE 202.—**A,** semirigid biopsy forceps extends from the end of the hysteroscopy operating sheath. This technique permits direct view during biopsies. **B,** biopsy of abnormal tissue performed under direct vision.

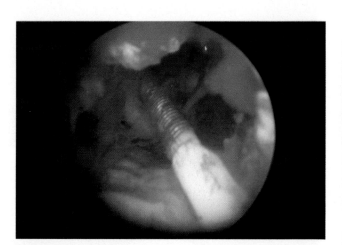

PLATE 203.—Copper 7 IUD lying in the uterus.

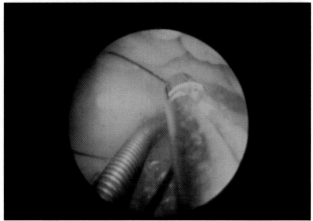

PLATE 204.—The filament of the IUD is grasped for direct removal.

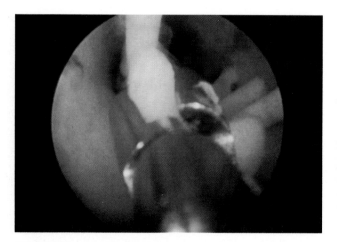

PLATE 205.—The entire hysteroscope and sheath together with the IUD are removed from the uterus.

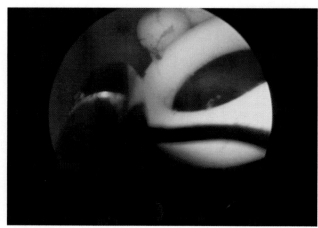

PLATE 208.—Easy removal under local anesthesia of a nonembedded loop device.

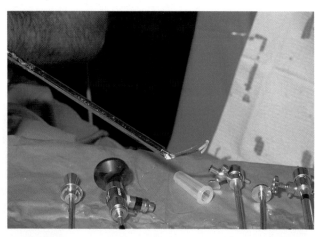

PLATE 206.—The stem of the device is firmly grasped by the hysteroscopic forceps prior to extraction.

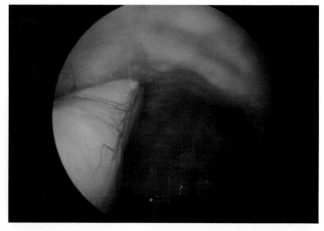

PLATE 209.—Nonfunctioning polyp with the pedicle originating on the anterolateral wall of the corpus.

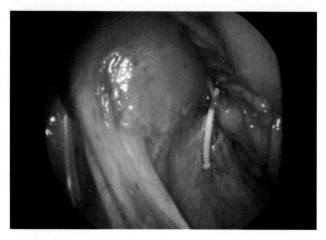

PLATE 207.—Not infrequently a portion of the device may penetrate the uterine serosa.

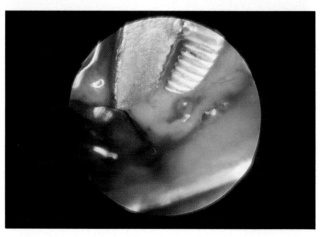

PLATE 210.—The pedicle of a uterine polyp is grasped within the jaws of semirigid scissors.

Color Plates

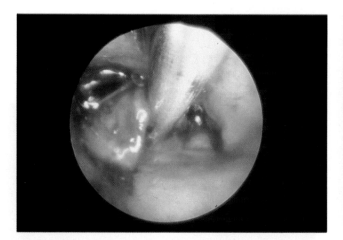

PLATE 211.—The base of the polyp has been transected.

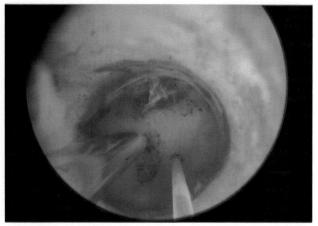

PLATE 212.—The Nd-YAG laser fiber has been inserted through the operating channel. The advantage of utilizing the laser fiber as an operating tool relates to its excellent hemostasis.

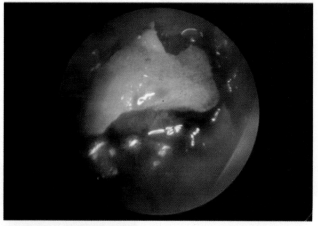

PLATE 213.—Endometrial ossification showing (above) a bone-like piece of calcified tissue penetrating the endometrium.

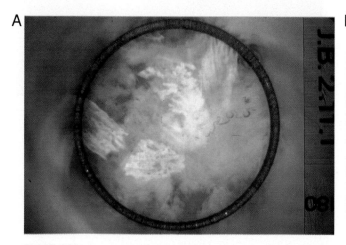

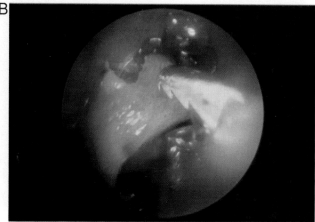

PLATE 214.—**A,** contact hysteroscopy detailing osteoid metaplasia with spicules of bone. **B,** osteoid is removed, under visual control, by forceps.

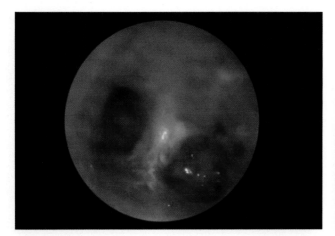

PLATE 215.—Central type of adhesion with broadening of the bases.

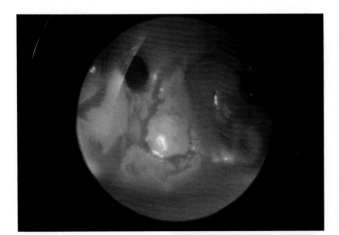

PLATE 216.—Column-shaped adhesion occluding the right uterine horn.

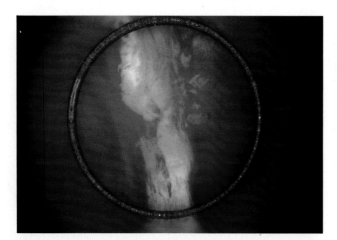

PLATE 217.—Contact hysteroscopy shows a column-shaped adhesion stretching between the anterior and posterior walls of the uterus.

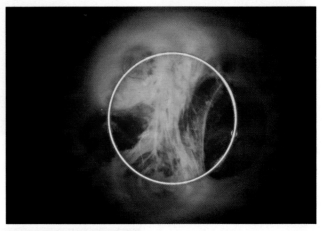

PLATE 218.—A second pattern of central type adhesions. Note the cavity on either side of the lesion.

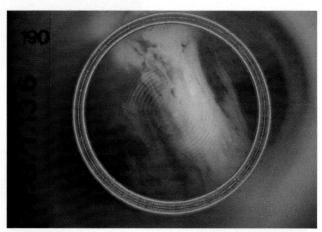

PLATE 219.—A central, columnar adhesion is seen by contact hysteroscopy.

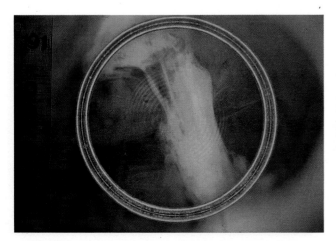

PLATE 220.—The tip of the hysteroscope applies pressure and the adhesion begins to separate (same patient as Plate 219).

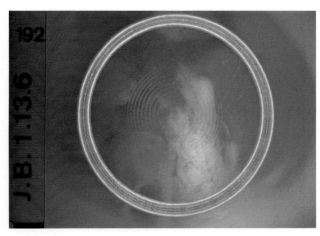

PLATE 221.—As the adhesion snaps, the retracted end can be seen.

A

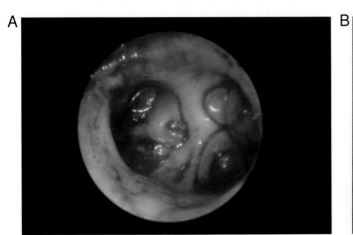

B

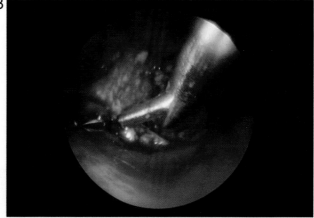

PLATE 222.—**A,** uterine adhesions secondary to tuberculosis. They form alveoli in the uterine fundus. **B,** dissection of uterine synechiae.

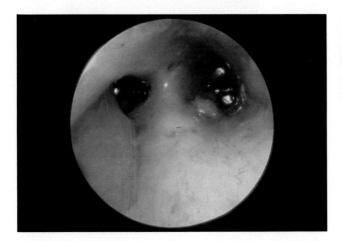

PLATE 223.—Septate uterus with endometrial hyperplasia and a small polyp at the entrance of the left horn.

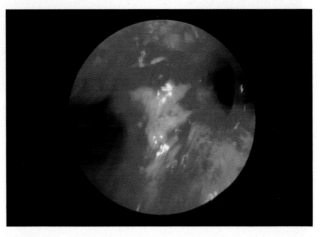

PLATE 224.—Broad septum associated with irregular bleeding and pregnancy loss.

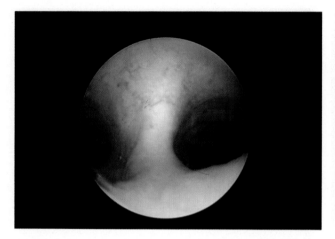

PLATE 225.—Hysteroscopy confirms the presence of the uterine septum.

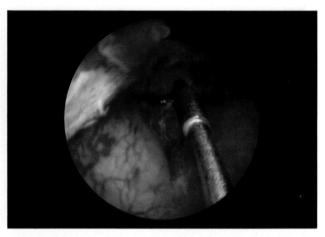

PLATE 227.—The septum is bloodlessly transected.

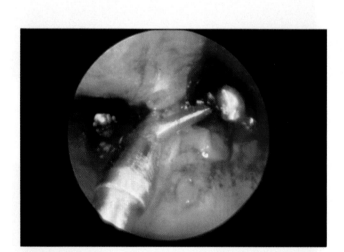

PLATE 226.—Semirigid scissors is poised at the central portion of the septum.

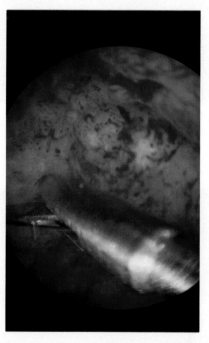

PLATE 228.—The septum has been excised. The myometrium is reddish and has a tendency to bleed. The muscle bundles are apparent. The transected septum on each side is white and does not bleed.

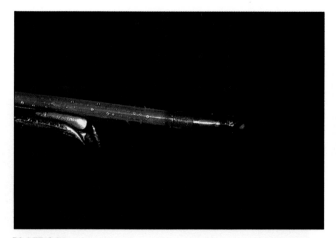

PLATE 229.—Nd-YAG fiber with a sapphire lens mounted or the distal extremity.

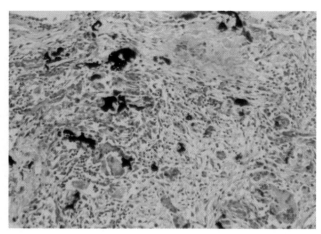

PLATE 230.—Histologic section of the uterine wall taken 8 weeks after laser ablation. Carbon particles surrounded by foreign body giant cells and collagen are all that remain of the endometrium.

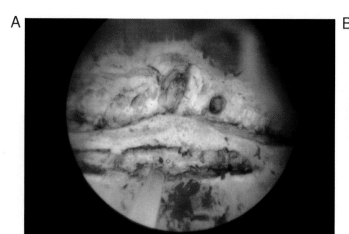

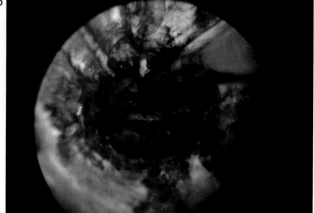

PLATE 231.—**A,** the Nd-YAG fiber is dragged across the endometrium, scooping out a furrow of tissue as it traverses. **B,** much of the endometrium is ablated. Only a small area of tissue (lower) remains to be treated.

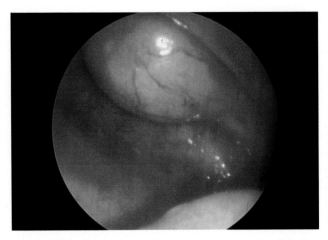

PLATE 232.—Submucous myoma as seen by panoramic hysteroscopy. The myoma is located on the anterior wall.

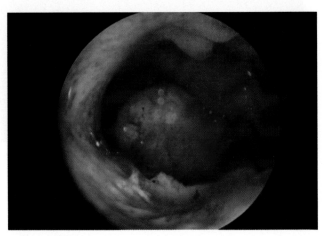

PLATE 235.—Submucous myomas characteristically tend to bleed since they have a very thin mucosal covering and are associated with chronic endometritis.

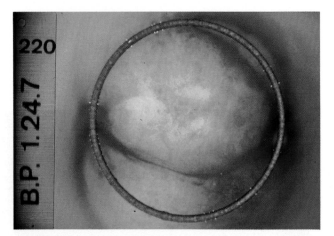

PLATE 233.—Contact hysteroscopy of the submucous myoma shown in Plate 232.

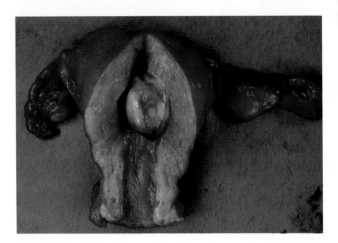

PLATE 234.—Gross specimen of the myoma seen in Plate 232, Plate 233, and Figure 20–22.

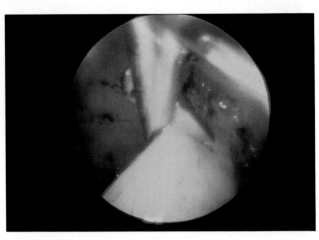

PLATE 236.—Transection of a pedunculated myoma with scissors. The pedicle is rather narrow, and this is easily performed by operative hysteroscopy.

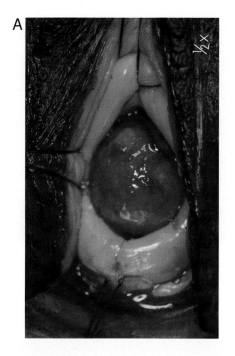

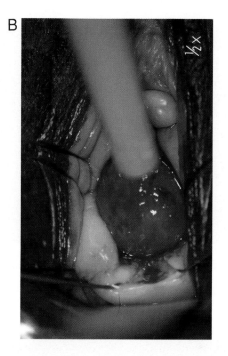

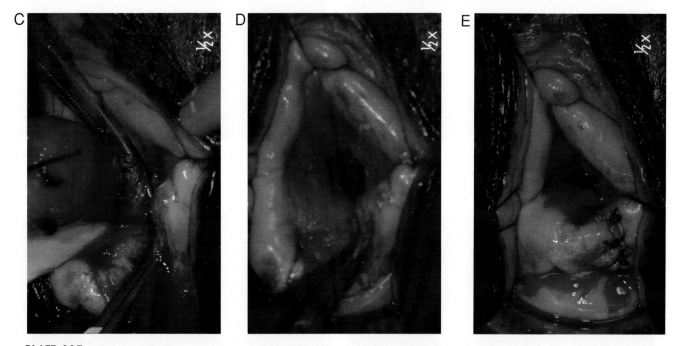

PLATE 237.—A, large submucous myoma prolapsed through the cervix. **B,** the cervix has been injected with Pitressin, and the posterior cervical lip is cut by means of CO_2 laser. **C,** the broad pedicle of the myoma is exposed. The base is clamped and the myoma cut off. **D,** the myoma is gone. **E,** the posterior lip of the cervix is sutured.

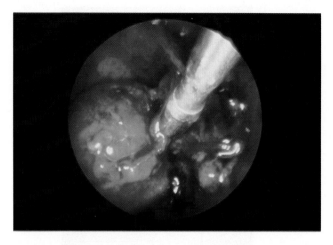

PLATE 238.—Excision of a sessile variety of submucous myoma. This procedure is much more difficult. The tumor is cut to the plane of the endometrial surface.

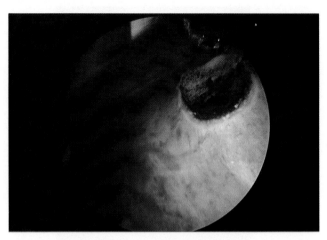

PLATE 241.—The procedure is terminated when the myoma is reduced to the level of the surrounding endometrium or just below surface level.

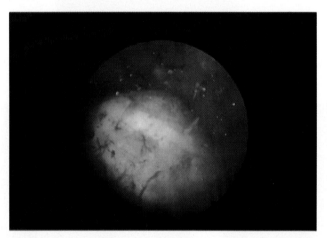

PLATE 239.—The myoma to be resected is identified at the time of operative hysteroscopy.

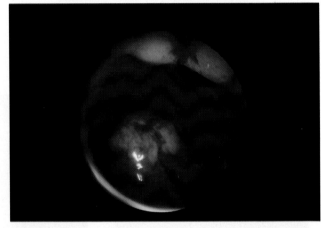

PLATE 242.—Two subcutaneous myomas are seen. The larger is noted on the right side wall; the smaller, on the left side wall.

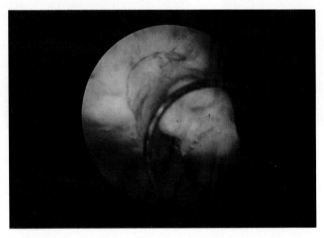

PLATE 240.—The loop of the resectoscope begins to shave the myoma plane by plane.

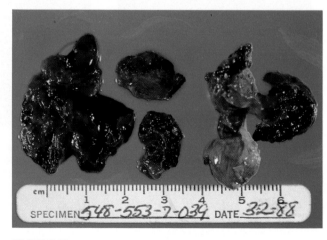

PLATE 243.—Submucous myomas removed in pieces.

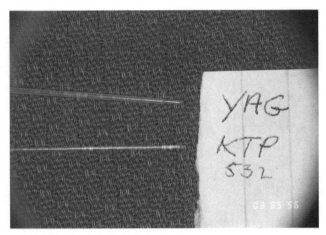

PLATE 244.—Both the Nd-YAG and KTP 532 laser light can be transmitted by fine, flexible, quartz fibers.

A

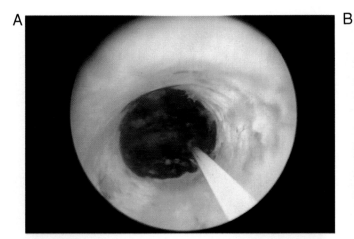

B

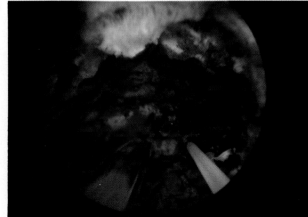

PLATE 245.—**A,** view from the cervix shows Nd-YAG fiber entering the endometrial cavity. **B,** ablation completed by the touch technique. The surface of the endometrium is entirely ablated.

The quartz laser fiber is seen at upper right. An aspirating cannula is noted at upper left (double channel laser hysteroscope).

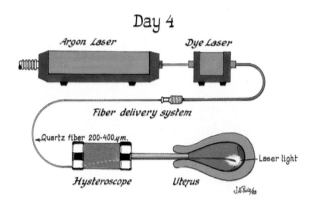

PLATE 246.—After three days the hematoporphyrin derivative has cleared normal cells. Dye laser light (630 nm) is delivered by fiber to the tumor.

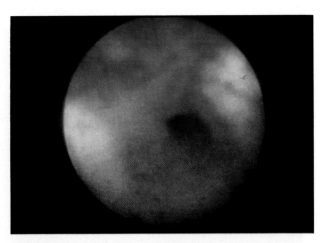

PLATE 247.—Tubal ostium at hysteroscopy.

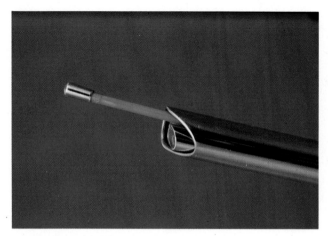

PLATE 248.—Insulated electrode protruding from the distal end of the operating sheath.

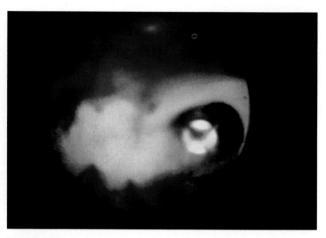

PLATE 251.—Hysteroscopic view of tubal plug(s) in place within the baboon uterus. (Courtesy of Dr. A. Hosseinian.)

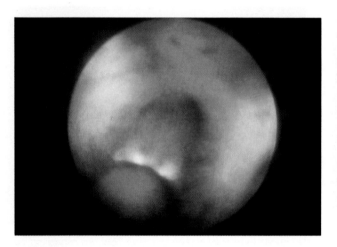

PLATE 249.—Electrode (from Plate 248) at the proximal portion of the intramural oviduct.

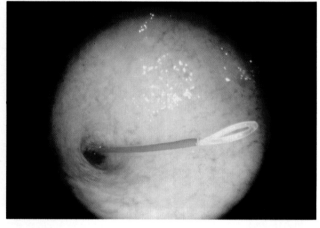

PLATE 252.—Photograph of intratubal device in situ. (Courtesy of Dr. J. Hamou.)

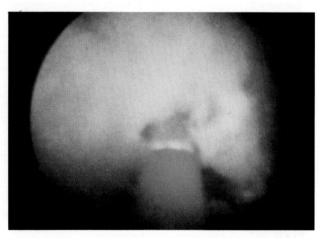

PLATE 250.—Blanching of tissue produced by transmission of the electric current as electrode is activated.

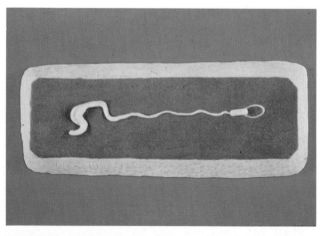

PLATE 253.—Silicone plug as devised by Erb.

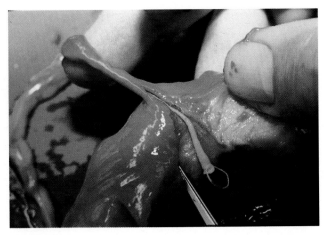

PLATE 254.—Evaluation of plug placed in rabbit horn and removed 284 days later.

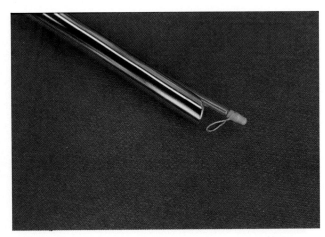

PLATE 257.—Obturator tip on end of guide assembly as it exits through the hysteroscope sheath.

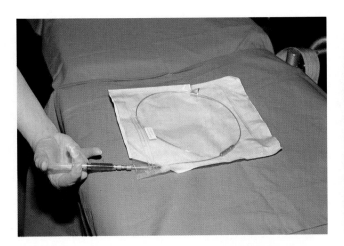

PLATE 255.—Guide assembly with syringe attached.

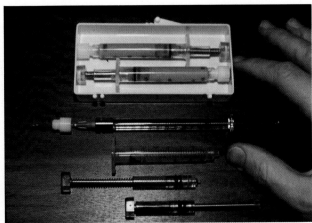

PLATE 258.—Non-air-entraining mixer-dispenser containing liquid silicone and catalyst.

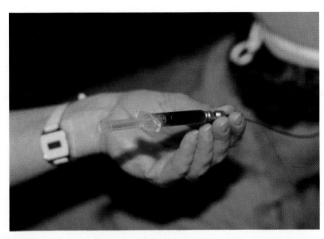

PLATE 256.—Methylene blue dispenser attached to guide assembly.

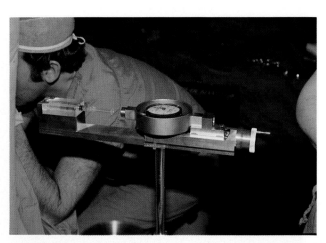

PLATE 259.—Fluid flow actuator.

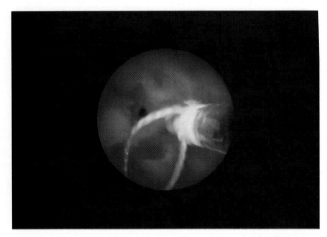

PLATE 260.—The guide assembly (cannula) approaches the ostium. A test dose of methylene blue is squirted through the assembly.

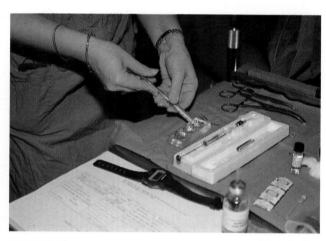

PLATE 263.—The nurse (assistant) squirts a sample of silicone onto the test plate.

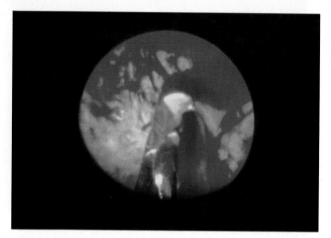

PLATE 261.—Liquid silicone is injected, and the operator watches for an air bubble in cannula.

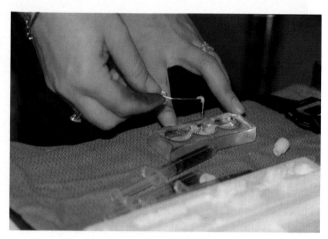

PLATE 264.—The "cure" of the silicone is tested.

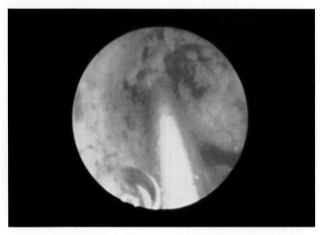

PLATE 262.—White liquid silicone now flows into the tube.

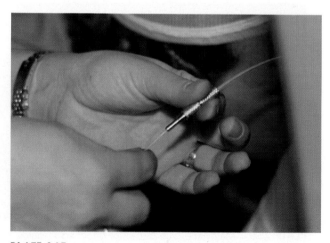

PLATE 265.—The tip is separated from the guide assembly.

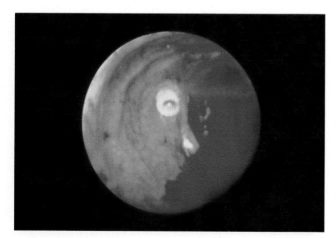

PLATE 266.—The plug is correctly in place.

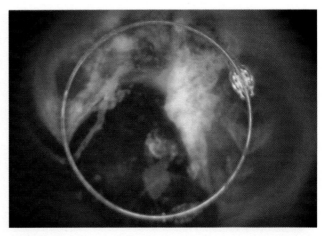

PLATE 269.—An amniotic window can be located in 70% to 80% of cases.

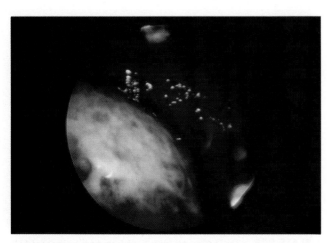

PLATE 267.—Panoramic view of the gestational sac.

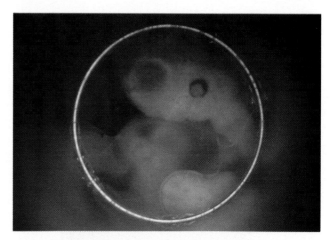

PLATE 270.—A 4-week embryo with bulbous cranial pole and paddlelike upper limb bud.

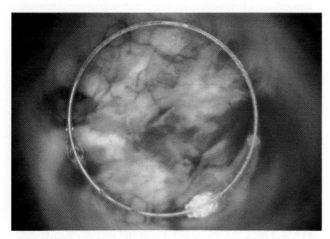

PLATE 268.—The chorionic sac shows white decidua interspersed with blue chorion.

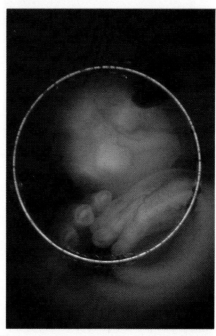

PLATE 271.—Fusion of cranial bulbs occurs at 5 to 6 weeks. This view details the ridge-like dorsum of the newly fused skull.

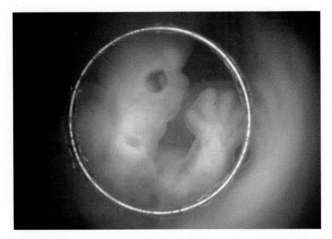

PLATE 272.—A 4 to 5 week embryo showing the first branchial cleft.

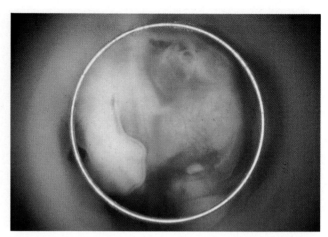

PLATE 274.—Paddlelike arm rests on the large (pink) embryonic heart.

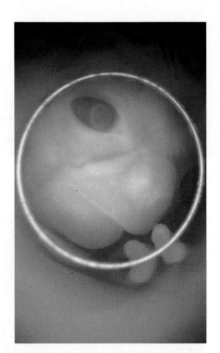

PLATE 273.—A 6 to 7 week embryo, full face view. A retinal reflex may be seen in the right eye.

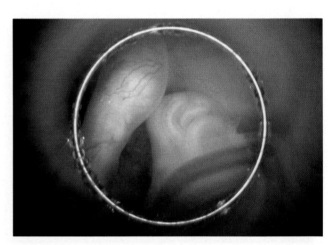

PLATE 275.—The embryo's arm is above and to the right. The border of the abdomen is to the left. Below and center are the intestines prolapsed into the cord.

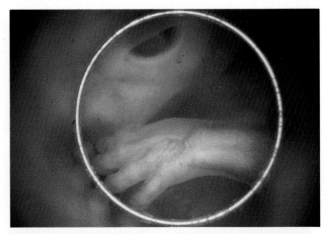

PLATE 276.—The upper extremities are well developed by 7 to 8 weeks, but the lower limbs lag behind by approximately 2 weeks.

A
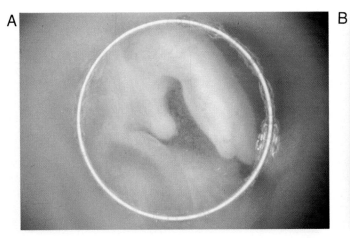

B
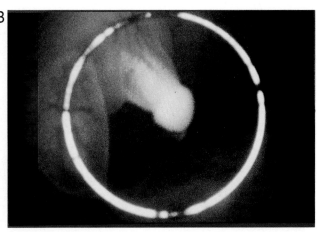

PLATE 277.—A, the indifferent phallus is seen between flipper-like lower limb and a piece of umbilical cord. **B,** detail of phallus and labial scrotal folds.

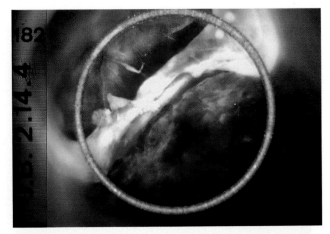

PLATE 278.—Incomplete abortion is identified by the presence of blue chorion, white decidua, and reddish-brown placental tissue.

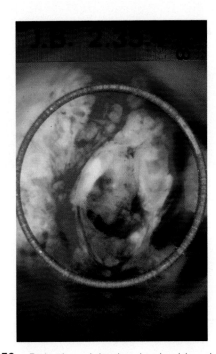

PLATE 279.—Early placental polyp showing blue chorionic tissue.

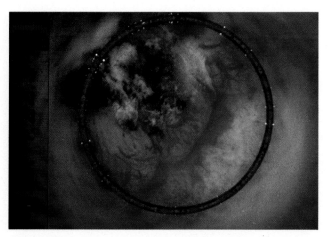

PLATE 280.—Older placental polyp illustrating typical color change from blue to green secondary to aging.

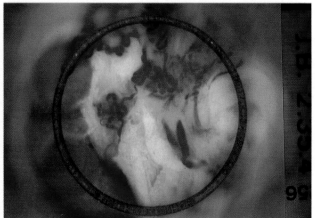

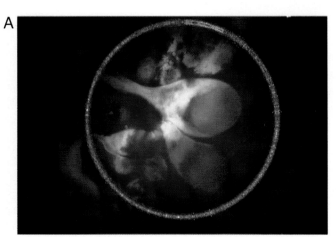

PLATE 281.—Most of the placental tissue has been resorbed or expelled after 1 month. The coiled, large vessels mark the site of retention.

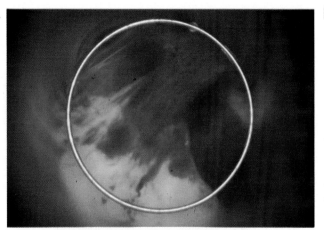

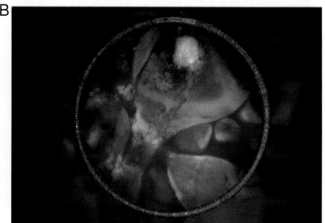

PLATE 282.—Retained membranes located by contact hysteroscopy during investigation for a major postpartum hemorrhage.

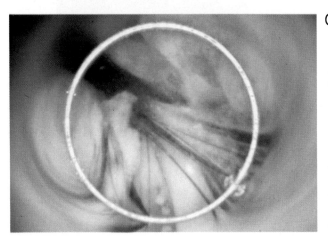

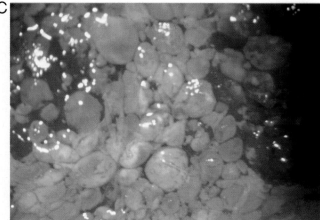

PLATE 283.—Amnioscopy showing clear fluid, fetal hair, and vernix.

PLATE 284.—**A,** molar vesicles appear as blue, edematous chorionic villi. **B,** close-up view of molar vesicles. **C,** panoramic view of hydatidiform mole.

History of Hysteroscopy

Jacques Barbot, M.D.

Looking back at the history of hysteroscopy enables one to better understand the scope of difficulties encountered when examining the uterine cavity, to see how these different problems were solved, and to track the evolution of hysteroscopy. The history of hysteroscopy can be divided into three periods:

1. An early period during which, for technical reasons, contact hysteroscopy was a necessity.
2. A middle period during which panoramic hysteroscopy with a distending medium was the only technique in use.
3. A later period during which panoramic hysteroscopy, as well as contact hysteroscopy and microhysteroscopy with modern technology, offered new advantages in visualization of the uterine cavity.

THE FIRST HYSTEROSCOPES: THE NEED FOR CONTACT HYSTEROSCOPY

Endoscopy had its beginnings in the early 19th century when Bozzini, in 1805, invented a hollow tube through which to observe natural human cavities such as the nose, the urethra, the vagina, and the rectum. The source of illumination was the light of a candle reflected by a mirror. The first satisfactory endoscope was presented to the Imperial Academy of Medicine in Paris by Desormeaux in 1853. His method of illumination was a lamp that burned a mixture of alcohol and turpentine. The flame was further stimulated by a chimney mounted at the top of the lamp. The endoscopic sleeve used to explore the cavity was a plain, hollow tube that attached to the light source. At the other extremity was the observer's eye (Fig 1–1). Desormeaux used his apparatus mainly for the examination of the urethra and the bladder, but he also mentioned a possible use in the uterus.

The first successful hysteroscopy was reported by Pantaleoni in the "Medical Press and Circular" of July 14, 1869. He described how, with the endoscope of Desormeaux, he examined a 60-year-old woman with an endometrial polyp and was able to destroy the polyp and cure the woman of her postmenopausal bleeding. It is amusing to note that 3 years earlier he cured the same woman, with the same endoscope, of a nasal polyp from which she had suffered for 30 years. Unfortunately, Pantaleoni's success did not lead to the promising future he anticipated. Although the uterus appeared to be an accessible organ for the newborn endoscope, others using the endoscope of Desormeaux (more or less modified) complained that they hardly saw anything. Endoscopy of the uterus, because of its peculiar anatomy, was indeed very difficult.

Difficulties in Endoscopic Examination of the Uterine Cavity

The uterine cavity is entered through a narrow passage, the internal os and isthmus. This passage must be dilated (Fig 1–2), and the operation is painful. Pantaleoni initiated dilatation through the isthmus with a sponge *(Laminaria),* which he placed in the cervical canal 24 hours before the operation.

The uterine cavity is rendered potential by the effect of the thick and rigid muscular walls. Inside the cavity, the extremity of the endoscopic tube necessarily comes into contact with the uterine walls and mucosa. When contact hysteroscopy is carried out, the field of vision is limited to the diameter of the tube (Fig 1–3).

The uterine mucosa is extremely fragile and bleeds at the slightest touch. The blood penetrates into the hollow tube and interferes with the endoscopist's vision (Fig 1–4).

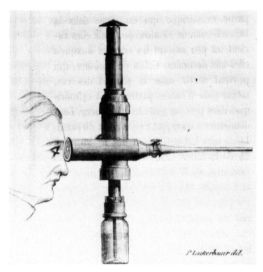

FIG 1–1.
The apparatus of Desormeaux. The alcohol lamp is attached to a vertically mounted chimney-like stack. The hysteroscope is a tapered metal tube.

Possible Solutions

1. It is possible to seal the distal extremity of the tube with a piece of glass, thus keeping the blood out. This is the method of modern contact hysteroscopy (Fig 1–5).

2. It is possible to flush the uterine cavity with water and/or to use a suction channel similar to that used in bronchoscopy.

To achieve a panoramic view of the uterus, it is necessary to separate the uterine walls. Blondel in 1893 utilized two tubes, one fitting into the other. The outer tube was opened and designed to separate the walls, while the inner tube was reserved for vision. With the exception of this purely mechanical attempt, the uterine cavity must be inflated with a gas or a liquid under pressure in order to be visualized (Fig 1–6).

Two difficulties remained: The field of vision, despite the distention of the cavity, was narrow because the tube itself was of limited diameter; and the illumination coming from an external light source was of poor quality. A possible remedy was to provide the tube with optical lenses in order to widen the field of vision, to magnify the images, and to place the source of illumination at the internal extremity of the tube (Fig 1–7). All of these improvements were introduced by Maximilian Nitze, but in the area of cystoscopy rather than hysteroscopy. Nitze (Fig 1–8), who may be considered the father of modern endoscopy, published an article in the "Wiener Medizinische Presse" in 1879 describing his new instruments: a cystoscope and a urethroscope (Fig 1–9). He used a platinum loop which was energized by

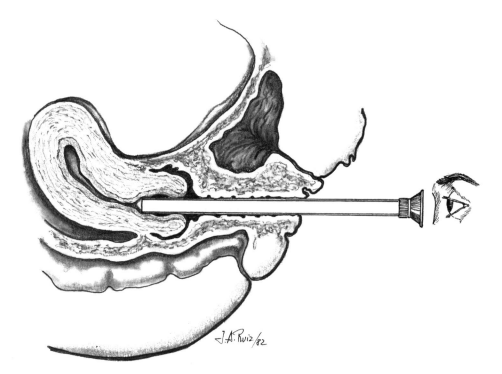

FIG 1–2.
The upper portion of the endocervix where it joins the lower corpus uteri is narrowed, the so-called internal os. For intrauterine visualization to occur, this isthmus must be passed by the hysteroscope.

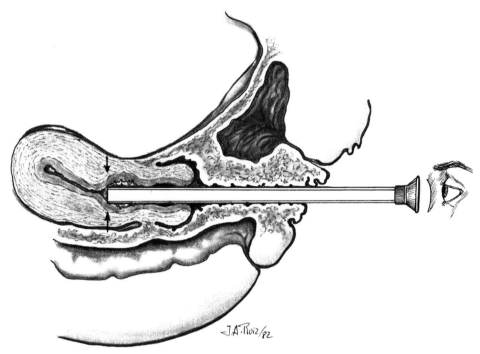

FIG 1–3.
Because of the muscular walls of the uterus (myometrium), the endometrial cavity is really a potential cavity with the anterior and posterior walls in close apposition.

electric current for distal illumination, and cooled the instrument with circulating water. An optical system was built into the tube. The bladder was inflated with water or air. Unfortunately the new principles of Nitze, which led to the rapid worldwide success of cystoscopy, were not applied to hysteroscopy because of the different anatomy of the uterus.

In 1898, Clado, a French surgeon, published an important treatise on hysteroscopy in which he described several instrument models. All were still composed of a

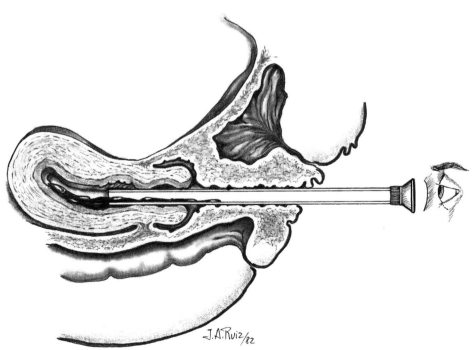

FIG 1–4.
Contact with the fragile endometrium will invariably result in bleeding and interfere with the endoscopist's vision.

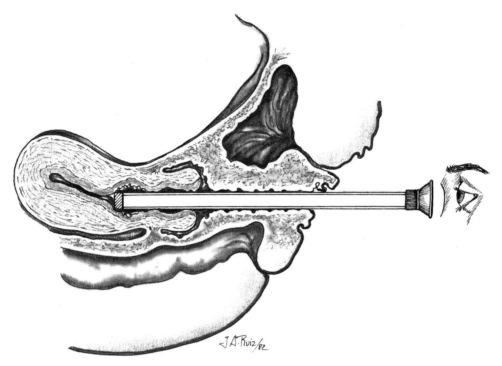

FIG 1–5.
Sealing the distal extremity of the hysteroscope with transparent glass keeps blood out of the hollow tube.

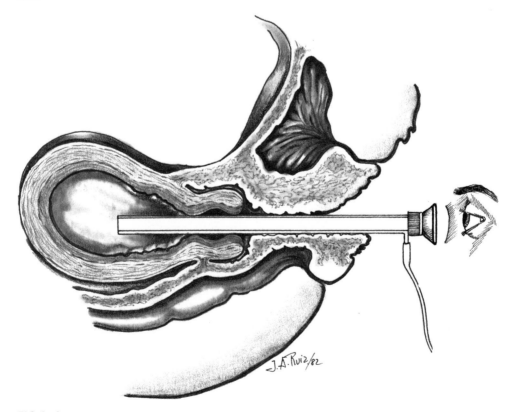

FIG 1–6.
Visualization of the uterine cavity may be accomplished by distending the cavity with a fluid medium in order to separate the thick walls.

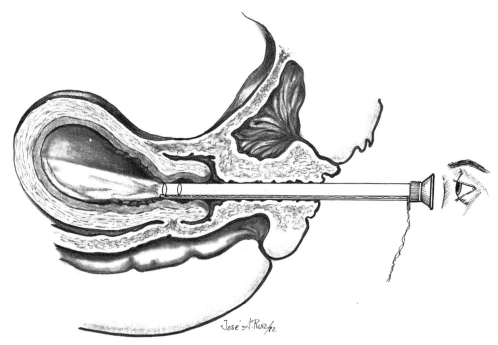

FIG 1–7.
Improved illumination may be obtained by placing the light source at the distal extremity of the hysteroscope behind the glass-sealed end of the tube. Additionally, a lens at the proximal portion of the instrument produces a magnified image.

hollow tube and a separate external source of illumination. The only progress was the introduction of the incandescent lamp invented by Edison in 1879 (Fig 1–10). Figure 1–11 illustrates a hysteroscopic examination conducted according to Clado's methods. A reflecting mirror was used with a central perforation for viewing. However, uterine bleeding continued to be a vexing problem, and visualization in the presence of blood was impossible.

It was not until 1907 that the innovations of Nitze were applied to hysteroscopy by Charles David, who wrote a treatise of hysteroscopy. David improved illu-

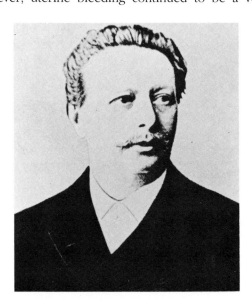

FIG 1–8.
Maximilian Nitze, the father of modern endoscopy, who described the contemporary cystoscope in 1879.

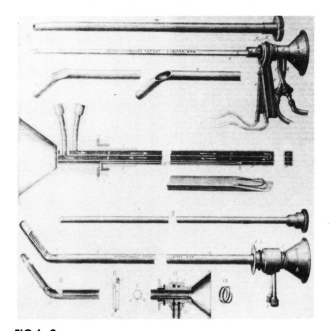

FIG 1–9.
Nitze's instruments are shown in an illustration from his 1879 article. Above, a urethroscope; below, a cystoscope.

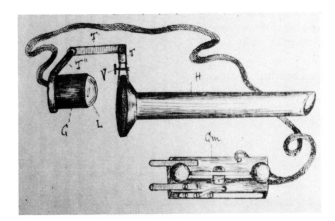

FIG 1–10.
Clado's hysteroscope with an incandescent light source.

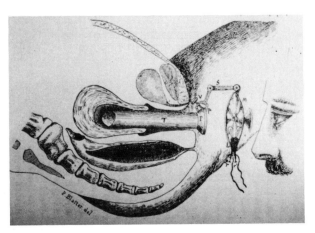

FIG 1–11.
Hysteroscopic examination according to the technique of Clado (1898).

mination by placing an electric incandescent bulb at the intrauterine end of his endoscope. But his most important modification was sealing the distal end of the tube with a piece of glass. Thus, not only was blood not permitted to penetrate the tube, but the pressure of the glass on the uterine wall also forced the blood out, allowing clear vision, regardless of the quantity of hemorrhage (Fig 1–12). The endoscope used by David is

shown in Figure 1–13. The endoscopic examination performed by David is a typical contact hysteroscopy. As demonstrated in Figure 1–14, the cavity is virtual, that is, the two uterine walls are touching. One can see the anterior wall, posterior wall, and the cavity between them through the endoscope. Examination required moving the endoscope about the two walls and over the fundus

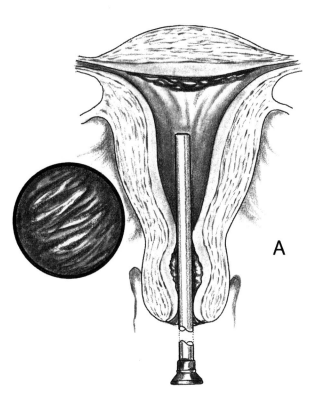

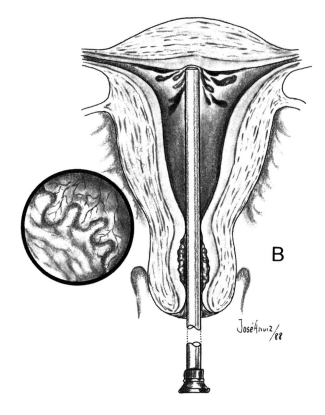

FIG 1–12.
David's contact hysteroscopic technique of forcing blood out of the field to be examined. **A,** view prior to contact. **B,** contact

made and blood excluded from the visual field.

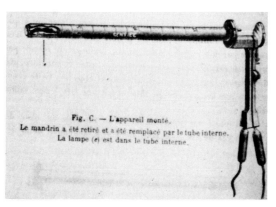

FIG 1–13.
The hysteroscope of Charles David. The instrument is equipped with transparent glass which sealed the hysteroscope's tube and an incandescent light source.

until the whole cavity was explored. The variety of lesions that David observed with his apparatus are shown in Plate 1. His endoscope was simple but effective and solved the major problem of hysteroscopy: visualization in the presence of blood. However, David's endoscope could show only what was seen at the extremity of the tube, and the desire to see beyond this—a more global view—led people to design more complex devices.

USE OF DISTENDING MEDIA

Rubin, who had described tubal insufflation in 1919, noticed that the uterine cavity could be distended under the pressure of a gas. In 1925, he combined the use of a cystoscope with carbon dioxide insufflation of the uterine cavity. He performed 42 examinations utilizing this technique. In several cases, patients were affected adversely by the pneumoperitoneum, and the method was abandoned. It was renewed in 1970 by Lindemann in Germany and Porto in France.

In 1928, Gauss (in Germany) investigated the use of water, not only to flush blood from the cavity but also to distend the uterus. It was necessary to raise the bottles containing water 50 cm above the patient to obtain the required distending pressure (Fig 1–15). Gauss was enthusiastic about the beautifully colored views of the uterine cavity that he obtained and called upon a German academic painter, Heinrich Hoheisel-Neisse, to reproduce them (Plate 2). Unfortunately, difficulties arose and retarded development of the technique. First, blood was not forced out of the field of vision by the interposition of David's glass, resulting in soiling of the optical system which, in turn, clouded the water. Frequent cleaning and rinsing were required to get rid of the

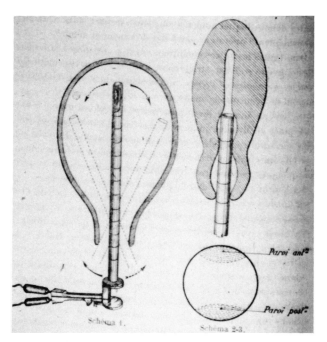

FIG 1–14.
Examination of the uterus by David's hysteroscope illustrates the "collapsed" state of the endometrial cavity (i.e., the anterior and posterior walls are in proximity with a narrow space between them).

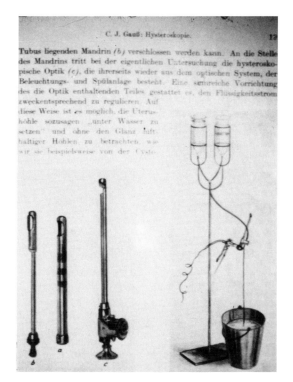

FIG 1–15.
Gauss utilized bottles of water raised 50 cm above the patient to obtain sufficient pressure to distend as well as to irrigate the uterine cavity.

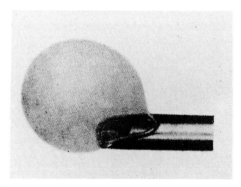

FIG 1–16.
The transparent balloon technique of Silander.

blood, and several liters of water were necessary for each examination. The second difficulty arose from the rigidity of the uterine cavity. To separate the walls, high pressure had to be developed; as a result, the distending medium passed through the oviduct into the peritoneal cavity and had the potential to enter the vascular system. The hazards of infection, cell dissemination, and embolism now existed.

Schroeder tried to determine the lowest pressure of water that allowed a clear view without tubal passage. When the pressure reached 55 mm Hg, the liquid flowed into the tubes. It was later demonstrated that it was impossible to prevent the distending medium from passing into the peritoneal cavity. Silander, in 1962, used a transparent rubber balloon mounted on the endoscope and inflated it within the uterine cavity (Fig 1–16). This technique was a compromise between panoramic and contact hysteroscopy, since it made a panoramic view possible without the danger of dissemination of the medium. The pressure of the balloon on the uterine walls also prevented blood from obscuring vision.

MODERN APPROACHES

Modern panoramic hysteroscopy has now overcome most of these difficulties. The illumination source is a powerful, cold light produced by fiberoptic transmission. As a result of advances in optics, several endoscopes have calibers of 6 mm or less and can easily be inserted into the uterine cavity without dilation of the cervix; larger models are available for intrauterine surgery. Several distending media are now available, including dextran (32%) and dextrose (5%) in water, and carbon dioxide (CO_2). The risk of infectious dissemination into the peritoneum by way of the tubes can easily be avoided by respecting the classic contraindications.

The risk of metastatic dissemination of cancer cells is difficult to prove. The use of carbon dioxide requires a tight fit to prevent cervical leakage, and occasionally a special cervical suction adapter is required. The surgeon must be particularly careful to respect the proper pressure-flow relationships, because a massive vascular passage of carbon dioxide can lead to arrhythmia and even cardiac arrest. This may be prevented by using proper insufflators, such as those developed by Semm and Lindemann.

Dextran is a high-viscosity polysaccharide that retains transparency over a long period and reduces peritoneal spillage. However, rare anaphylactic reactions have been reported with the use of this material. Modern panoramic hysteroscopy can require the use of rather complex and expensive equipment in order to obtain a satisfactory view and to reduce the risks of the procedure. The accesories include a fiberoptic light source with its cable, an irrigating system or a special insufflator with a suction generator, plus their connections. In the presence of mucus, clots, or endometrial debris, visualization becomes difficult and requires frequent cleaning of the distal lens and washing or aspiration of the cavity. A well-trained operator is needed to reduce the manipulation time. In the case of significant bleeding, visualization may be very poor.

In 1966, Marleschki in East Germany concluded that hysteroscopy, despite its hundred years of history, was not as widespread a technique as it deserved to be. He thought that this might be somehow related to the increasing complexity of the equipment, making manipulations delicate and the advantages of the procedure doubtful. He advocated abandoning the separation of the walls and a return to contact hysteroscopy. He developed a simple apparatus in which the extremity was placed directly on the uterine mucosa. The history of the contact endoscope has been connected to the invention in 1952 by Vulmiere, a French optical engineer, of a revolutionary illumination process in endoscopy; the "cold light" process. The idea of Nitze to place the illumination source inside the cavity was revolutionary. Subsequently, no progress has been reported in the development of illumination. The reasons for the limited intensity of light were: (1) the electric bulb must be small in order to penetrate into the cavity to be examined; (2) the emission of heat by the bulb can be dangerous for the uterine tissues. The components of cold light are twofold and consist of (1) a powerful external source, which is transmitted through (2) a special optical guide into the endometrial cavity. Therefore, the power of the light source is no longer limited by space, and the heat is eliminated by an infrared filter before

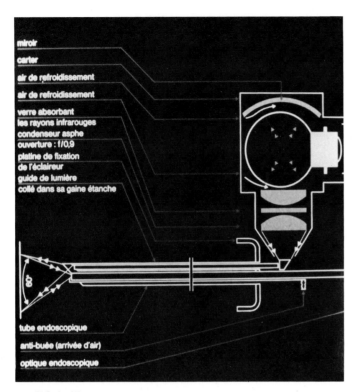

FIG 1–17.
Schematic view of the universal endoscope.

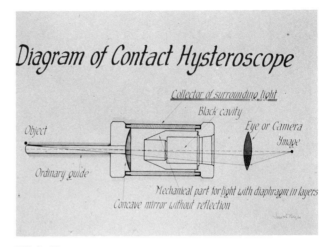

FIG 1–19.
The quality of the image seen with the contact hysteroscope is excellent, because the image is transmitted without distortion (i.e., the angle of entry and exit of the light rays is equal).

the light passes through the guide. Thus, illumination can be as strong as desired and remain harmless.

Most optical guides now consist of a fiberoptic cord. However, from the beginning, Vulmiere utilized a rigid, one-piece, mineral-glass guide (Fig 1–17). He noticed that the mineral-glass guide, when properly treated, could not only transmit light (i.e., illuminate an object) but also bring back the magnified image of the object when the extremity of the guide was in contact with the object. The first application of his principle, in 1963, was an optical trochar, contained in a metallic sheath, which was used in neurosurgery to penetrate the brain tissue and which under direct visual control could reach the ventricles (Fig 1–18). Then, the optical trochar could be removed and replaced by a classic endoscope. This simple endoscope was perfected and, in 1973, Barbot began

its use in France, jointly with Dr. B. Parent, for the examination of the uterine cavity. Baggish, in 1979, reported the first experience with the instrument in the United States (Fig 1–19).

Hamou combined the principles of modern panoramic hysteroscopy with a variation of contact hysteroscopy in a single endoscope, the microcolpohysteroscope (1980). Most recently, Baggish (1987) invented a focusing panoramic hysteroscope and a four-channel operating sheath particularly advantageous for neodymium-yttrium–aluminum-garnet (Nd-YAG) laser hysteroscopic procedures.

BIBLIOGRAPHY

Baggish MS: Contact hysteroscopy: A new technique to explore the uterine cavity. *Obstet Gynecol* 1979; 54:350.

Blondel R: *CR Soc Obstet* December, 1907.

David C: De l'endoscopie de l'uterus apres avortement et dans les suites de couches a l'etat normal et a l'etat pathologique. *Bull Soc Obst Paris* December 1907.

Desormeaux AJ: *Del'Endoscope et de ses Applications au Diagnostic et au Traitement des Affections de l'Uretre et de la Vessie*. Paris, Balliere, 1865.

Gauss CJ: Hysteroskopie. *Arch Gynaekol* 1928; 133:18.

Hamou J: Microhysteroscopy: A new procedure and its original applications in gynecology. *J Reprod Med* 1981; 26:375.

Lindemann HJ: The use of CO_2 in the uterine cavity for hysteroscopy. *Int J Fertil* 1972; 17:221.

Lindemann HJ: Pneumometra fur die hysteroskopie. *Geburtsch Frauersheilk* 1973; 33:18.

Marleschki V: Die moderne zervikoskopie und hysteroskopie. *Zentralbl Gynakol* 1966; 20:637.

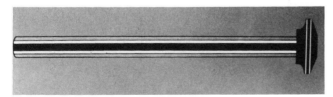

FIG 1–18.
The contact cerebroscope.

Nitze M: Uber eine neue behandlungs—methode de hohlen des menslichen korpers. *Med Press Wien* 1879; 26:851.

Pantaleoni D: On endoscopic examination of the cavity of the womb. *Med Press Circ* 1869; 8:26–27.

Parent B, Barbot J, Doerler B: *L'hysteroscopie de Contact.* Paris, Documentation Scientifique Lab Roland-Marie, Diffusion Edition Publicité, 1976.

Porto R: *Une Nouvelle Methode d'Hysteroscopie.* Marseille, These, 1972.

Rubin C: Uterine endoscopy. Endometroscopy with the aid of uterine insufflation. *Am J Obstet Gynecol* 1925; 10(3):313.

Semm K, Rimkus V: Technische bemerkungers zur CO_2—hysteroskopie. *Geburtsch Frauersheilk* 1974; 34(6):451.

Seymour HF: A method of endoscopic examination of the uterus with its indications. *Proc R Soc Med* 1926;19:74.

Silander T: Hysteroscopy through a transparent rubber balloon. *Surg Gynecol Obstet* 1962; 114(1):125.

2

Embryology and Histology of the Uterus

Leslie B. Arey, Ph.D., Sc.D., L.L.D.†

EMBRYOLOGY

The Bisexual Primordia

The human embryo of 8 weeks is provided with two pairs of potential genital ducts. The male pair originate as the mesonephric ducts of the provisional midkidneys but because at this stage gonadal sex is becoming established, these ducts soon regress, leaving remnants near the ovaries and the so-called Gartner's ducts in regions between the ovaries and hymen. The female ducts, by contrast, are created specifically for genital purposes.

The first indication of each female duct is a groove on the lateral surface of each mesonephros that appears in embryos of nearly 6 weeks' development (Fig 2–1). This groove indents the superficial epithelium, and its lips promptly close, thereby creating a detached tube that advances caudally within the mesonephric ridge. This female duct was originally named the müllerian duct but is now known officially as the paramesonephric duct (Fig 2–2,A–C). Near the cloaca of the embryo the two ridges bearing the ducts swing toward the midplane and fuse into a cylindrical mass called the genital cord (Fig 2–3). At this time (7 weeks) the two internal tubes are still separate but have nearly reached the cloaca.

Uterine Morphogenesis

In embryos of 10 weeks the general plan of the female duct system is evident (Fig 2–4). The cranial segments of both ducts persist as uterine tubes. Slanting, middle segments of both ducts will soon merge and give rise to the fundus of the uterus. The caudal segments of the ducts, already fused, become the corpus cervix and much of the vagina. The caudal end of the

†Deceased.

now single tube presses against the urogenital subdivision of the cloaca, the joint membrane then representing the future hymen. The early uterus lacks a fundus as such, and hence is bicornuate (Figs 2–4 and 2–5,A). After a time the cranial walls of the slanting segments bulge in a cranial direction, so that their original angular junction (Fig 2–5,A) becomes flat (Fig 2–5,B) and finally a dome (Figs 2–5,C and 2–6).

The uterine epithelium buds off glands by the 7th prenatal month, and this establishes the endometrium; yet, they remain small until the child reaches puberty. A distinction between uterus and vagina becomes evident at the middle of the 4th month when the fornices appear. The muscular wall, or myometrium, of the uterus is indicated at 3 months by mesenchyme of the genital cord condensing into smooth muscle fibers that invest the endometrium. The perametrium differentiates from the exterior of the genital cord into a peritoneal covering (mesothelium and connective tissue). The uterus grows rapidly in the final months of fetal development, and the cervix becomes the longest segment by far. Shortly after the child's birth, the uterus loses one half of its length, mostly at the expense of the cervix. It does not recoup this loss until the onset of puberty. The state of the female genitals at birth is shown in Figure 2–6.

The Uterine Ligaments

These supports are logical survivors in relation to the development of the uterus itself. The two genital ridges, containing the paired müllerian ducts, swing together and meet, thereby providing a horizontal shelf that bridges between the right and left body walls (Fig 2–7). It contains the uterus in its midportion. The shelf itself persists as the sheetlike broad ligaments, fibromembranous in composition (see Fig 2–7). Portions of

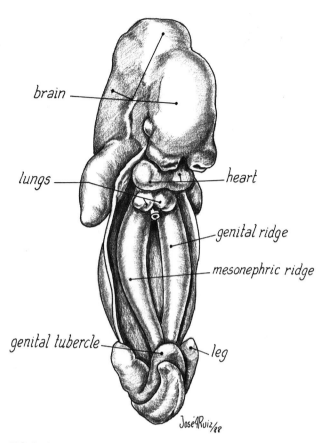

FIG 2–1.
Urogenital ridge of the human embryo; 9-mm ventral view. (After Arey LB: *Developmental Anatomy,* ed 7. Philadelphia, WB Saunders, 1974.)

the genital ridges unite the caudal end of each ovary to the slanting segments of the genital ridges that become the cranial end of the uterus. The sites of uterine attachment are lateral. These bands become fibromuscular and are known as the proper ligaments of the ovaries (Figs 2–7 and 2–8). By the beginning of the 3rd fetal month, continuous cords extend from the upper lateral regions of the uterus into the swellings that become the labia majora. They represent the linkage of two strands: the inguinal ligaments to the body wall at the sites of the future inguinal canals; and the labial ligaments extending into the labia majora. The total lengths of the compound cords become fibromuscular and are named the round ligaments (see Fig 2–8). The cardinal ligament develops as a fibrous sheet of fascia embedded in the lateral wall of the cervix; it is a deeper continuation of the broad ligament. The uterosacral ligament differentiates from mesenchyme as a fascial band extending from the cranial part of the cervix to the sacrum.

Uterine Anomalies

The most common departure of the uterus from its normal configuration result from failures of the müllerian ducts to unite completely or to form a fundus. Figure 2–9,A illustrates the conditions affecting both the uterus and the vagina; Figure 2–9,B shows a double uterus alone; Figure 2–9,C illustrates a largely bipartite uterus with a variably persistent median septum; Figure

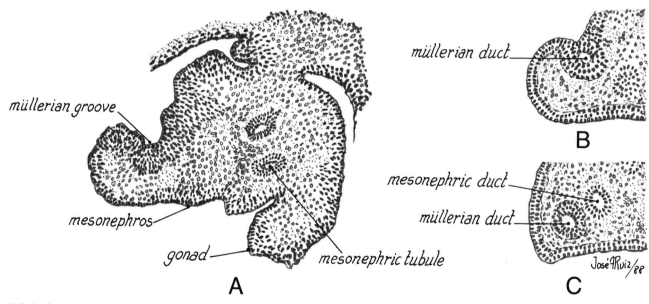

FIG 2–2.
Origin of the Müllerian ducts, illustrated by transverse sections through the early urogenital ridge. **A,** infolding of the peritoneum (mesothelial lining); **B,** narrowing of the neck of the invaginated mesothelium; **C,** the neck is pinched off and a free tube is formed. (After Arey LB: *Developmental Anatomy,* ed 7. Philadelphia, WB Saunders Co, 1974.)

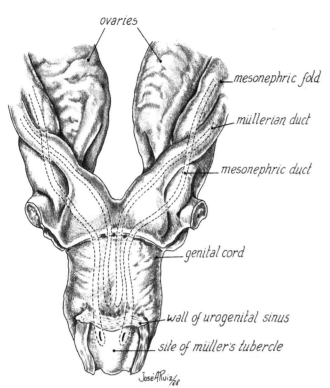

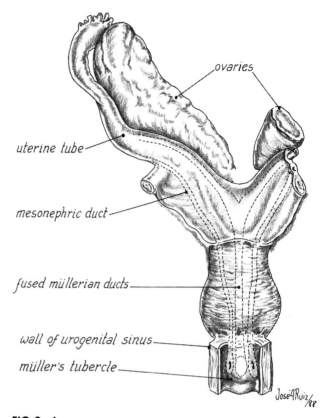

FIG 2–3.
Course of the Müllerian ducts and formation of the genital cord at 2 months. (After Arey LB: *Developmental Anatomy*, ed 7. Philadelphia, WB Saunders, 1974.)

FIG 2–4.
Female genital tract at 10 weeks. (After Arey LB: *Developmental Anatomy*, ed 7. Philadelphia, WB Saunders, 1974.)

2–9,D shows a bicornuate uterus in which the domed fundus fails to form. All of these differences are incorporated in the final adult states of various subprimate mammals. Retention of the infantile size of the uterus results from an inadequate supply of puberal estrogen or a failure of normal tissue response. Congenital absence of the total uterus is rare.

HISTOLOGY

General Plan

The uterus adheres to the general plan for hollow visceral organs. Bordering the lumen is a mucous membrane (tunica mucosa), known clinically as the endo-

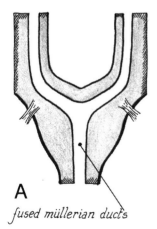

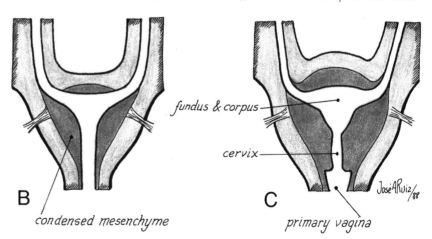

FIG 2–5.
Diagrams of the later progress of the transverse limbs and fused Müllerian ducts. (After Arey LB: *Developmental Anatomy*, ed 7. Philadelphia, WB Saunders, 1974.)

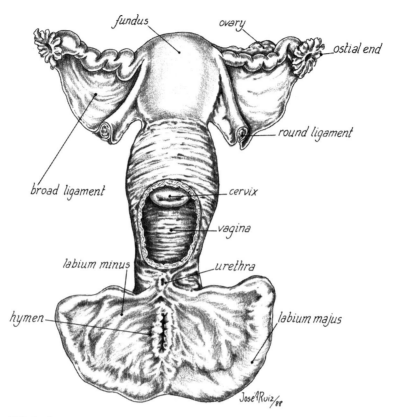

FIG 2–6.
Female genital tract at birth. (After Arey LB: *Developmental Anatomy*, ed 7. Philadelphia, WB Saunders, 1974.)

metrium. It is enveloped by the tunica muscularis, known clinically as the myometrium. At the exterior is an investment of peritoneum, the tunica serosa, known clinically as the perimetrium. Lacking from a complete assembly of mucosa components are a muscularis mucosae at the base of the tunica mucosa and a tunica submucosa, intervening between the tunica mucosa and the tunica muscularis.

Tunica Mucosa (Endometrium)

Surface Epithelium
In the fundus and corpus of the endometrium the epithelium is a simple columnar layer containing groups of ciliated cells. In the cervix the cells are taller; some are ciliated, but most contain so much mucigen that the nuclei are displaced to the cell base.

Glands
The uterine glands extend the full depth of the mucosa and are spaced apart about four times their breadths. There are two regional types: fundus-corpus and cervical.

Fundus-corpus glands.—These make a vertical palisade of tubules that may branch slightly at their deep ends. The component cells are like those on the surface. Their secretion is mucoid and contains glycogen. They undergo marked periodic changes during the menstrual cycle.

Cervical glands.—These are highly branched glands composed of tall mucous cells (Fig 2–10; Plates 3 and 4). Sometimes they occlude and dilate, producing so-called nabothian follicles. These glands undergo relatively slight cyclic changes, but the secretion is thinner and much more profuse at midcycle. In pregnancy the glands both enlarge and proliferate.

Membrana Propria (Basement Membrane)
The epithelium rests upon an inconspicuous membrane of double origin. The basal lamina is an amorphous layer, collagenous in structure and elaborated by the epithelium. A deeper component contains a meshwork of reticular fibers embedded in an amorphous ground substance. This double layer is commonly called the basement membrane, or membrana propria.

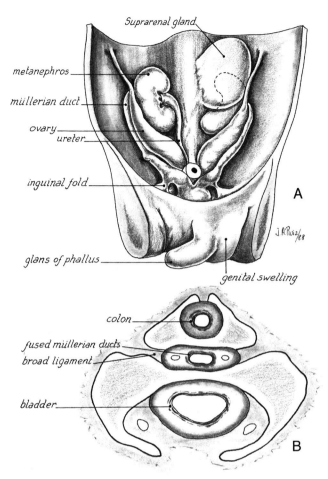

FIG 2–7.
A, union of the paired genital ridges producing the broad ligaments. **B,** transverse section through the lower trunk at approximately 3 months. (After Arey LB: *Developmental Anatomy,* ed 7. Philadelphia, WB Saunders Co, 1974.)

Lamina Propria Mucosae

A connective tissue framework is a mesh of delicate tissue composed of reticular fibers. Infiltrating the meshwork densely are characteristic stromal cells. They are small, angular elements containing a large, ovoid nucleus. Lymphocytes and other leucocytes also occur. In the first half of pregnancy these stromal cells may enlarge and make up the decidual cells of the placenta. In the cervix the stroma is firmer, more fibrous, and less cellular.

Tunica Muscularis (Myometrium)

The muscular coat of the fundus-corpus is relatively massive. It consists of three layers, not sharply demarcated. The inner layer, or stratum submucosum, is mostly longitudinal. The middle layer, or stratum vasculare, is obliquely circular and is the thickest of the three; many large blood vessels give it a spongy texture. The outer layer, or stratum supravasculare, is the thinnest layer. Its component smooth muscle fibers are arranged in bundles, separated by connective tissue. Individual fibers of the tunic are large and vary cyclically in length from 0.040 to 0.090 mm. In pregnancy they elongate to nearly ten times these lengths; they also increase in number, new fibers differentiate, and some old fibers perhaps subdivide.

The cervical musculature is relatively deficient and is arranged in irregular bundles; many collagenous and elastic fibers produce a definite firmness. An outer layer, fairly longitudinal, continues into the vagina.

Tunica Serosa (Perimetrium)

The outermost coat is a covering of peritoneum continuous with that of the broad ligament. It is lacking caudally on the anterior uterine wall, where the urinary bladder abuts.

Vessels and Nerves

Blood vessels enter from the broad ligament and reach the middle layer of muscle. From here one set of short arteries distributes to the relatively inert basal layer of the endometrium. Another set of vessels differentiates into coiled arteries and extends to higher levels, eventually branching into terminal tufts of arterioles. Veins in the endometrium form a varicose meshwork that drains into a venous plexus in the so-called vascular stratum of the myometrium. These vessels then pass into the broad ligament.

Lymphatic vessels form abundant plexuses in all three uterine tunics but are wholly absent in the superficial endometrium. Unmyelinated nerve fibers supply uterine blood vessels and muscle bundles. Myelinated nerve fibers enter the endometrium, but the specific sites of their endings are not known.

Cyclic Changes

Menstrual Cycle

Five stages can be recognized in the typical menstrual cycle of the fundus-corpus. During this period of 28 days, the first day of flow is designated as day 1, and later days are numbered sequentially.

1. *Resurfacing (day 5 or 6).* Repair begins even before all bleeding ceases. Epithelial cells leave the remnants of eroded glands, glide over the denuded surface, and restore a new surface covering (Plate 5,A and B).

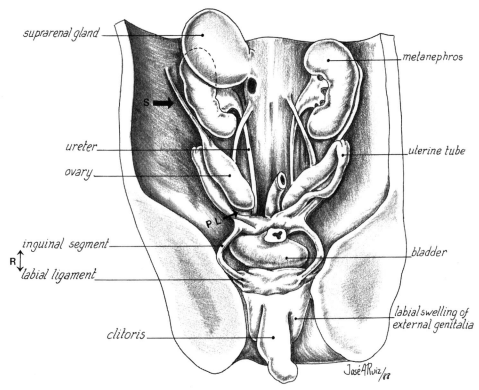

FIG 2—8.
The genital ligaments at 10 weeks. *R* = round ligament of the uterus; *S* = suspensory ligament of the ovary; *PL* = proper ligament of the ovary. (After Arey LB: *Developmental Anatomy*, ed 7. Philadelphia, WB Saunders, 1974.)

2. *Proliferation (days 7 to 10).* Also called the pre-ovulatory or follicular stage, the proliferation stage extends and completes the postmenstrual repair through a period of growth in thickness that coincides with the growth of ovarian follicles; it is induced by estrogen. The glands lengthen rapidly; glycogen accumulates in the cells; and a thin, mucoid secretion is expelled (Plate 6,A and B). Connective tissue rebuilds the lamina propria, and coiled arteries are regrowing into this layer.

3. *Secretion (days 15 to 26).* Also called the premenstrual or luteal stage; the secretion stage is constant in length, in contrast to the proliferative stage, which differs in length in short or long cycles. The glands cease proliferating but they become wavy, tortuous, and swollen (Plate 7,A and B). The coiled arteries spiral into tighter coils and nearly reach the surface epithelium.

4. *Ischemia (days 27 and 28).* Local groups of

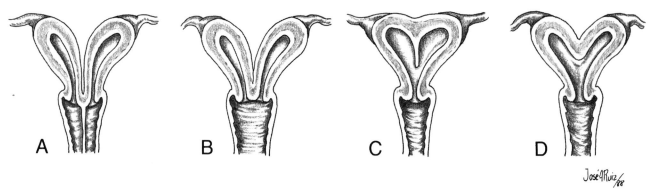

FIG 2—9.
Uterine anomalies. **A,** double uterus and vagina. **B,** double uterus. **C,** bipartite uterus. **D,** bicornuate uterus. (After Arey LB: *Developmental Anatomy*, ed 7. Philadelphia, WB Saunders, 1974.)

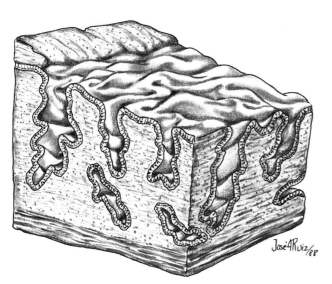

FIG 2–10.
A, (above), section through the cervix at the squamocolumnar junction. **B,** (see Plate 3), detail of endocervical mucous epithelium. **C,** (see Plate 4), endocervical papillae and surface mucous secreting epithelium with extensive squamous metaplasia.

coiled arteries constrict intermittently, and blood flow ceases for an hour or more. The endometrium pales and shrinks, losing glandular secretion and stromal tissue-fluid.

5. *Menstruation (days 1 to 4 or 5).* All levels except the basal layer undergo necrosis. Blood cells slip through the walls of intact capillaries and escape from injured capillaries whose blood supply has failed. At times the coiled arteries relax locally, and blood escapes from bursting vessels. Patches of blood-soaked tissue separate away and accumulate in the uterine lumen.

The superficial compact layer of the endometrium and a variable amount of the spongy layer slough off (Plate 8,A and B). A deeper portion of the spongy layer and all of the basal layer are regained. The short, straight arteries, the sole supply to the basal layer, do not constrict intermittently; hence, this layer does not become ischemic and consequently suffer damage.

Anovular Cycle

Sometimes ovulation fails, and no corpus luteum forms. Menstruation can then occur in an endometrium that advances only through the proliferative (estrogen) state and then lacks further endocrine support.

BIBLIOGRAPHY

Arey LB: *Developmental Anatomy,* ed 7, revised. Philadelphia, WB Saunders, 1974, pp 317–318, 326–330.

Fawcett DW: *A Textbook of Histology,* ed 11. Philadelphia, W B Saunders, 1986, pp 877–886.

Hamilton WJ, Boyd JD, Mossman HW: *Human Embryology,* ed 4. Baltimore, Williams & Wilkins, 1972, pp 287–291.

Keibel F, Mall FP: *Manual of Human Embryology.* Philadelphia, JB Lippincott Co, 1912, vol 2, pp 911–920, 924–933.

Von Moellendorff W: Harn- und Geschlechtsapparat. Berlin, Springer, 1930, pp 419–468.

Weiss L: *Histology,* ed 5. New York, Elsevier North-Holland, Inc, 1983, pp 931–940.

3

Anatomy of the Uterus

Michael S. Baggish, M.D.

GROSS ANATOMY

The uterus is a hollow, pyriform, muscular structure measuring 7 to 8 cm in length, 4 to 5 cm in width at its upper portion, and 2 to 3 cm in thickness. It weighs between 50 and 80 gm. The uterus is divided into three portions: cervix; corpus; and fundus. The narrowed area between the cervix and body is called the isthmus and corresponds to the level of the internal os or the opening between the cervical canal and the uterine cavity (Fig 3–1).

The cervix appears cylindrical in shape and measures 2.5 to 3 cm in height and in its posterior extent; it is covered with peritoneum which is reflected from the back of the vagina. The anterior portion of the supravaginal cervix is separated from the bladder by endopelvic fascia. Laterally the cervix is bounded by the structures lying within the broad ligament (Fig 3–2).

The vaginal portion of the cervix projects into the vaginal canal and is surrounded by four vaginal fornices. The terminus of the cervix is rounded and is punctuated with a circular or transverse opening, the external os (Plate 9). Two lips are identified; these are termed the anterior, which is shorter and thicker, and the posterior, which is longer and thinner. Nearly half of the cervix lies within the vagina. The portio vaginalis cervix usually enters the vagina obliquely from ventral to dorsal, pointing to the posterior wall of the vagina.

The canal of the cervix is for all practical purposes spindle-shaped. Longitudinal crests of endocervical mucosa protrude into the cavity anteriorly and posteriorly as the plicae palmatae (Fig 3–3). Secondary oblique branching of the mucosa gives the appearance of a tree and constitutes the arbor vitae. The endocervical mucosa is whitish pink in color and, as noted, is thrown

into numerous folds or papillae interspersed with clefts (Plate 10). Not infrequently small bluish-grey bubbles or retention cysts are visible within the canal (Plate 11). The lumen of the cervix ranges between 3 and 10 mm in diameter depending on individual variation and parity. There is, however, some resiliency to light pressure that may allow 1 to 2 mm additional space with stretching. During stretching, the mucosal folds appear flat and white. During contact and low-pressure-CO_2 panoramic hysteroscopy the pink, papillary mucosal pattern with its plentiful fine vessels are appreciated. However, with higher CO_2 pressure and fluid media hysteroscopy, the endocervical canal appears as a flat, white cylindrical structure because the mucosal pattern has been smoothed and the vasculature occluded.

The isthmus is a flattened, narrowed, short canal between the upper portion of the cervix and the corpus. The mucosa is smooth compared with the highly folded endocervix. The isthmus measures about 1 cm in length and is marked by a construction (internal os) where it meets the cervix. The isthmus is very narrow in the nulliparous woman, but expands to approximately 1 cm after delivery. The anterior and posterior walls of the uterus are in close opposition and are best appreciated in the natural state during contact hysteroscopy (Plate 12).

The corpus forms the main mass of the uterus, and is usually bent anteriorly on the isthmus and usually tipped slightly to the right. The convex posterior wall of the uterus is covered with peritoneum (Plate 13,A). Two thirds of the flattened anterior aspect is covered with peritoneum as it reflects off the urinary bladder (Plate 13,B). The walls are heavily musculatured and measure about 2 cm thick.

The potential cavity of the uterus is flattened and

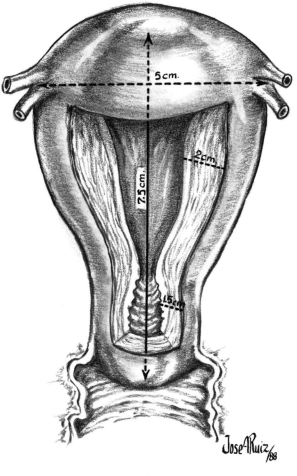

FIG 3–1.
The anterior wall of the uterus has been cut out. The three major subdivisions of the uterus are clearly identified: cervix; corpus; fundus. The thickest musculature is seen in the corpus and fundus. The narrowed area between the internal os of the cervix, and the wider corpus is the isthmus.

A

B

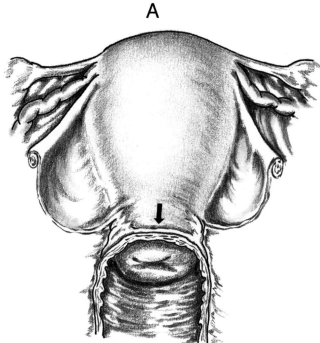

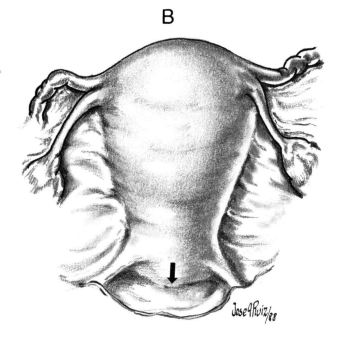

FIG 3–2.
The cervix measures approximately 2.5 cm in height. Anteriorly **(A)** the cervix is separated from the bladder by the endopelvic fascia *(arrow)*. Posteriorly **(B)** the cervix lies below the uterosacral ligaments and is covered with peritoneum, which reflects off the posterior vagina (cul de sac).

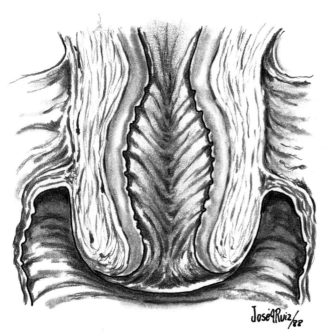

FIG 3–3.
Open view of the cervix. The endocervical mucosa projects into the canal and fans out as the plicae palmatae. Laterally the cervix is bordered by the lateral fornices of the vagina and the bases of the broad ligaments. The internal os leads into the uterine cavity *(i)*.

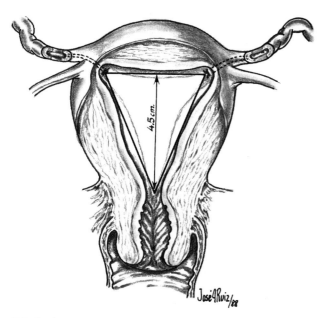

FIG 3–4.
The cavity of the uterus forms an inverted triangle with the base formed by a line drawn between the two tubal ostia and the vertex at the isthmus.

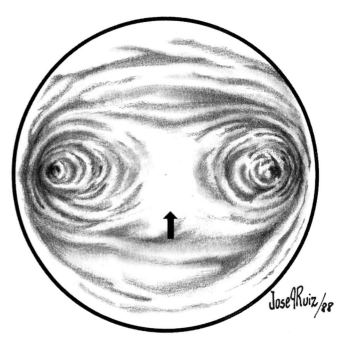

FIG 3–5.
The tubal ostia enter the fundus with great variation as to angle and appearance. The anatomic landmark where the paired müllerian ducts have fused creates a pillar *(arrow)* separating the cornua. This may be mistaken for a septum.

has the shape of an inverted triangle with base formed by a line drawn between the two tubal ostia and the apex at the isthmic opening. From top to bottom this space measures 4–5 cm (Fig 3–4). Hysterovolumetric studies of the uterus have been reported by Davis and Israel.

Anteriorly the corpus lies in close proximity to the urinary bladder. Posteriorly the uterus relates to the sigmoid colon and small intestine. The lateral margins of the uterus are convex and juxtapose the interior of the broad ligament where the ascending branch of the uterine artery ascends from the isthmus to the fundus in a coiled pattern. The mucosa of the corpus, i.e., the endometrium, varies in thickness depending on the phase of the menstrual cycle and ranges between 1 and 4 mm. On gross examination it appears smooth, orange-tan, and is usually thickest in the cornual areas (Plate 14,A and B).

During hysteroscopic examination the normal endometrium exhibits hues ranging from orange-red to pink and appears rather flattened when viewed during the proliferative phase (see Plate 12).

The endometrium becomes velvety and reddish during the secretory phase and under contact hysteroscopy shows irregular polypoid-like patterns that protrude into the cavity, analogous to stalactites and stalagmites (Plate 15).

The thick fundus lies above a line drawn between the two tubal ostia. Frequently, the anatomic site is marked with a central ridge identifying the point where the müllerian ducts have fused. This normal variant must not be confused with the more exaggerated subseptate uterus. The tubal ostia lie recessed in shallow depressions at either extremity of the fundus (i.e., the cornua; Plates 16,A and B). During hysteroscopy there is some variation in the appearance of the ostia as well as in the depth and position of the cornual recesses. For example, at two extremes, the cornua may be recessed almost horizontally in one instance and approximately 30% to 40% off the vertical in the other (Fig 3–5). Likewise, there is great variety in the relative locations of the tubal ostia. They may be seen as flat slits or circles or appear elevated on papilla-like pedestals or look completely flat (Fig 3–6). During Hyskon hysteroscopy the tubal ostia frequently demonstrate a bluish tint.

Regardless of the phase of the menstrual cycle, the endometrium is highly vasculatured and bleeds with the slightest touch of the endoscope. When one is using a focusing magnified telescope, the submucosal capillaries are disposed to form a netlike, intricate vascular pattern covering the entire endometrial surface (Plate 17). Additionally the depth of the endometrium may be estimated either intentionally or accidentally by allowing the pressure of the endoscope to impact the posterior wall, producing a groove into the mucosa.

When using a magnifying or contact hysteroscopy depressions representing the mouths of the endometrial

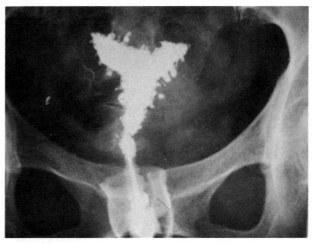

FIG 3–7.
A (see Plate 18), contact hysteroscopy may reveal small holes or diverticula in the otherwise intact endometrium. **(B)** (above), hysterogram demonstrates the diverticula illustrated in **A.**

glands are readily apparent. Occasionally, small holes (diverticulae) may also be observed in otherwise intact interior mucous membrane of the uterus (Fig 3–7 and Plate 18).

POSITIONS OF THE UTERUS

Characteristically, the uterus is anteflexed over the urinary bladder; the cervix is angulated toward the axis

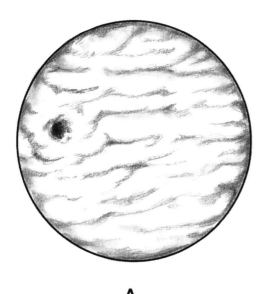

A

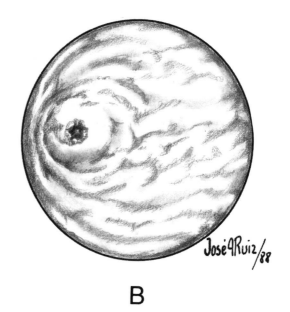

B

FIG 3–6.
Two common variants of tubal ostium appearance as viewed during hysteroscopy: **(A)** the ostium is flat, **(B)** the ostium is seated on a papilla-like pedestal.

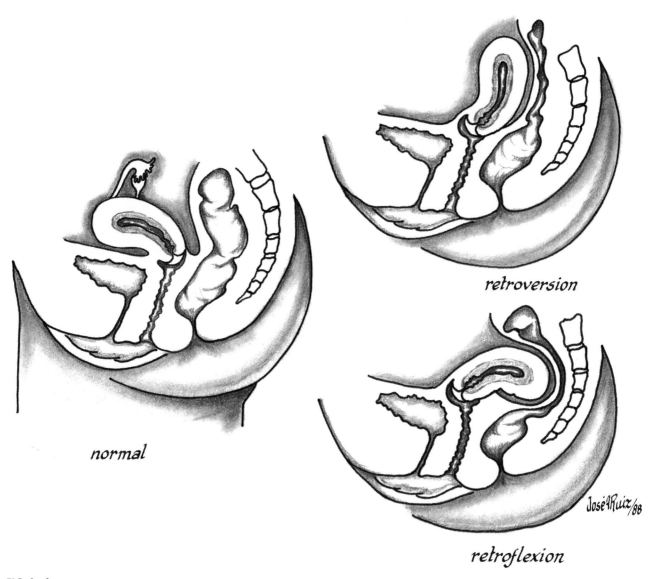

retroversion

Jose9Ruiz/88

retroflexion

normal

FIG 3–8.
The uterus is most frequently flexed over the bladder (anteflexed). Other common positions which are ascertained by bimanual ex-

amination are retroversion and retroflexion.

TABLE 3–1.

Uterine Positions in 200 Random Pelvic Examinations*

Position	Age of Subject (yr)	
	<50	>50
Anteflexed, no. (%)	150 (90)	13 (43)
Retroflexed, no. (%)	12 (5.3)	2 (7)
Retroversion, no. (%)	8 (4.7)	15 (50)
Total	170 (100)	30 (100)

*Data from Health Science Center, State University of New York, Syracuse. Used by permission.

of the vagina or directed slightly to the posterior of that axis. As a result of childbearing and stretching of the main ligamentous supports, the uterus may be displaced backward toward the sacrum, a condition referred to as retroversion (Fig 3–8). Occasionally, the uterus is flexed posteriorly on itself (retroflexion; Fig 3–8). At the time of vaginal examination a severe anterior or posterior pointing of the cervix should alert the practitioner to suspect a displacement. In an analysis of 200 random pelvic examinations, the anteflexed or normal variant was detected in 150 (90%) of women under the age of 50 years (Table 3–1). Of 30 women over 50 years of age, over 50% demonstrated retroversion. Accurate determi-

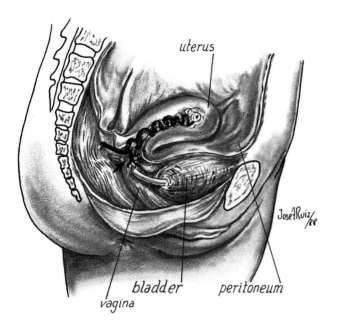

uterus

bladder

vagina

peritoneum

JoséARuiz/88

FIG 3–9.
A (see Plate 19), the uterine artery arises from the hypogastric artery (seen lateral to the ureter) *(arrow).* **B** (left), the uterine artery crosses the ureter and ascends the lateral aspect of the corpus after giving off a descending branch to the cervix *(arrow).*

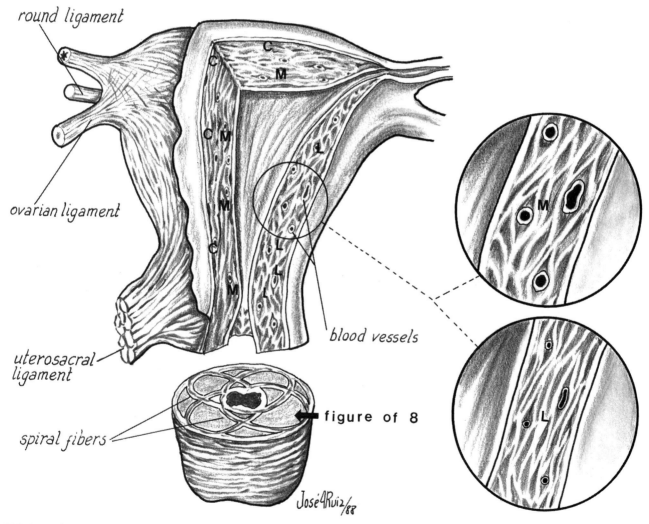

round ligament

ovarian ligament

uterosacral ligament

spiral fibers

blood vessels

figure of 8

JoséARuiz/88

FIG 3–10.
The myometrium is indistinctly arranged in three layers: an outer longitudinal *(L),* an oblique middle *(M)* layer, and an inner circular *(C)* layer just beneath the endometrium. The middle layer is oriented to compress the traversing blood vessels during muscular contraction.

nation of the position of the uterus is definitely essential to performing a successful hysteroscopic examination.

BLOOD SUPPLY

The uterine artery, which arises from the anterior division of the hypogastric artery, is the main blood supply of the uterus (Plate 19). The vessel arrives at approximately the level of the isthmus after crossing above the ureter. The uterine artery gives off a large branch to the

cervix, then proceeds upward in a coiled pattern along the edge of the uterus between the layers of the broad ligament until it reaches the uterotubal junction, where it anastomoses with the ovarian artery (Fig 3–9). Veins are large and abundant, forming thin-walled plexuses within the myometrium and beneath the peritoneum. Usually two or more veins accompany the uterine artery and anastomose with tributaries of the hypogastric, vaginal, and ovarian veins. Branches of uterine artery pierce the myometrium, circle that structure, and anastomose with similar branches derived from the opposite uterine

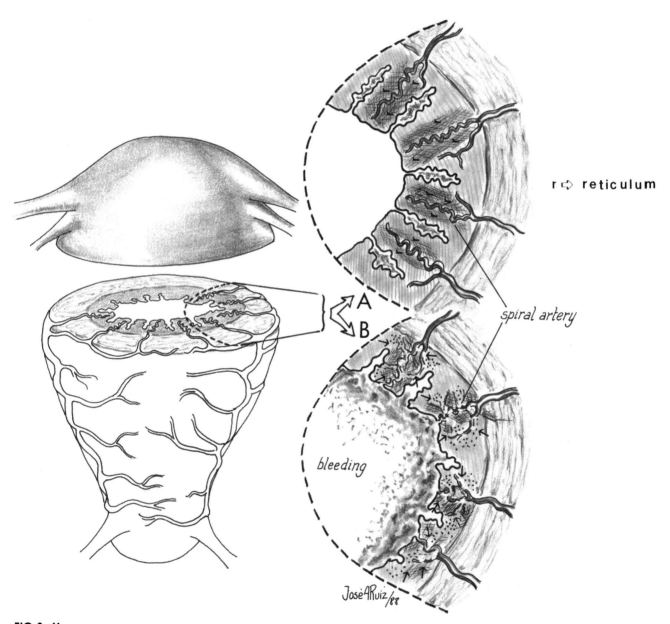

r ⇨ **r e t i c u l u m**

spiral artery

bleeding

José A Ruiz/88

FIG 3–11.
The spiral arteriole is surrounded by a reticulum network as illustrated in Plate 20. Breaks in this reticulum network result in collapse of the supporting endometrial stroma and diapedesis.

artery. These circling vessels in turn give off numerous branches that pass inward to the inner muscle layers at right angles. These in turn branch again into a short, basal arteriole, which supplies the basalis, and a spiral arteriole, which supplies the remainder of the endometrium.

SEROSA AND MUSCULARIS

The serosa of the uterus, which is derived from the peritonerium, covers 100% of the posterior surface but only two thirds of the anterior surface. The layers of smooth (involuntary) muscle are indistinctly arranged in three layers: a thin outer longitudinal layer; an interfacing middle layer; and a submucosal circular layer (Fig 3–10). The musculature is thickest at the level of the fundus and corpus and thinnest at the orifices of the tube. Within the muscularis are numerous veins and arteries. The coats of the vessels are intimately adherrent to the muscularis and connective tissue such that even thin-walled veins are patulous on cross section. Most importantly, when the crisscrossing muscle fibers contract strongly, they squeeze off the vessels in a fashion similar to a figure-of-8 ligature.

MICROANATOMY

The mucosa of the uterus constitutes the endometrium. This consists of endometrial glands interspersed in a stromal matrix which in turn is supported by a reticular network (Plate 20,A). The surface of the endometrium is covered by a single layer of low columnar cells, the capsule. The endometrium may in turn be subdivided into a more or less static portion, the basalis, and a dynamically changing portion, the functionalis (Plate 20,B). The latter undergoes morphologic changes in response to the activity of ovarian hormones during the menstrual cycle. Following the menopause, the endometrium consists essentially of a sparsely populated basalis with a thin capsule consisting of a single layer of cuboidal cells. Lymphocytes are frequently observed within the endometrium throughout the cycle and should not be considered pathologic (i.e., chronic endometritis). Likewise, reserve cells may be observed immediately beneath and within the lining cells of the endometrial glands and capsule. These totipotential cells have been seen to wander through the endometrial stroma and to first initiate regeneration of the endometrium following menstruation by a process akin to squamous metaplasia. Similarly, the application of reticulum stains to sections of the endometrium just prior to and during early menstruation demonstrates the collapse of these fibers preceding the disruption of the endometrial glands and stroma. Interestingly, the small arterial leaks (diapedesis) can also be attributed to the disruption of reticulum surrounding the spiral arterioles (Fig 3–11).

BIBLIOGRAPHY

Baggish MS, Pauerstein CJ, Woodruff JD: Role of stroma in regeneration of endometrial epithelium. *Am J Obstet Gynecol* 1967; 99:459.

Brash JC: *Cunningham's Manual of Practical Anatomy,* ed 11. London, Oxford University Press, 1948, vol II.

Cullen TS: *Cancer of the Uterus.* Philadelphia, W B Saunders, 1909.

Davis HJ, Israel R: Uterine cavity measurements in relation to design of intrauterine contraceptive devices. Proceedings of the 2nd Internal Conference on Intrauterine Contraception. Amsterdam, Excerpta Medica Foundation, 1964.

Fluhmann FC: Histology of the cervix uteri, in Meigs JV, Sturgis SH (eds): *Progress in Gynecology.* New York, Grune & Stratton, 1963, vol IV pp 3–16.

Gray H, in Goss CM (ed): *Anatomy of the Human Body,* ed 26. Philadelphia, Lea & Febiger, 1954.

Jewett C: *Practice of Obstetrics.* New York, Lea Brothers, 1901.

Jordan J, Singer A: *The Cervix.* London, W B Saunders, 1976.

Kelly HA: *Operative Gynecology.* New York, D Appleton, 1898, vol 1.

Netter FH: *Reproductive System.* The CIBA Collection of Medical Illustrations, vol 2. Summit, New Jersey, CIBA, 1954.

Sabotta J, Uhlenhuth E: *Atlas of the Descriptive Human Anatomy.* New York, Hafner, 1954, vol II.

4

Physiology of the Uterus

Shawky Z. A. Badawy, M.D.

The objectives of this chapter are directed toward understanding the normal menstrual cycle. The following aspects are discussed:

1. The normal interplay between the hypothalamic pituitary system and the ovary to produce ovulatory cycles.
2. The ovarian changes during the cycle.
3. The uterine and endometrial changes resulting from the secretion of ovarian steroids during the cycle.

Endometrial changes represent the end result of the entire cascade of events that occur cyclically during a woman's reproductive years. Hysteroscopic evaluation of the uterine cavity, therefore, varies according to the stage of the cycle. In addition, learning the normal events will help the hysteroscopist to diagnose the abnormalities that are sometimes present and lead to abnormal uterine bleeding, discharge, and/or infertility.

PHYSIOLOGY OF THE NORMAL MENSTRUAL CYCLE

Cyclic shedding of the endometrium occurs regularly during the reproductive years of women with normal sexual development. This is the result of the effect of ovarian hormones on the endometrium, leading to certain cyclic changes. Such normal function requires an intact hypothalamic pituitary system, a normal ovary with functioning follicles and stroma, and a healthy endometrium with the necessary receptors for both estrogen and progesterone.

The hypothalamus secretes gonadotropin-releasing hormone (Gn-RH) from certain nuclei in the median eminence, arcuate, preoptic, and supraoptic areas. The secretion of this hormone is under the complex control

of neurotransmitters that are affected by the internal hormonal milieu of the woman as well as other factors such as stress, weight, exercise, and drugs. Gn-RH is a decapeptide that reaches the pituitary gland through the portal circulation. Gn-RH attaches to receptors on the gonadotropes to stimulate the synthesis and release of both follicle stimulating hormone (FSH) and luteinizing hormone (LH). Both FSH and LH are needed for the process of follicle growth, maturation, and ovulation, and normal functioning of the corpus luteum of the ovary (Fig 4–1).

THE OVARIAN CYCLE

The changes in the ovary in each menstrual cycle can be divided into the follicular phase, ovulatory phase, and luteal phase.

Follicular Phase

As a result of the decline in the secretion of ovarian steroids at the end of the preceding cycle, the negative feedback effect on the hypothalamic pituitary gonadotropin system is abolished. Both FSH and LH start to rise during the first 5 to 7 days of the menstrual cycle. A group of follicles start to grow due to the proliferation of granulosa cells under the effect of FSH. By the mid-follicular phase, the dominant follicle is identified and continues to grow, and the other follicles undergo atresia. The growing follicles stimulate estrogen secretion. Ovarian stroma, and especially theca cells under the effect of LH, secrete androstenedione. The granulosa cells, on the other hand, aromatize androstenedione under FSH stimulation to produce estradiol-17β. Estradiol enhances the sensitivity to FSH by increasing FSH receptors on the follicle. FSH induces LH receptors, which

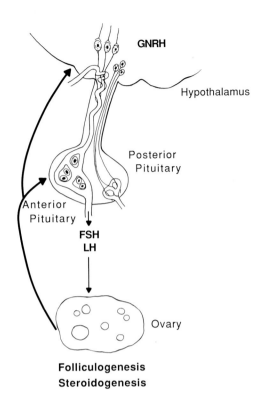

FIG 4–1.
Schematic representation of the hypothalamic-pituitary-ovarian hormonal axis.

process is also enhanced by estradiol. As a result of these changes the follicle continues to grow until it reaches maturity in the preovulatory stage. Estrogen secretion increases, and a preovulatory serum level of 200 to 300 pg/ml is reached. With the increase in estrogen levels during the late follicular phase, there is a slight decline in FSH, but LH secretion continues to increase (Fig 4–2,A).

Ovulatory Phase

The high estrogen peak at the end of the follicular phase of the cycle leads to a positive-feedback effect on the hypothalamic pituitary system. It stimulates the secretion of Gn-RH with more frequent pulses. It also sensitizes the gonadotropes to the effect of Gn-RH. The end result is the production of an LH peak. The LH peak is the result of the estrogen-positive effect on the hypothalamic pituitary axis. The low progesterone levels at that stage play a facilitatory role with estrogens. The peak of LH stimulates biologic changes in the follicle, including numerically more LH receptors and maturation of the oocyte. In addition, the LH peak stimulates prostaglandin secretion in and around the follicle and increases collagenase in the stroma at the surface of the follicle.

As a result of all these changes, the muscle fibers around the graafian follicle contract, owing to the prostaglandin effect. The softening of the stroma near the stigma allows for follicle rupture and ovulation, which occur about 24 hours following LH peak. These changes have been described by Wallach as a result of in vitro studies of the perfused rabbit ovary. He postulates that LH surge prior to ovulation activates the cyclic AMP (adenosine prime monophosphate) system in the follicle. This leads to an increase in plasminogen and plasmin in the follicle. This process also leads to conversion of procollagenase to collagenase. This collagenase leads to lytic changes in the wall of the follicle and adjacent ovarian wall; thus effecting thinning down of the wall in the future stigma of ovulation. At the same time the meiotic division of the oocyte is resumed to lead to ovum maturation. The increase in prostaglandin F_2 (PGF_2) and noradrenalin locally in the ovary causes the contraction of the smooth muscle fibers around the follicle to initiate the ovulation process (Fig 4–2,B).

Luteal Phase

With ovulation, the remaining granulosa and theca cells of the follicle become luteinized to form the corpus luteum. Increased vascularity occurs during the first half of the luteal phase when the secretion of progesterone and estrogen reach a peak. The function of the corpus luteum continues for 12 to 14 days if pregnancy does not occur. The role of intraovarian prostaglandins in the function and survival or demise of the corpus luteum is still under study in humans. It is fair to say that during the active stage of the corpus luteum there is a high ratio of PGE_2 to $PGF_{2\alpha}$. If there is no pregnancy, the corpus luteum starts its decline, which may be due to an increased $PGF_{2\alpha}/PGE_2$ ratio.

THE UTERINE CYCLE

The uterus is a target organ for the action of ovarian steroids. It is located in the pelvic cavity in the nonpregnant woman. During pregnancy, the uterus enlarges as a result of myohyperplasia to accommodate the growing fetus and becomes a pelvic abdominal organ. During the postpartum period, the uterus involutes gradually to reach a prepregnancy size within 6 weeks after delivery of the fetus. The process of myohyperplasia during pregnancy is the result of the effect of both estrogen and progesterone acting on specific receptors in the wall of the uterus. In the nonpregnant state, the uterus measures 7 cm in length, 6 cm in width at the fundus, and 5 cm in anteroposterior diameter. The uterus has three

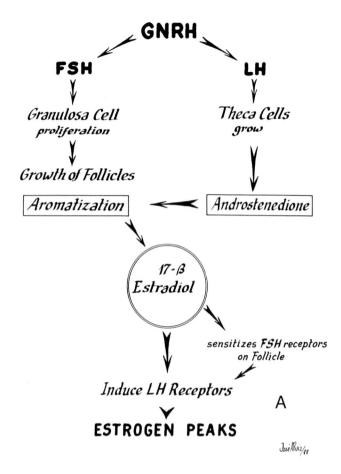

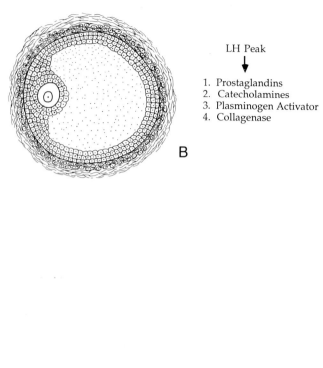

FIG 4–2.
A, factors controlling estrogen secretion. **B,** the graafian follicle and events at the LH peak.

muscle layers: outer longitudinal, inner circular, and middle intermingled layer of muscle fibers. The anterior and posterior walls of the uterus lie in opposition of each other with almost no cavity between. So the uterine cavity is a potential cavity that becomes apparent when it is distended with Sinografin (diatrizoate meg-

lumine and iodipamide meglumire) during hysterosalpingography, or with Hyskon during hysteroscopy, or physiologically during pregnancy.

The endometrium is the mucus membrane lining of the uterine cavity. It is lined with columnar epithelium. It has both glands and stroma. The endometrium is another end organ that is subject to the effects of both estrogen and progesterone secreted by the ovary. The changes that occur in the endometrium during the menstrual cycle can be classified into three phases: menstrual phase, proliferative phase, and luteal phase. For the sake of discussion of these phases in a sequential manner, the proliferative and luteal phases of the cycle will be presented first (Fig 4–3).

Proliferative Phase

Following shedding of the endometrium during menstruation, a process of regeneration starts. The epithelium regenerates from the basal portions of the endometrial glands that are embedded superficially in the inner muscular layer of the uterine wall. This basal endometrial layer does not shed during menses. Under the effect of estrogen secreted by the ovary at this stage (es-

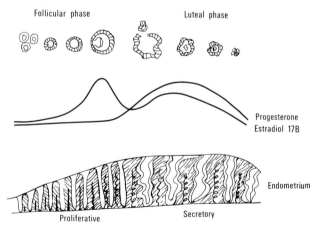

FIG 4–3.
Diagram representing ovarian and endometrial changes during the normal menstrual cycle.

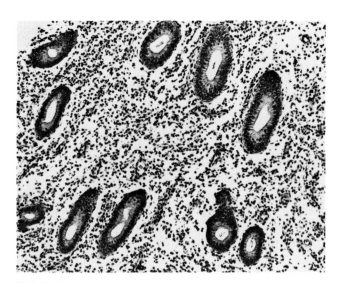

FIG 4–4.
Proliferative endometrium; ×125.

tradiol-17β), proliferation of the glands and stroma takes place. This process continues until ovulation occurs. The glands are straight, tubular structures lined with columnar epithelium without any evidence of secretion (Fig 4–4). The stroma is abundant and composed of small cells. The endometrium also increases in thickness to about 5 to 7 mm at the end of the proliferative stage. Estrogen acts as a growth hormone for the endometrium. To produce such changes, estrogen induces estrogen receptors in the endometrial cells. Estradiol-17β attaches to these receptors, leading to an estrogen-receptor complex which is translocated to the nucleus of

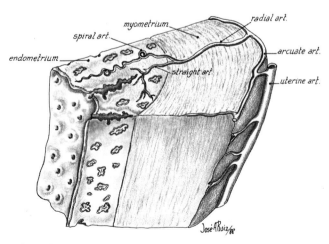

FIG 4–5.
The blood supply to the endometrium emanates from the uterine artery; which enters the myometrium by first giving off circumferential arteries; which in turn penetrate the muscle with radial branches. The latter supply the endometrium with basal (straight) and spiral arterioles.

the cell where estrogen stimulates messenger RNA (mRNA). The mRNA is transferred to the cell mitochondria, where it stimulates protein synthesis and cell growth during that stage. Estradiol also induces progesterone receptors in the endometrium. Thus, the estrogen-primed endometrium will be ready for the effect of progesterone following ovulation.

In cases of anovulatory cycles, the endometrium—under the unopposed effect of estrogen—will continue to proliferate. In some long-standing cases a process of endometrial hyperplasia may occur, which can predispose the endometrium to malignant change at some time in the future. These continued proliferative changes occur in postpubertal and premenopausal women. They also occur in anovulatory women as a result of obesity, polycystic ovarian syndrome, and conditions of hypothalamic pituitary dysfunction.

The tributaries of the uterine vessels supplying the basal endometrium also regenerate, leading to vessels supplying and draining the entire thickness of the endometrium during the proliferative phase (Fig 4–5).

Secretory Phase

Following ovulation and the formation of the corpus luteum, progesterone levels in the circulation start to rise and reach a peak about 5 to 7 days later. The level of estradiol-17β drops sometime around ovulation, to rise again to a lesser peak than the preovulatory estrogen peak. This estrogen peak coincides with the progesterone peak in the luteal phase.

Progesterone attaches to intracellular receptors in the endometrial cells. This progesterone receptor complex is translocated to the nucleus. Progesterone then stimulates mRNA, which moves to the mitochondria and stimulates the secretory changes in the endometrium. These secretory changes have been described by Noyes et al. for endometrial dating. These changes occur in both the glands and stroma. In the early secretory phase, subnuclear secretory vacuoles occur in the cells lining the glands. These secretory vacuoles then move to be supranuclear, and these are secreted into the lumen of the glands at the acme of the corpus luteum function. The glands become tortuous. The stroma cells enlarge to be mosaic shaped, with edema of the endometrium (Fig 4–6). These changes are associated with tortuous changes in the blood vessels supplying the endometrium. The changes occur in preparation for the process of implantation if pregnancy happens. If pregnancy does not happen, the corpus luteum function declines 12 to 14 days after ovulation. With the corpus luteum demise, the serum levels of estradiol and progesterone decline, and menstruation starts.

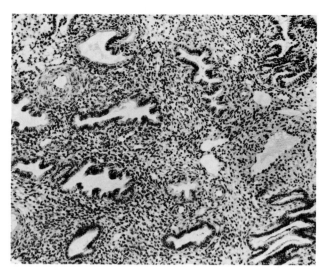

FIG 4–6.
Secretory endometrium; ×125.

Menstrual Phase

As a result of the decline in ovarian steroids, prostaglandin synthesis in the endometrium increases. This results from activation of phospholipase, which leads to formation of arachidonic acid—the precursor of the prostaglandins. These prostaglandins cause constriction of the endometrial capillaries, with resultant degeneration and necrosis of endometrium. Subendometrial hemorrhage occurs from these vessels (Fig 4–7). The endometrial tissue and accompanying blood are discharged through the cervical canal as the menstrual flow. The duration of the flow normally is from 3 to 7 days. The amount of flow under normal conditions is about 80 ml. The prostaglandins also cause contractility

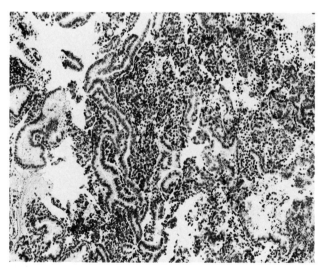

FIG 4–7.
Menstruating endometrium; ×125.

of the uterine wall, and thus control the amount of bleeding from the endometrial vessels during menstruation. This process is usually associated with a sense of cramping in lower abdomen in some women. In some women this process is exaggerated and is known as dysmenorrhea. Studies have shown that there is excess prostaglandins in the menstrual fluid of dysmenorrheic women as compared with controls. This explains the increased uterine contractility in these women. Furthermore, the systemic effect of the increased prostaglandins may lead to gastrointestinal problems such as nausea, vomiting, and diarrhea. It also may lead to vascular problems, such as syncopal attacks and headaches, which sometimes accompany menstruation in such women. These symptoms are successfully treated by antiprostaglandins.

BIBLIOGRAPHY

Aksel S, Schonberg DW, Hammond CB: Prostaglandin $F_2\alpha$ production by the human ovary. *Obstet Gynecol* 1977; 50:347.

Chan WY, Hill JC: Determination of menstrual prostaglandin levels in non-dysmenorrheic and dysmenorrheic subjects. *Prostaglandins* 1978; 15:365.

Ferenczy A, Bertrant G, Gelfand MM: Proliferation kinetics of human endometrium during the normal menstrual cycle. *Am J Obstet Gynecol* 1979; 133:859.

Fritz MA, Speroff L: The endocrinology of the menstrual cycle: The interaction of folliculogenesis and neuroendocrine mechanisms. *Fertil Steril* 1982; 38:509.

Harrison RJ: The structure of the ovary, in Zukerman S, Mandl AM, Eckstein P (eds): *The Ovary.* London, Academic Press, 1962, pp 143–182.

Hodgen GD: The dominant ovarian follicle. *Fertil Steril* 1982; 38:281.

Lundstrom V, Green K, Svanborg K: Endogenous prostaglandins in dysmenorrhea and the effect of prostaglandin synthetase inhibitors (PGSI) on uterine contractility. *Acta Obstet Gynecol Scand* [Suppl] 1979; 87:51.

Mikhail G: Hormone secretion by the ovary. *Gynecol Invest* 1970; 1:5.

Noyes RW, Hertig AW, Rock J: Dating the endometrial biopsy. *Fertil Steril* 1950; 1:3.

Tsany BK, Moon YS, Simpson CW, et al: Androgen biosynthesis in human ovarian follicles: Cellular source, gonadotropic control, and adenosine 3'5' monophosphate mediation. *J Clin Endocrinol Metab* 1979; 48:153.

Yen SSC: Neuroendocrine regulation of gonadotropin and prolactin secretion in women: Disorders in reproduction, in Vitukaitis JL (ed): *Current Endocrinology.* Clinical Reproductive Endocrinology series. New York, Elsevier Biomedical Press, 1982, pp 137–176.

Yoshimura Y, Wallach EE: Studies of the mechanisms of mammalian ovulation. *Fertil Steril* 1987; 47:22.

5

Uterine Estrogen and Progesterone Receptors

Margaret A. Thompson, Ph.D

GENERAL CONSIDERATIONS

Cyclicity of the endometrium of the premenopausal uterus in response to the circulating hormones estrogen and progesterone requires the presence of steroid hormone receptors in the tissue. Steroid receptors are intracellular proteins that bind their respective hormones specifically and with high affinity. An estrogen receptor, by definition, is a protein that binds with high affinity only estrogens from the group of compounds known as steroid hormones. High affinity implies that avidity of the receptor for the hormone is sufficiently great that changes in circulating concentrations of hormones are reflected by variation in the portion of receptors occupied by hormones. Affinity of a receptor for its hormone is usually presented as a dissociation constant, a molar concentration. The dissociation constant is equal to the hormone concentration at which any population of the receptor is one-half filled.

Mechanistic models of steroid hormone action are the same for all species, all steroids, and all target tissue. Recent developments, elucidating steroid hormone mechanisms of action, have emphasized that biochemical models evolve over time. It is helpful to remember that any model is only a tool to assist in the management of practical problems. Currently, there are two different models to explain how steroids bind to their receptors and elicit a response by target tissues (Fig 5–1). In all studies published prior to 1984, data were interpreted in accordance with the original model developed in the pioneering work of the laboratories of Drs. Elwood Jensen and Jack Gorski (Fig 5–1,A). Studies published subsequent to 1984, although similar in design and identical in method to earlier studies, report data interpreted in accordance with both models. The second model has

gained a great deal of acceptance recently and may soon supercede the original. This second model was originally proposed by Sheridan et al. in 1979. A review of the historical development of both of these models was presented by Walters in 1985.

STEROID RECEPTORS OF THE HUMAN UTERUS

Elucidation of receptor dynamics associated with endometrial histology was complicated by an array of technical considerations unique to humans. Studies prior to 1976 struggled to demonstrate intracellular proteins in uterine tissue with characteristics of estrogen and progesterone receptors. Values reported for the quantity of receptor and dissociation constants varied widely. The major factor confounding measurement of estrogen receptors was the plasma protein, sex steroid binding globulin (SHBG). The dissociation constant of estrogen receptors for estradiol is only ten-fold lower than that of SHBG. SHBG, therefore, interfered substantially, because it was present at higher concentrations than estrogen receptors in tissue homogenates and varied with the amount of blood in the tissue. A similar problem was experienced with measurement of progesterone receptors. Plasma corticosteroid binding globulin (CBG) has a high affinity for progesterone. The specificity of each receptor for its own hormone was exploited to overcome the problem of interference by plasma proteins. SHBG has a high affinity for both estrogen and androgen and, therefore, an accurate quantitation of estrogen receptors could be obtained in the presence of

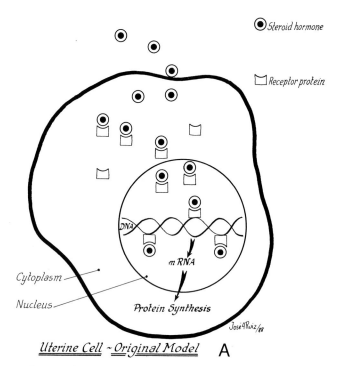

Uterine Cell ~ Original Model   **A**

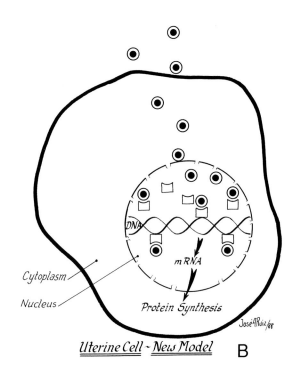

Uterine Cell ~ New Model   **B**

FIG 5–1.

A, steroid enters the cell by diffusion and binds to receptor protein, which is soluble in the cytoplasm. Steroid, bound to protein, which is soluble in the cytoplasm. Steroid, bound to cytoplasmic receptor, undergoes a biochemical transformation that permits passage of the steroid-receptor complex thorugh nuclear pores, and the complex binds to nuclear DNA. The binding of the steroid-receptor complex results in synthesis of new messenger RNA *(mRNA)* and protein synthesis. **B,** steroid enters the cell and the nuclear compartment by diffusion. Steroid binds receptor protein, which is a constitutive component of the nuclear compartment but is not securely attached to the DNA in the absence of steroid. The steroid receptor complex than forms a secure attachment to the DNA and stimulates synthesis of new *mRNA* and protein synthesis.

sufficient androgen to block the binding of estrogen to SHBG. Similarly, progesterone receptors could be accurately determined in the presence of cortisol. Androgen, by definition, does not bind to estrogen receptors, and cortisol, a glucocorticoid, does not bind to progesterone receptors with high affinity.

Distribution of estrogen and progesterone receptors within the human uterus is not uniform. The quantity of both receptors in myometrium has been reported as two to ten times less than in endometrium. The biochemical properties of the myometrial steroid receptors, however, do not differ from those of endometrial receptors. It has also been reported that there is an uneven distribution of estrogen and progesterone receptors within the endometrium. A steep decrease, approximately ten-fold, in both receptors exists from fundal to cervical sections. This steep receptor gradient persists throughout the menstrual cycle and after menopause. Tissue obtained for steroid receptor measurement should, therefore, always be taken from the uterine fundus, where the greatest quantity of receptors are located, for consistent results. However, even with this precaution, variation in absolute concentration of these

receptors remains a problem. Investigators have reported differences as large as five-fold among women on the same day of their cycle. The absence of a predictable value for each day of the menstrual cycle limits the usefulness of estrogen and progesterone receptor measurement for routine clinical management.

There is a cyclic pattern in the quantity of uterine estrogen and progesterone receptors present during the menstrual cycle. In humans, as in other species, the progesterone receptor is an estrogen-induced protein. The uteri of postmenopausal women contain normal to high levels of estrogen receptors. However, because there is a general absence of circulating estrogen, progesterone receptors are not present. To demonstrate the cyclicity of steroid receptors in premenopausal uteri, endometria from regular menstrual cycles were used for receptor assays, and a portion of the tissue was saved to confirm dating with histologic methods. In the original studies only cytosol receptors were measured. Later workers were able to measure nuclear and cytosol receptors, because assays were developed which enabled exchange of endogenous hormones bound to the receptor for radiolabeled hormones in vitro. The original model of the steroid hormone mechanism of action (see Fig 5–1,A) led investigators to reason that receptors in the nuclear fraction of tissue homogenates represented receptors bound to endogenous hormones. It was expected that the fraction of receptors found in the nucleus would increase with increasing circulating concentration of estrogen and progesterone during the menstrual cycle. Measurement of receptors in both compartments was, therefore, necessary to obtain an accurate total. Surprisingly, conclusions reached did not prove significantly different, regardless of the method employed.

In a large study by Levy et al. in 1980, endometrial estrogen and progesterone receptors were measured in 101 cases of normal menstrual cycles. Both empty sites and those filled with endogenous hormones were quantitated. During the preovulatory phase, there was a constant elevated level of cytosol estrogen receptors while nuclear receptor sites more than doubled. Cytoplasmic estradiol receptor sites decreased early in the secretory phase, with the decrease in nuclear sites occurring later. These data and those of others have been interpreted to support a stimulatory role for estradiol in the synthesis of new estrogen receptors by the endometrium. Cytoplasmic progesterone receptors also increase in response to the rise in circulatory estradiol during the proliferative phase of the cycle. Cytoplasmic progesterone receptors show a large decrease immediately after ovulation. At that time, nuclear progesterone receptors are at their highest level. The total cellular concentration of both receptors is lowest during the late luteal phase. Any stimulatory effect of the luteal-phase rise in circulating estradiol on receptor levels is inhibited by progesterone. Progesterone is thought to have a negative, receptor-mediated effect on the tissue concentration of both receptors. It also has an indirect effect, which is expressed as an increase in activity of the enzyme that converts estradiol to estrone, 17 β-hydroxysteroid dehydrogenase. The human estrogen receptor, unlike that of some other species, has a much lower affinity for estrone than for estradiol, and this metabolic conversion hastens termination of the effectiveness of estradiol.

The presence of unoccupied nuclear estrogen receptors was first detected in the tumor cell lines MCF-7 (1973) and HEC 1B (1978). MCF-7 is a breast cancer cell line, and HEC 1B is an endometrial cancer cell line. It was initially proposed that cancer cells were defective in their mechanism of hormone action because unoccupied receptors were translocated to the nucleus. Unoccupied nuclear estrogen receptors, however, were not a unique property of carcinoma cells. Several reports published in 1980 demonstrated available (not occupied by hormone) estrogen receptors in nuclei of normal endometrium. Available receptors constituted almost all of the nuclear receptors in proliferative tissue and approximately 50% in the secretory phase. Further confirmation of the nuclear localization of estrogen receptors in vivo came in 1984 when a series of monoclonal antiestrophilin (estrogen receptor) antibodies were developed. These antibodies were used with an indirect immunoperoxidase technique to locate estrogen receptors in frozen sections of normal human endometrium. Specific staining for estrogen receptors was always limited to nuclei, and cytoplasmic staining was not observed. Although immunohistochemical assessment of estrogen receptor distribution in endometrium is not quantitative, qualitatively these methods have confirmed the cyclic pattern of estrogen receptors in endometrium, which was established earlier with biochemical methods. Monoclonal antibodies for the purified progesterone receptors are currently being developed. More recent biochemical experiments carried out with nonaqueous methods of subcellular fractionation have also found 86% of the estrogen receptors in the nuclear karyoplasts. Similar nonaqeous fractionation methods have demonstrated in animal tissues that progesterone receptors and glucocorticoid receptors were also nuclear proteins.

PHARMACOLOGIC MANIPULATION OF UTERINE ESTROGEN AND PROGESTERONE

There are reproductive disorders, such as luteal phase defects, for which it might be helpful to modify steroid receptor levels in the uterine endometrium with exogenously added hormones. Natural steroids, however, are poorly absorbed through the gastrointestinal tract, and that portion which does cross into the circulation is rapidly inactivated by the liver. Synthetic compounds, which are more readily absorbed, were developed to serve as substitute ligands for estrogen and progesterone receptors. Several of these compounds are used extensively to modulate reproductive function. Some are derivatives of the natural hormone in which a portion of the molecule has been chemically modified. Others have no structural relationship to the steroid configuration. Ethinyl estradiol and diethylstilbesterol are both potent estrogens. Ethinyl estradiol is a derivative of estradiol, and diethylstilbesterol is a diphenolic compound that structurally does not resemble a steroid.

Generally, it was not difficult to design synthetic ligands for estrogen and progesterone receptors with appropriate affinity. However, specificity has been a substantial problem. For example, recent, carefully designed receptor-binding studies demonstrated that danazol, which is used to treat endometriosis, competed with endogenous hormones for binding sites on SHBG, CBG, estrogen receptors, progesterone receptors, and androgen receptors. This is an extreme example, but most synthetic compounds do cross over to receptor systems other than those for which they were developed. This is particularly a problem when high dosage is administered. Most synthetic ligands for steroid receptors are also metabolized in the hepatic circulation. However, the loss with first pass through the liver is less than 100%. Uptake of natural steroids and synthetic ligands by tissue is very rapid and thought to occur by diffusion. Therefore, survival of one pass of the liver is often sufficient for retention of activity. Sometimes it is the metabolite of a compound that is active, and an initial pass through the liver enhances biologic activity. For example, mestranol, the estrogenic component of some oral contraceptives, is systemically metabolized to ethinyl estradiol, which is active at target tissues. The use of animal models to test new ligands for estrogen receptors and progesterone receptors has been questioned because of species differences in metabolism. Generalization of data from animal models to human endocrinology can be difficult.

Metabolic conversion is still incompletely understood for some of the receptor ligands used to modify reproductive function. This is particularly true of the triphenylethylene antiestrogens tamoxifen and clomiphene. Although these compounds are generally referred to as antiestrogens, they often act as agonists or partial agonists, depending on the target tissue investigated. Four major metabolites of tamoxifen have been identified in the plasma of women. Of these four, it is the hydroxylated compound, 4-hydroxytamoxifen, which is thought to be active at the estrogen receptor. Clomiphene is very similar in structure to tamoxifen (Fig 5–2). In spite of this similarity, they were reported to have very different effects on the steroid receptor concentration of uterine endometrium and on plasma hormones when administered from day 3 to day 23 of the menstrual cycle. Clomiphene increased plasma luteinizing hormone (LH), follicle stimulating hormone (FSH), estradiol, and progesterone. Elevated LH and FSH reflected an antiestrogenic effect of clomiphene at the pituitary, and elevated estradiol and progesterone was a response of the ovary. The concentration of estradiol receptors and progesterone receptors was reduced in the endometrium. In contrast, tamoxifen administered during the same period resulted in no change in plasma LH and FSH, while plasma estradiol and progesterone were elevated as after clomiphene. Tamoxifen treatment resulted in no loss of estrogen receptors or progesterone receptors in the endometrium. The overall effect of these drugs include mechanisms in addition to

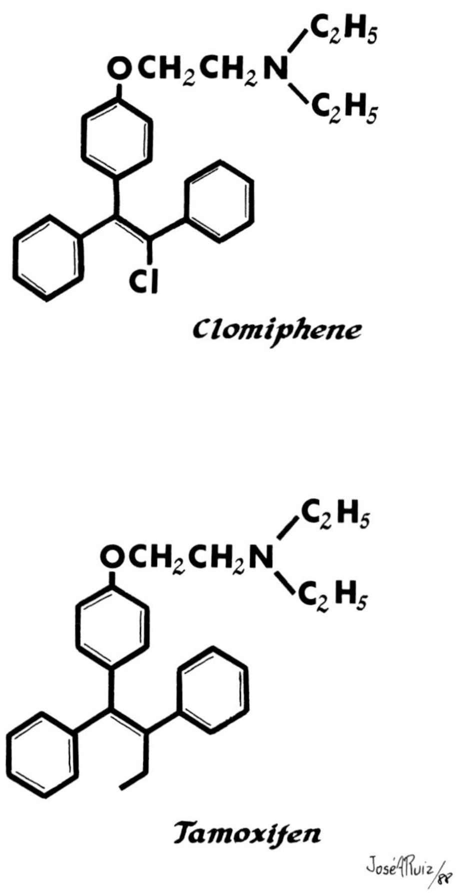

FIG 5–2.
Chemical structures show similarity of clomiphene and tamoxifen.

steroid receptor activation. Separate binding sites, specific for these antiestrogens, have been described in microsomal fractions of uterine cells. The physiologic relevance of specific antiestrogen receptors is presently unclear.

Current efforts for pharmacologic manipulation of the endocrine system include development of better delivery systems for natural hormones. Grinding crystalline progesterone to a fine powder, in which the size of each particle is a micron or less, enhances its absorption through the gastrointestinal tract. While liver clearance remains a serious problem, several investigators have been successful in increasing circulating progesterone with this method. Transdermal delivery of the steroids is also being explored. That method allows steroid access to the circulation without an initial pass through the liver. Steroid entering plasma through the skin is taken up by SHBG, which prolongs its retention in the circulation. Further investigation of the endocrine physiology of the human uterus will be greatly assisted by new methods that deliver natural hormones in a controlled manner.

BIBLIOGRAPHY

Bayard F, et al: Cytoplasmic and nuclear estradiol and progesterone receptors in human endometrium. *J Clin Endocrinol Metab* 1978; 46:635.

Fleming H, Gurpide E: Available estradiol receptors in nuclei from human endometrium. *J Steroid Biochem* 1980; 13:3–11.

Fritz MA, Westfahl PK, Graham RL: The effect of luteal phase estrogen antagonism on endometrial development and luteal function in women. *J Clin Endocrinol Metab* 1987; 65:1006–1013.

Gravanis A, Gurpide E: Enucleation of human endometrial cells: Nucleo-cytoplasmic distribution of DNA polymerase alpha and estrogen receptor. *J Steroid Biochem* 1986; 24:469–474.

Gurpide E, Marks C: Influence of endometrial 17β-hydroxysteroid dehydrogenase activity on the binding of estradiol to receptors. *J Clin Endocrinol Metab* 1981; 52:252.

Jordan VC: Biochemical pharmacology of antiestrogen action. *Pharmacol Rev* 1984; 245–276.

Kokko E, Jänne O, Kauppila A, et al: Effects of tamoxifen, medroxyprogesterone acetate, and their combinations on human endometrial estrogen and progestin receptor concentrations, 17 beta-hydroxysteroid dehydrogenase activity, and serum hormone concentrations. *Am J Obstet Gynecol* 1982; 143:382–388.

Levy C, Robel P, Gautray JP, et al: Estradiol and progesterone receptors in human endometrium: Normal and abnormal menstrual cycles and early pregnancy. *Am J Obstet Gynecol* 1980; 136:646–651.

Press MF, Nousel-Goebl N, King WJ, et al: Immunohistochemical assessment of estrogen receptor distribution in the human endometrium throughout the menstrual cycle. *Lab Invest* 1984; 51:495–503.

Sheridan PJ, Buchanan JM, Anselmo VC, et al: Equilibrium: The intracellular distribution of steroid receptors. *Nature* 1979; 282:579–582.

Tamaya T, Wada K, Fujimoto J, et al: Danazol binding to steroid receptors in human uterine endometrium. *Fertil Steril* 41:732–735.

Tsibris JC, Cazenave CR, Cantor B, et al: Distribution of cytoplasmic estrogen and progesterone receptors in human endometrium. *Am J Obstet Gynecol* 1978; 132:449–454.

Walters M: Steroid hormone receptors and the nucleus. *Endocrine Rev* 1985; 6:512.

6

Pathology of the Endometrium

W. Dwayne Lawrence, M.D.

Robert E. Scully, M.D.

THE NORMAL ENDOMETRIUM

The typical 28-day menstrual cycle can be divided into menstrual, proliferative, and premenstrual secretory phases without a distinct demarcation between the end of one phase and the beginning of the next. The first day of menstrual bleeding is designated day 1 of the cycle. The menstrual phase lasts for an average of 4 days, during which a variable amount of tissue is sloughed and fluid is lost from the residual endometrial tissue; regeneration of the glands and surface epithelium has already begun before the midpoint of the menstrual phase. During the proliferative phase—which averages 10 days, but can vary considerably in length from one individual to another and from one cycle to another in the same individual—the endometrial glands and stroma proliferate under the influence of rising levels of estrogens secreted by developing graafian follicles. Ovulation occurs typically on day 14 with the formation of a corpus luteum; progesterone secretion by the corpus luteum induces the onset of the secretory phase of the cycle. During this phase, the endometrium is primed for reception of the fertilized ovum. Glandular secretion is at its height from days 20 to 23, and progressive transformation of stromal cells into large predecidual cells dominates the last third of the secretory phase. If implantation does not occur, the corpus luteum degenerates, with progressively decreasing production of estrogens and progesterone. When these hormones have fallen to very low levels the spiral arterioles of the endometrium undergo spasm followed by dilation; the endometrial tissue undergoes degeneration, and menstruation begins. Evaluation of the architectural and cytologic variations in the glands, stroma, and spiral arterioles of the endometrium permits accurate assessment of its phase of development.

Gross Examination

Hysteroscopic examination has demonstrated that menstruation usually begins in the cornual and fundal regions; in one study, sloughing was occasionally noted before the clinical onset of menstrual bleeding. Fragments of desquamated endometrial tissue appear gray-white, while the remaining mucosa is red and focally covered by white necrotic tissue. The late menstrual endometrium is thin and congested, with multiple punctate hemorrhages. Proliferative endometrium is pink-gray, smooth, and glistening; it increases progressively in height from 1 or 2 mm to 3 or 4 mm and occasionally is 6 or 7 mm just prior to ovulation. Secretory endometrium is yellow-white and glistening and may attain a thickness of 5 mm or more. About 5 days before the onset of menstruation, or sometimes earlier in the cycle, the endometrium may have a polypoid appearance, simulating hyperplasia (Plate 21). Around day 24 the endometrium begins to shrink, and by the time of onset of menstruation it is only one half to three quarters of its maximum height. This loss of tissue volume, resulting in a premenstrual thickness of about 2 mm, is caused principally by a loss of stroma fluid. If fertilization occurs the endometrium continues to thicken. The ovum, which usually implants on the 20th day of the cycle, may be visible on the endometrial surface as a slightly elevated red spot less than 1 mm in diameter.

The postmenopausal endometrium may be paper

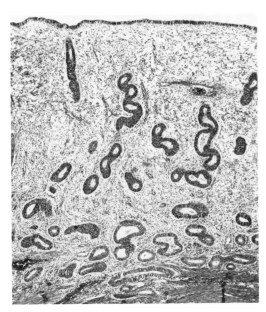

FIG 6–1.
Proliferative phase. The endometrium is relatively thin with straight or slightly tortuous glands; ×64.

thin if glandular atrophy with fibrosis of the stroma have occurred; however, if, as often occurs during the first 10 or more years after the onset of the menopause, atrophy is less marked or irregular in its distribution, the endometrium may be 1 or 2 mm in thickness. Thin-walled cystic glands are occasionally visible and are generally more numerous in elderly women.

Microscopic Examination

In the early proliferative phase, the glands are small, straight, and tubular and are lined by low columnar cells with basal nuclei, which may be slightly pseudostratified. Mitotic figures are uncommon. The stroma is composed of delicate stellate and spindle cells with sparse cytoplasm. As the endometrium continues to proliferate, mitotic activity increases in both the glands and the stroma, and pseudostratification of the epithelial nuclei and enlargement and slight tortuosity of the glands are evident (Fig 6–1).

In the early secretory phase the first morphologic evidence of ovulation appears within 36 to 48 hours in the form of subnuclear vacuoles in the glandular epithelium. Mitotic activity and pseudostratification of nuclei disappear within approximately 3 days after ovulation as secretion begins to appear in the gland lumens; maximal glandular secretion and stroma edema are achieved during the 20th through the 22nd days (6 to 8 days after ovulation). The beginning of the late secretory phase is heralded by prominence of the spiral arterioles, around

which mitotic activity recommences in the endometrial stromal cells on the 23rd day. The arterioles coil extensively and the stromal cells acquire increasing amounts of pale cytoplasm, becoming predecidual cells. This change spreads throughout the upper part of the endometrium, and the glands assume a sawtooth configuration (Fig 6–2). Subsequently, fluid escapes from the stroma, and the endometrium decreases in thickness. Endometrial granulocytes, mainly of stromal origin, accumulate in increasing numbers as menstruation approaches. If implantation occurs, the endometrium becomes increasingly congested, the secretion and edema persist, and the predecidual cells become progressively larger to form decidual cells.

The postmenopausal endometrium varies from a relatively thick layer with glands of varying sizes lined by mitotically inactive pseudostratified epithelium and abundant fibrous stroma, to a very thin layer containing small glands lying in a sparse component of fibrotic stroma (Fig 6–3). The atrophic glands may be cystically dilated and lined by flattened epithelium. Varying combinations of these changes may be seen within individual endometria after the menopause. In general the thicker endometria, which have been designated as showing inactive hyperplasia, are seen in the earlier postmenopausal years; simple atrophy (predominance of small atrophic glands), in later years; and cystic atrophy (predominance of cystic atrophic glands), in the most elderly age group.

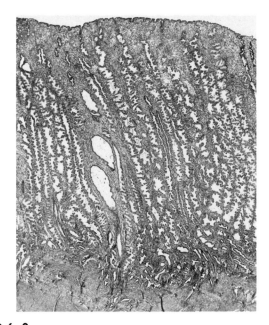

FIG 6–2.
Secretory endometrium. The endometrium is thick and its glands are tortuous with serrated borders; ×24.

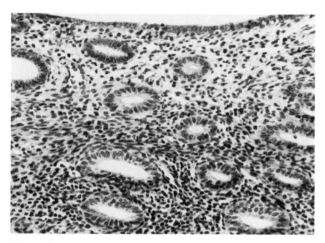

FIG 6–3.
Atrophic endometrium. Small and inactive-appearing glands are set in a fibrotic stroma; ×64.

ENDOMETRIAL HYPERPLASIA

Diffuse hyperplasia of the endometrium results from a continuous exposure to estrogens unopposed by progesterone. This disorder may be encountered in women of wide age ranges in a variety of clinical conditions. Women of reproductive age with anovulatory cycles, perimenopausal and postmenopausal women on estrogen therapy, obese women with a high rate of peripheral conversion of androgens to estrogens, and women of all ages with estrogen-producing ovarian tumors are among those subject to the development of endometrial hyperplasia. Focal hyperplasia, differing only in its extent from diffuse hyperplasia, is occasionally seen within an otherwise normal endometrium. The pathogenesis of this lesion is unclear; presumably, it results from a localized exaggerated response to estrogens or deficiency of progesterone receptors. Most examples of endometrial hyperplasia can be assigned to one of two major categories: cystic hyperplasia, and the complex forms. The latter are known by various terms, among which are adenomatous hyperplasia, atypical hyperplasia, atypical adenomatous hyperplasia, architectural atypicality, cellular atypicality, and carcinoma in situ. Cystic hyperplasia is thought to have a very low malignant potential, whereas the more severe forms of complex hyperplasia are regarded as significantly precancerous.

Gross Pathology

The hyperplastic endometrium may retain the glistening, mucoid, pink-gray appearance of the normal proliferative endometrium, but is usually thicker and is occasionally polypoid (Plate 22). Small cysts may be visible, and dilated congested sinusoids may be seen just beneath the surface; although small red foci of hemorrhage and yellow foci of necrosis are sometimes seen, the latter finding should raise the suspicion of focal carcinoma.

Microscopic Pathology

Cystic hyperplasia has a characteristic Swiss-cheese appearance on low-power magnification. Variably sized dilated glands, lined by flattened to pseudostratified columnar epithelium, are found either diffusely or focally on the background of a proliferative endometrium (Fig 6–4). The stroma appears abundant and active with naked nuclei. Mitotic figures vary from few to numerous.

The complex forms of hyperplasia may be superimposed on cystic hyperplasia, but are also encountered in pure or almost pure form. This category includes a variety of architectural abnormalities (sometimes referred to as adenomatous hyperplasia) and cytologic atypicality (sometimes designated atypical hyperplasia) in various combinations and varying degrees of severity. Some investigators use the term "adenomatous hyperplasia" and others "atypical hyperplasia" to embrace the entire spectrum of cytologic and architectural abnormalities—including the most severe form, which still others refer to as "carcinoma in situ."

In most cases, architectural and cellular abnormalities coexist. The most common mild manifestation of the former is the presence of outpouchings from cystic glands creating a so-called finger-in-glove pattern; the outpouchings may appear as small glands pinched off by

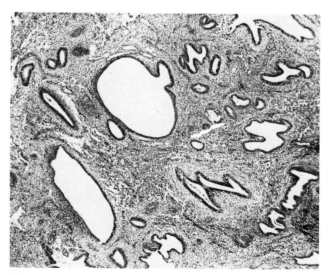

FIG 6–4.
Cystic hyperplasia. Variably sized generally rounded cystic glands lie in a cellular endometrial stroma; ×64.

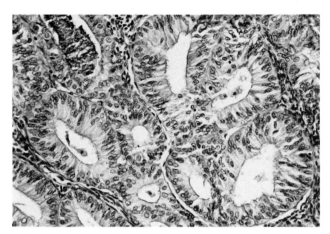

FIG 6–5.
Endometrial hyperplasia with severe architectural and cytologic atypia. The glands are crowded and most are separated by only thin wisps of stroma. The nuclei are stratified and many are rounded and vesicular; ×250.

stroma from the adjacent cystic glands. Despite varying degrees of glandular crowding, clearly recognizable stroma remains between the glands. With increasing severity of architectural atypia, epithelial stratification and glandular crowding become more prominent until only thin wisps of stroma separate thick-walled glands of distorted shapes (Fig 6–5). Rarely the lumina of the gland are obliterated focally by proliferation of the lining cells. Another form of architectural atypicality is the presence of papillae with fibrovascular stalks within dilated glands. Cytologic atypicality is characterized by nuclear rounding, hyperchromatism, pleomorphism, and loss of polarization. Mitotic activity is usually but not invariably increased, and nucleoli may be enlarged and prominent.

A variety of metaplastic changes may be encountered in the complex forms of hyperplasia including the acquisition of abundant eosinophilic cytoplasm (eosinophilic metaplasia), the appearance of cilia on the cell surfaces (ciliated cell metaplasia), and squamous metaplasia (acanthosis), with the formation of "morules" of small, immature squamous cells, which may be centrally necrotic. These alterations do not of themselves indicate a premalignant state, but alert the pathologist to scrutinize closely the architecture and nuclear characteristics of the associated glandular epithelium.

In our laboratory the architectural and cellular abnormalities within a specimen of endometrium are graded separately as mild, moderate, or severe, and the extent of the lesion within the entire specimen is determined. When the cytologic and architectural features are indistinguishable from those of adenocarcinoma but the lesion forms a single small focus or disseminated small foci without obvious invasion of the surrounding

stroma, the designation "carcinoma in situ" is used. The definition of carcinoma in situ of the endometrium is controversial, however, and many pathologists do not use the term, including the lesion in the category of severe atypical or adenomatous hyperplasia.

ENDOMETRIAL POLYPS

Although endometrial polyps have been reported to occur in young girls before puberty, they are encountered almost always in older patients, particularly those in their 5th decade. These lesions may be asymptomatic or may be associated with abnormal uterine bleeding. Their frequency is increased in cases of endometrial carcinoma.

Gross Pathology

Endometrial polyps occur singly in about three fourths of cases. Although they may occur at any location within the endometrial cavity, they are found most often in the fundus, particularly in the cornual areas. They range from barely perceptible lesions less than a few millimeters in diameter to large masses that occupy the entire endometrial cavity and simulate cancer. Some of them are broad-based and sessile, whereas others have long, slender stalks (Plates 23 and 24). Occasionally a large one protrudes through the external cervical os and very rarely through the introitus, mimicking procidentia. Most polyps are pink-gray to white with smooth, glistening surfaces, beneath which small cysts may be visible. Occasionally the entire polyp or only its tip is hemorrhagic or infarcted. It must be emphasized that a variety of lesions other than glandular polyps may have a polypoid configuration, including carcinomas, sarcomas, carcinosarcomas, adenosarcomas, leiomyomas, fragments of retained placenta (placental polyps), and even secretory endometrium.

Microscopic Pathology

The endometrial glands within polyps may have a variety of appearances, which depend in part on the age and hormonal status of the patient. In women in the reproductive age group they are often out of phase with those of the adjacent endometrium. Although they may be secretory during the luteal phase of the cycle, more typically they have a weakly proliferative pattern, and often they are cystically dilated. In postmenopausal patients, cystic glands lined by low cuboidal to flattened epithelium are most frequently encountered (Fig 6–6). The stroma within polyps may resemble that of a prolif-

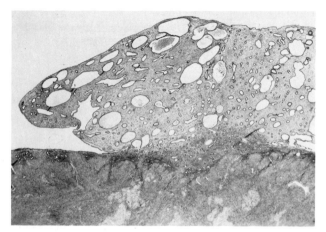

FIG 6—6.
Endometrial polyp containing numerous variably sized glands, many of which are dilated, within a fibrous stroma. The adjacent endometrium is thin and atrophic.

erative endometrium but is often fibrotic instead. A consistent feature of a fully developed polyp is the presence of large, thick-walled blood vessels throughout its core. Occasionally smooth muscle is present within the stroma of a polyp; if it is the predominant component, the term adenomyomatous polyp or polypoid adenomyoma may be appropriate.

Various types and degrees of glandular atypicality, carcinoma in situ, and even frank carcinoma may be encountered within otherwise benign polyps. When glandular atypicality, usually associated with acanthosis, occurs within an adenomyomatous polyp, the term atypical polypoid adenomyoma has been used. In a curettage specimen this lesion is distinguishable from a low-grade adenocarcinoma or adenoacanthoma that has invaded the myometrium by the pattern of its smooth muscle, which lacks the orientation of bundles seen in the normal myometrium.

ENDOMETRIAL CARCINOMAS

Carcinoma of the endometrium occurs over a wide age range of patients. Exceptional examples have been encountered in prepubertal girls, and fewer than 10% are seen in women of reproductive age; the great majority occur in postmenopausal women. Just as in cases of endometrial hyperplasia, unopposed estrogenic stimulation has been shown by numerous investigators to increase significantly the risk of endometrial carcinoma. Many of these tumors arise on a background of severe cytologic and architectural atypicality, but some originate within an otherwise normal-appearing endometrium.

Gross Pathology

Endometrial carcinomas may be localized or involve the entire endometrium; when they are diffuse they typically terminate abruptly at the internal cervical os. Localized tumors may be polypoid, and either sessile or pedunculated (Plates 25 and 26). Although small carcinomas may be occult within a normal or hyperplastic endometrium or an endometrial polyp, the typical tumor is composed of irregularly heaped up tissue, which often has a pebbly or granular surface (Plate 27). In contrast to the glistening, mucoid, grey, elastic features of proliferative or hyperplastic endometrium, carcinomatous tissue tends to appear opaque, dry, pale-yellow or white, and friable. Dark-yellow areas are often conspicuous as a result of necrosis or the accumulation of lipid-filled cells of stromal origin between the neoplastic glands. Hemorrhage and ulceration are common, particularly when the tumor is poorly differentiated, and abnormal vascular patterns may be seen on the surface of the tumor.

Microscopic Pathology

Although they have not been correlated to any significant extent with specific gross features, a variety of histologic patterns and cell types may be encountered in cases of endometrial carcinoma. Adenocarcinomas of the usual type, characterized by the presence of tubular glands lined by stratified, mucin-free or mucin-poor epithelial cells, account for the majority of cases (Fig 6–7). The criteria for separating severely atypical hyperplasia

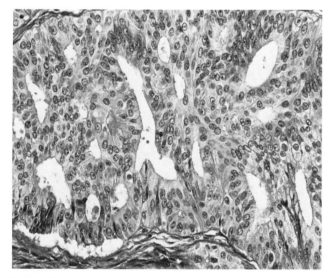

FIG 6—7.
Grade 1 adenocarcinoma with cribriform arrangement of glands, which are closely packed without intervening stroma; ×400.

from adenocarcinoma in situ and low-grade adenocarcinoma of the endometrium are not sharply defined, but atypical glandular proliferations that have the following features are accepted as adenocarcinomas by almost all observers: a back-to-back arrangement of glands without recognizable intervening stroma; a cribriform pattern (bridging of epithelial lining cells to form multiple lumina within an enlarged gland); a complex papillary architecture; stratification, loss of polarity, rounding and pleomorphism of nuclei; irregular clumping of chromatin alternating with clear foci within the nuclei; mitotic figures, which may be relatively few in well-differentiated tumors; and a desmoplastic reaction of the stroma separating the glands. One or more of these features may be absent in individual cases.

Squamous cell differentiation is often encountered in endometrial carcinomas, particularly in low-grade tumors, in which rounded nodules of cytologically benign, small, immature squamous cells partially occupy or replace varying numbers of the neoplastic glands (Fig 6–8). The presence of these nodules or "morules" in an adenocarcinoma has given rise to the designation "adenoacanthoma." When the squamous component is cytologically malignant and typical of that seen in squamous cell carcinoma, and also invades the stroma independently of the glandular component of the tumor, the term "adenosquamous carcinoma" has been used (Fig 6–9). This tumor is typically associated with a less well differentiated glandular component than the adenoacanthoma, and has a much worse prognosis. Some investigators have concluded that the presence of malignant squamous cells per se in the adenosquamous carcinoma

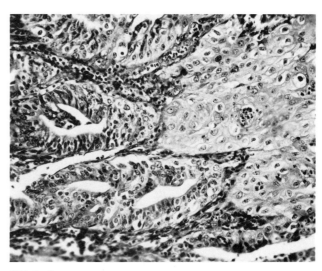

FIG 6–9.
Adenosquamous carcinoma. Grade 2 (of 4). Sheets of malignant squamous cells (right portion of figure) abut malignant glands; ×256.

explains its poor prognosis, whereas others attribute the latter to the typically higher grade of the accompanying glandular component.

Rarer subtypes of endometrial carcinoma are also encountered. The clear cell carcinoma closely resembles that found in other portions of the genital tract such as the ovary, cervix, and vagina. This tumor may have a papillary, tubular, cystic, or solid pattern. It is characterized by two predominant cell types: (1) polyhedral or rounded clear cells with abundant intracytoplasmic glycogen (Fig 6–10,A) and (2) hobnail cells, characterized by scanty cytoplasm and bulbous, hyperchromatic nuclei that protrude into the glandular lumina (Fig 6–10,B). The serous papillary carcinoma has microscopic features similar to those of the serous papillary carcinoma of the ovary (Fig 6–11). This tumor has a poor prognosis, related to the frequent presence of deep invasion of the myometrium and peritoneal implantation. Other rare forms of endometrial carcinoma include the secretory type, a well-differentiated adenocarcinoma with subnuclear vacuolization similar to that observed in normal early secretory endometrium, and the mucin-rich carcinoma, characterized by the presence of abundant mucin, which is primarily intraluminal but may be additionally present in the apical portions of the cytoplasm of the neoplastic cells. In contrast, in mucinous carcinomas, which are relatively common in the cervix but extremely rare in the endometrium, mucin fills the cytoplasm of many of the tumor cells. Another very rare type of endometrial carcinoma is the pure squamous cell form, which may arise on a background of pyometra and squamous metaplasia.

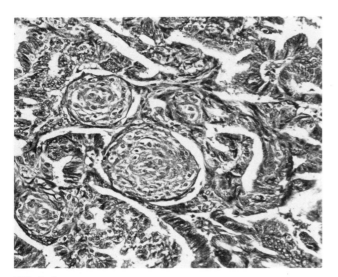

FIG 6–8.
Adenoacanthoma. Grade 1 (of 4). Malignant endometrial glands contain rounded nodules (morules) of small cytologically benign squamous cells; ×256.

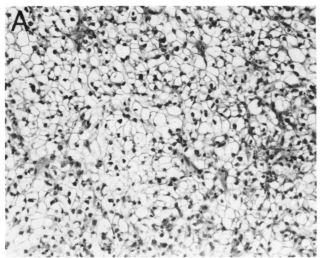

FIG 6–10.
A, clear cell carcinoma. Grade 2 (of 4). The solid pattern is composed of polygonal and rounded cells with clear cytoplasm and relatively small dark eccentric nuclei. The clear cytoplasm stains positively for glycogen; ×256. **B,** clear cell adenocarci-noma. Variably sized glandular spaces are lined by prominent hobnail cells with scanty cytoplasm and large, bulbous nuclei which protrude into the lumina × 260.

In the grading of endometrial carcinomas, we utilize both a four-grade system similar to that developed by Broders for squamous cell carcinoma of the skin, and a three-grade system modified from that proposed by the International Federation of Gynecology and Obstetrics (FIGO). Accordingly, well-differentiated tumors composed almost entirely of well-formed glands lined by slightly to moderately atypical cells fall into the Broders grade 1 and 2 and the FIGO grade 1 categories. In moderately differentiated tumors (Broders grade 3 and FIGO grade 2), glands are prevalent but significant areas are composed of solid nests or masses of tumor cells, and cellular atypicality and mitotic activity are more marked. Poorly differentiated adenocarcinomas (Broders grade 4 and FIGO grade 3) contain mostly solid areas composed of poorly differentiated tumor cells with an absent or minor glandular component (Fig 6–12). A problem with utilization of the unmodified FIGO criteria, which are based entirely on the architecture of

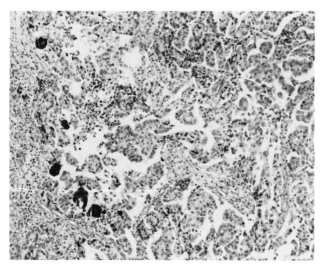

FIG 6–11.
Serous papillary adenocarcinoma. Grade 2 (of 4). The tumor contains delicate papillae with small buds of neoplastic cells appearing to lie free within the lumen. Psammoma bodies are present in the left portion of the micrograph; ×160.

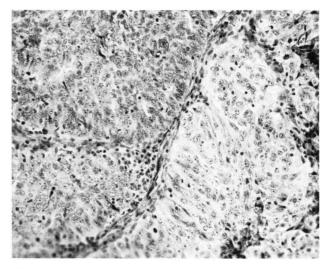

FIG 6–12.
Adenocarcinoma. Grade 4. The tumor is composed of sheets of poorly differentiated cells with rare to absent glandular differentiation; ×256.

the tumor, is that some carcinomas such as adenoacanthomas and clear cell carcinomas may have a predominantly solid pattern and yet be well differentiated, whereas an occasional adenocarcinoma with little or no solid growth may be poorly differentiated. It must be emphasized also that the grade assigned to a tumor in an endometrial curettage specimen is often lower than that revealed by thorough examination of a subsequently removed uterus.

SMOOTH MUSCLE TUMORS

Leiomyomas are the most common tumors of the uterus, occurring most often in women of reproductive age, especially those in their 4th and 5th decades. In the postmenopausal period these tumors typically undergo atrophy, often accompanied by extensive calcification; but occasionally they enlarge progressively. Leiomyosarcomas, which are much rarer, but account for about 45% of sarcomas and carcinosarcomas of the uterus, reach their peak incidence in a woman's 5th and 6th decades.

Gross Pathology

Leiomyomas may occur in any portion of the myometrium and present as intramural, subserosal, or submucosal masses. They vary in size from microscopic to massive. Submucosal leiomyomas appear as rounded masses that bulge to varying extents into the endometrial cavity; they may also form pedunculated tumors on stalks, sometimes presenting as soft or firm polypoid masses protruding through the external cervical os, or rarely through the introitus (Plate 28). The overlying endometrium may be atrophic, congested, ulcerated, or hemorrhagic. The tumor tissue itself may undergo a variety of degenerative changes, including infarction and cyst formation.

Leiomyosarcomas are typically softer and more often necrotic and hemorrhagic than leiomyomas. Approximately 20% are predominantly submucosal, protruding into the endometrial cavity in polypoid fashion.

Microscopic Pathology

The typical leiomyoma is composed of interlacing bundles of spindle-shaped cells with eosinophilic cytoplasm and cigar-shaped pale nuclei (Figs 6–13,A and B). Focal or diffuse hyalinization and edema are common. Calcification is a frequent finding, particularly after the menopause. The leiomyoblastoma, sometimes referred to as an epithelioid or clear cell leiomyoma, is composed predominantly or exclusively of smooth muscle cells resembling epithelial cells, with abundant eosinophilic or clear cytoplasm, and growing diffusely or in cords or trabeculae.

The diagnosis of leiomyosarcoma is usually obvious but may be difficult in borderline cases. Heightened mitotic activity and invasion of the adjacent myometrium are the most useful criteria. The presence of ten or more mitotic figures per ten high-power microscopic fields almost always indicates malignancy, whereas tumors with four or fewer mitotic figures are almost al-

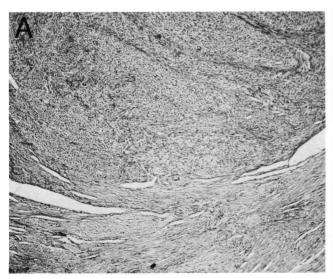
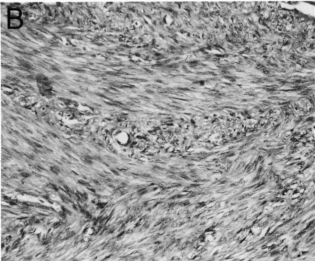

FIG 6–13.
Leiomyoma. The tumor is well demarcated **(A)** and composed of interlacing bundles of well-differentiated spindle-shaped cells **(B)**. **A,** ×64; **B,** × 256.

ways benign. Problems in diagnosis arise in the evaluation of tumors with intermediate mitotic rates. The term "smooth muscle tumors of uncertain malignant potential" has been suggested to designate these neoplasms. Important criteria for the diagnosis of leiomyosarcoma are the degree of nuclear atypicality (Fig 6–14) and invasion of the adjacent myometrium. Leiomyoblastomas are benign in the great majority of cases; the histologic criteria for malignancy of these tumors are even less clear-cut than those for neoplasms composed of spindle-shaped smooth muscle cells.

ENDOMETRIAL STROMAL TUMORS

Endometrial stromal tumors include benign forms, low-grade sarcomas, and high-grade sarcomas. The benign tumors are the very rare stromal nodules, 75% of which occur in women of reproductive age. Endometrial stromal sarcomas account for 10% to 15% of uterine sarcomas and carcinosarcomas. The low-grade variety (endolymphatic stromal myosis; endometrial stromatosis) occur over a wide age range of patients, but are encountered in women of reproductive age in over half the cases, with a mean age in the woman's early 40s. High-grade sarcomas occur in slightly older women, with the average age being approximately 50 years.

Gross Pathology

Although most stromal nodules are intramural, approximately 20% form soft polypoid masses that bulge into the endometrial cavity. The uterus is typically enlarged in cases of endometrial stromal sarcoma regardless of its grade. The low-grade tumors usually form smooth-surfaced polypoid masses that fill the endometrial cavity (Plate 29); in the underlying myometrium, they grow as yellow-tan, serpiginous and nodular masses or as wormlike structures protruding from the lumina of myometrial vessels. Sectioning of the broad ligament and adnexal structures may reveal extrauterine extension, including intravascular wormlike prolongations. In some cases, the tumor appears to blend imperceptibly with the surrounding myometrium, and a clearly defined mass is not appreciated.

High-grade stromal sarcomas characteristically form large polypoid masses that fill the endometrial cavity. They are more apt to exhibit hemorrhage and necrosis than the low-grade tumors and are less prone to extend as wormlike structures within the uterine and extrauterine vessels.

Microscopic Pathology

The stromal nodule is composed of bland cells closely resembling the stromal cells of normal proliferative endometrium. The diagnostic feature of this tumor is its sharp demarcation from the adjacent myometrium. The mitotic rate is generally very low. In contrast, the low-grade stromal sarcoma invades the myometrium in a serpiginous fashion, typically extending within vascular spaces (Fig 6–15). Numerous small blood vessels, similar in appearance to the spiral arterioles of a secretory endometrium, are a characteristic feature, and

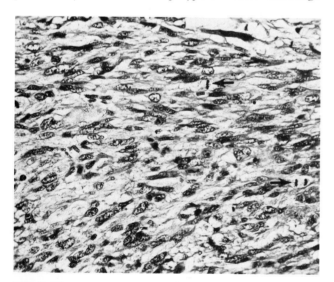

FIG 6–14.
Leiomyosarcoma. The tumor is composed of spindle cells with enlarged pleomorphic nuclei. Mitotic figures are numerous *(arrows)*; ×256.

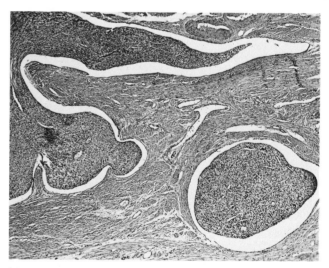

FIG 6–15.
Low-grade stromal sarcoma (endolymphatic stromal myosis). Tongues of tumor permeate the myometrium and its vessels; ×44.

sharply etched foci of hyalinization may be present. The neoplastic cells are similar to those of the stromal nodule. Stromal sarcomas with more than 10 and usually more than 20 mitotic figures per 10 high-power fields are classified as high-grade. The cells of these tumors have less resemblance to the stromal cells of normal proliferative endometrium than those of a low-grade sarcoma and may assume nonspecific features of a round cell or spindle cell sarcoma.

MIXED EPITHELIAL AND STROMAL TUMORS

These tumors contain epithelial as well as stromal elements. The epithelial component is occasionally benign, but the stromal component is very rarely so. Adenosarcomas and the much more common malignant müllerian mixed tumors generally occur in postmenopausal women, although in one series of the latter tumors approximately one third of the patients were premenopausal, and three were 16, 17, and 22 years of age. Malignant müllerian mixed tumors account for about 35% of uterine sarcomas and carcinosarcomas.

Gross Pathology

Most mixed tumors partly or completely fill the endometrial cavity in the form of irregular single or multiple polypoid masses (Plates 30 and 31). They may be soft or firm depending on the degree of malignancy of either the epithelial or stromal component. Necrosis and hemorrhage are common in the more poorly differentiated tumors.

Microscopic Pathology

The very rare adenofibroma is characterized by club-shaped polypoid masses lined by low columnar or cuboidal epithelium projecting from the surface of the tumor or into cysts within it. The stroma is composed of cytologically benign cells, which may have the appearance of endometrial stromal cells or fibroblasts. Mitotic figures are extremely rare or absent in both the epithelium and the stroma. In contrast, the müllerian adenosarcoma contains benign or atypical appearing glands and a sarcomatous stroma that exhibits more than an occasional mitotic figure (Fig 6–16). A characteristic feature is collaring of the glandular component by cellular foci of stromal neoplasia. The epithelium may be endometrial, endocervical, or squamous in type.

In homologous malignant müllerian mixed tumors the sarcomatous component may be similar to that of an endometrial stromal sarcoma, but other types of sar-

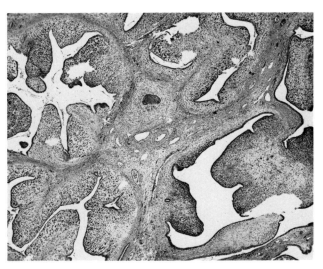

FIG 6–16.
Adenosarcoma. Irregularly branching cleft-like glands are surrounded by a cellular sarcomatous stroma imparting a collaring effect; ×28.

coma, such as leiomyosarcoma, are occasionally encountered. The malignant epithelial element is most commonly a carcinoma of müllerian type such as endometrioid, serous, clear cell, or squamous cell carcinoma (Fig 6–17). The malignant müllerian mixed tumor with heterologous elements may include rhabdomyoblasts, immature cartilage or immature bone, or a combination of these elements (Fig 6–18). In one series rhabdomyosarcoma was present in 68% of the patients, chondrosarcoma in 29%, and osteogenic sarcoma in the remainder.

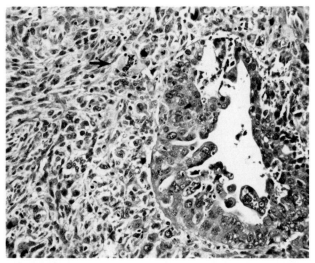

FIG 6–17.
Malignant müllerian mixed tumor; homologous (carcinosarcoma). A gland lined by irregularly stratified malignant cells is surrounded by a highly cellular stroma with numerous, often atypical mitotic figures (arrows); ×256.

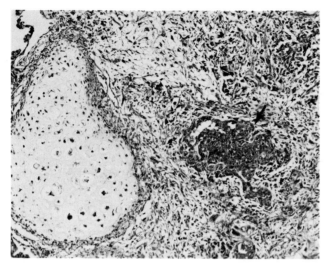

FIG 6–18.
Malignant müllerian mixed tumor; heterologous. A nest of carcinoma *(arrow)* is present within an area of spindle cell sarcoma. An island of malignant cartilage is present on the left; ×100.

GESTATIONAL TROPHOBLASTIC NEOPLASIA

The term gestational trophoblastic neoplasia encompasses the hydatidiform mole, chorioadenoma destruens (invasive mole), choriocarcinoma, and placental site trophoblastic tumor. The hydatidiform mole has been reported to occur in approximately one of every 2,000 pregnancies and choriocarcinoma in one of every 20,000 to 40,000 pregnancies. The choriocarcinoma, which is composed of cytotrophoblast and syncytiotrophoblast cells growing in concert, follows a hydatidiform mole in approximately one third to one half of the cases; in the remainder, it follows some other form of pregnancy, including a full-term delivery and a spontaneous or therapeutic abortion. Moles usually are detected in the first trimester of pregnancy, with vaginal bleeding. The uterus is larger than expected for the estimated age of the fetus in approximately half the patients; in the remainder, the uterus is either of normal size or smaller than normal. The placental site trophoblastic tumor (PSTT) is a recently described neoplasm composed of intermediate trophoblast cells of the type normally encountered in the implantation site. Patients typically present with amenorrhea and uterine enlargement and are often thought to be pregnant. The tumor generally secretes only small amounts of chorionic gonadotropin and has a benign clinical course, but occasional tumors, which typically contain numerous mitotic figures, have an aggressive clinical behavior with metastatic spread and a fatal outcome.

Gross Pathology

The uterus containing a hydatidiform mole is typically distended by a multitude of thin-walled, fluid-filled vesicles up to 1 to 2 cm in diameter; the vesicles are usually connected by thin strands of connective tissue. The invasive mole can be recognized grossly if intramyometrial vesicles are identified. The most characteristic gross features of a choriocarcinoma are hemorrhage and necrosis. The tumor may form a bulky, soft, friable mass filling the uterine cavity, with multiple nodules of hemorrhagic tumor involving the myometrium (Plate 32). The PSTT may present as a polypoid tumor protruding into the endometrial cavity or may primarily involve the myometrium, with extension to or beyond the serosa. Sectioning reveals soft, tan masses; hemorrhage and necrosis are usually not prominent features except in the occasional clinically malignant forms of the tumor.

Microscopic Pathology

The histologic hallmarks of the hydatidiform mole are hydrops of the chorionic villi and proliferation of the overlying trophoblastic cells. The villi are enlarged, generally avascular, and filled with pale, edematous tissue, which may form cysts of varying sizes. The degree of trophoblastic proliferation and atypicality determines the histologic grade of the tumor. Grade 1 has been assigned to those lesions with minimal hyperplasia of well-differentiated trophoblastic cells, grade 2 to those

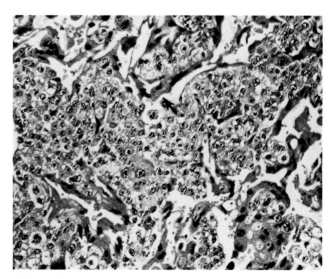

FIG 6–19.
Choriocarcinoma. The typical biphasic pattern is composed of a central core of cytotrophoblast with a rim of syncytiotrophoblast *(arrow)*; ×256.

with moderate to marked hyperplasia of well-differentiated trophoblast, and grade 3 to those with marked hyperplasia of atypical trophoblastic cells. The histologic features of invasive moles are generally similar to those of the noninvasive forms, although the villi within the myometrium may be relatively few and tend to exhibit less severe hydropic changes.

Choriocarcinoma is characterized by proliferation of cytotrophoblast and syncytiotrophoblast without associated hydropic villi. The better differentiated tumors grow in a typical biphasic pattern with a central core of cytotrophoblast rimmed by syncytiotrophoblast (Fig 6–19). In contrast, poorly differentiated forms are characterized by proliferation of large, bizarre cells with poor delineation between cytotrophoblast and syncytiotrophoblast cells, although the latter can be recognized in small numbers. Numerous typical and atypical mitotic figures can be identified, especially in the more poorly differentiated lesions. Extensive hemorrhage is a consistent finding.

The cells of the placental site trophoblastic tumor have features similar to those of the implantation site, appearing polygonal to fusiform, with abundant eosinophilic to amphophilic cytoplasm. The nuclei range from small, vesicular, and rounded to large, hyperchromatic, and pleomorphic. Some cells are binucleate, trinucleate, or multinucleate. The tumors characteristically invade the myometrium as single cells or as small groups of cells interposed between bundles of smooth muscle fibers or individual fibers (Fig 6–20). Studies utilizing immunoperoxidase have revealed that the cells of the PSTT typically stain strongly for placental lactogen (hPL) and only focally for chorionic gonadotropin (hCG). Conversely, most choriocarcinomas stain strongly for hCG and only focally for hPL. The staining pattern of the placental site trophoblastic tumor is similar to that observed in normal intermediate trophoblast, which contains predominantly hPL and only small amounts of hCG.

On the basis of an analysis of a small series of cases, mitotic activity appears to be the most reliable, but not exclusive, criterion for differentiating the clinically benign cases of PSTT from those with a malignant course. In the benign tumors, the mitotic rate is usually 4 or less per 10 high-power fields. In contrast, several tumors that have shown an aggressive clinical behavior have had mitotic rates ranging from 8 to 12 per 10 high-power fields.

NON-NEOPLASTIC GESTATIONAL DISORDERS

Non-neoplastic disorders associated with gestation that may occupy the endometrium include products of conception retained after an incomplete abortion, which occasionally take on the configuration of a polyp, and fetal remnants. Placental polyps are almost always found in women of reproductive age, but at least one example was not discovered until 5 years after the menopause. Abnormal uterine bleeding is a common presenting symptom and may be manifested as severe postpartum

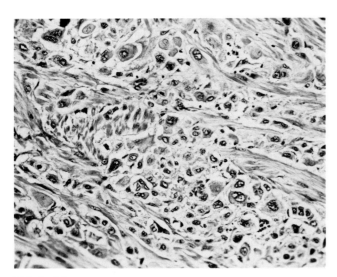

FIG 6–20.
Placental site trophoblastic tumor. Sheets and strands of polygonal trophoblastic cells invade the smooth muscle of the myometrium, splitting muscle bundles; ×256.

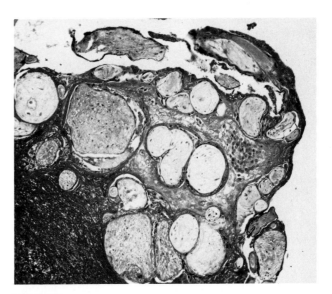

FIG 6–21.
Placental polyp. Hyalinized avascular chorionic villi are lined by a flat layer of trophoblast and enveloped in a mass of fibrin; ×100.

hemorrhage when the polyp is of recent origin, and menometrorrhagia in cases of longer duration. Occasionally fetal remnants, particularly fragments of bone, are found in the presence or absence of trophoblastic tissue.

Gross Pathology

Placental polyps appear as pedunculated firm or soft, mottled, red or yellow necrotic tissue, which may be located anywhere within the uterine cavity, although in one series over half of them occurred in the fundus or in a cornu (Plate 33). They may attain a diameter of 5 to 6 cm.

Microscopic Pathology

Placental polyps may contain either well preserved chorionic villi with viable appearing trophoblast and decidua, or hyalinized villi with degenerated trophoblast and decidua (Fig 6–21). In one series of 20 cases, the chorionic villi were not found within the myometrium, but in some reported cases their presence therein has suggested a focal process similar to placenta accreta. Sectioning of bony fragments in the endometrium generally reveals their fetal character (Plate 34). Very rarely, glial tissue is found within the endometrium and sometimes the myometrium; it is usually interpreted as retained fetal tissue, but in some cases, it is truly neoplastic and may even spread beyond the uterus.

BIBLIOGRAPHY

Baldwin WC: Placental polyps—an unusual cause of post-menopausal bleeding. *Am J Obstet Gynecol* 1956; 71:1126.

Bard DS, Zuna RE: Sarcomas and related neoplasms of the uterine corpus. A brief review of their natural history, prognostic factors and management. *Obstet Gynecol Annu* 1982; 45(5):783–5.

Broders AC: The microscopic grading of cancer. *Surg Clin North Am* 1941; 21:937–962.

Christopherson WM, Alberhasky RC, Connelly PJ: Carcinoma of the endometrium: I. A clinicopathologic study of clear cell carcinoma and secretory carcinoma. *Cancer* 1982; 49:1511.

Clement PB, Scully RE: Müllerian adenosarcoma of the uterus. A clinicopathologic analysis of ten cases of a distinctive type of müllerian mixed tumor. *Cancer* 1974; 34:1138.

Courpas AS, Morris JD, Woodruff JD: Osteoid tissue in utero. Report of three cases. *Obstet Gynecol* 1964; 24(4):634.

Dallenbach-Hellweg G: *Histopathology of the Endometrium*. New York, Springer-Verlag, 1971.

Driscoll SG: Gestational trophoblastic neoplasms: Morphologic considerations. *Hum Pathol* 1977; 8(5):529.

Dyer I, Bradbum DM: An inquiry into the etiology of placental polyps. *Am J Obstet Gynecol* 1971; 109(6):858–67.

Greenwald P, Caputo TA, Wolfgang PE: Endometrial cancer after menopausal use of estrogen. *Obstet Gynecol* 1977; 50:239.

Hammond CB, Weed JC, Barnard DE, et al: Gestational trophoblastic neoplasia. *CA* 1981; 31(6):322.

Hendrickson MR, Kempson RL: in, Bennington JL (ed): *Surgical Pathology of the Uterine Corpus*. Philadelphia, WB Saunders, 1980.

Hendrickson M, Ross J, Eifel P, et al: Uterine papillary serous carcinoma: A highly malignant form of endometrial adenocarcinoma. *Am J Surg Pathol* 1982; 6(2):93.

Kottmeier HL (ed): Annual report on the results of treatment in gynecological cancer. *Fed Gynecol Obstet Radiumhemmet* (Stockholm), 1982; vol 18.

Kurman R, Mazur MT: Benign diseases of the endometrium, in, Kurman RJ (ed): *Blaustein's Pathology of the Female Genital Tract,* ed 3. New York, Springer-Verlag, 1987, p 292.

Kurman RJ, Norris HJ: Mesenchymal tumors of the uterus: VI. Epithelioid smooth muscle tumors including leiomyoblastoma and clear cell leiomyoma. A clinical and pathologic analysis of twenty-six cases. *Cancer* 1976; 37:1853.

Kurman RJ, Scully RE, Norris HJ: Trophoblastic pseudotumor of the uterus. An exaggerated form of "syncytial endometritis" simulating a malignant tumor. *Cancer* 1976; 38:1214.

Kurman RJ, Young RH, Main CS, et al: Immunocytochemical localization of placental lactogen and chorionic gonadotropin in the normal placenta and trophoblastic tumors with emphasis on intermediate trophoblast and the placental site trophoblastic tumor. *Int J Gynecol Pathol* 1984; 3:101–121.

Lawrence WD, Qureshi F, Bonakdar M: Placental polyp: Light microscopic and immunohistochemical observations. *Hum Pathol* (in press).

Mazur MT: Atypical polypoid adenomyoma of the endometrium. *Am J Surg Pathol* 1981; 5(5):473–482.

Ng ABP, Reagan JW, Storaasli JP, et al: Mixed adenosquamous carcinoma of the endometrium. *Am J Clin Pathol* 1973; 50:765.

Norris HJ, Taylor HB: Mesenchymal tumors of the uterus: I. A clinical and pathological study of fifty-three endometrial stromal tumors. *Cancer* 1966; 19:755.

Novak ER, Woodruff JD: in, *Novak's Gynecologic and Obstetric Pathology,* ed 8. Philadelphia, WB Saunders, 1979.

Peterson EP: Endometrial carcinoma in young women. A clinical profile. *Obstet Gynecol* 1968; 31:702.

Schmidt-Matthiesen H (ed): in, *The Normal Human Endometrium*. New York-London, McGraw-Hill Book Co, 1963.

Swan RW, Woodruff JD: Retained products of conception. Histologic viability of placental polyps. *Obstet Gynecol* 1969; 34:506–14.

Tavassoli FN, Norris HJ: Mesenchymal tumors of the uterus: VII. A clinicopathological study of 60 endometrial stromal nodules. *Histopathology* 1981; 5:1.

Vellios F, Starder RW, Huber CP: Carcinosarcoma (malignant

mixed mesodermal tumor) of the uterus. *Am J Clin Pathol* 1963; 39:496.

Weiss NS, Szekely DR, Austin DF: Increasing incidence of endometrial cancer in the United States. *N Engl J Med* 1976; 294:1259.

Welch WR, Scully RE: Precancerous lesions of the endometrium. *Hum Pathol* 1977; 8:503.

Williamson E, Christopherson WM: Malignant mixed müllerian tumors of the uterus. *Cancer* 1972; 29:5.

Yoonis M, Hart WR: Endometrial stromal sarcomas. *Cancer* 1977; 40:898.

Young RH, Scully RE: Placental site trophoblastic tumor. Current status. *Clin Obstet Gynaecol* 1987; 27:248.

Zaloudek CJ, Norris HJ: Mesenchymal tumors of the uterus, in Kurman RJ (ed): *Blaustein's Pathology of the Female Genital Tract*, ed 3. New York, Springer-Verlag, 1987.

7

Optical Principles of the Endoscope

Fred M. Gardner, Ph.D.

An endoscope is an optical instrument that uses controlled light beams for gathering visual or photographic information about parts of the human body which are inaccessible or difficult to see by direct viewing. Various endoscopes such as bronchoscopes, laryngoscopes, laparoscopes, gastroscopes, hysteroscopes, and many others have been devised to serve the needs of physicians within the medical specialties. However, the optical principles and the basic features used in these different instruments are similar.

Basically an endoscope consists of an optical system to carry light in order to illuminate the object being viewed and either the same (as in the contact hysteroscope) or generally a different optical mechanism for conveying the image back to the eye or camera. The image may be conveyed through a series of lenses, in which case the endoscope tube is rigid, or it may be carried to the viewer by means of light trapped in a flexible fiberoptic bundle. In most modern endoscopes the illuminating light is carried to the object by an optical fiber bundle. In addition to illuminating and image capabilities, most endoscopes have channels that allow the passage of biopsy forceps, gas, liquids, laser radiation, and a variety of surgical tools.

FIBEROPTIC PRINCIPLES

The transmission of light through a glass fiber depends on the phenomenon of total internal reflection. If a fiber is straight or curved, light entering one end travels in a zigzag path, repeatedly reflecting off the internal surface of the fiber, until it emerges from the other end.

The transmission of visible light (0.40 μm to 0.70 μm) through fibers having diameters of 8 μm or more can be traced by the application of the principles of geometrical optics. In fibers smaller than 8 μm, diffraction losses occur, significantly reducing the intensity of the transmitted light. For this reason, endoscopes use fibers with diameters of approximately 10 μm.

Refraction of a Light Ray

When light is incident from air onto a transparent medium such as glass, part of the light intensity is reflected back into the air and part is transmitted into the glass, as shown in Figure 7–1. For the reflected component, the incident angle θ_i equals the reflected angle θ_i'. The transmitted ray, however, changes direction at the interface because of the difference of the speed of light in air and in glass. Because the speed of the ray slows down as it passes from the air into the glass, the ray bends toward the interface normal, and $\theta_i > \theta_r$. The amount of bending or refraction in passing from air into glass can be given as the index of refraction of the glass relative to air. This is defined as the ratio of the speed of light in air *(a)* to the speed of light in the glass *(g)*; $n = v_a/v_g$. Usually the index of refraction of a transparent medium is given relative to the speed of light in a vacuum ($C = 3.0 \times 10^8$ meters/sec) that is, $n = c/v$. Typical optical glasses have refractive indices between 1.5 and 1.7 for the visible spectrum.

The relationship between θ_i and θ_r is given by Snell's law:

$$n, \sin \theta_i = n_2 \sin \theta_r.$$

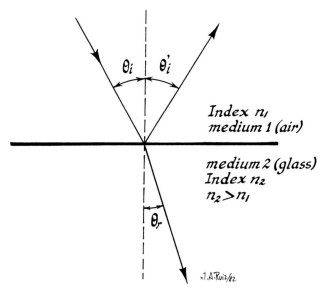

FIG 7–1.
Reflection and refraction of light at an interface between two transparent media.

Total Internal Reflection

If a ray travels from a higher refractive index medium to a lower index medium, as shown in Figure 7–2, Snell's law predicts that the ray will bend away from the interface normal, that is, $\theta_i < \theta_r$. As the incident angle is increased, the angle of refraction becomes larger until it finally reaches 90°. The angle of incidence for which the angle of refraction is 90° is called the critical angle. The critical angle has a value between 36° and 42° for typical optical glasses in air.

If the critical angle is exceeded, the ray reflects from the interface back into the higher index medium.

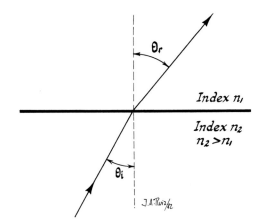

FIG 7–2.
A ray incident upon an interface from the higher index side bends away from the interface normal.

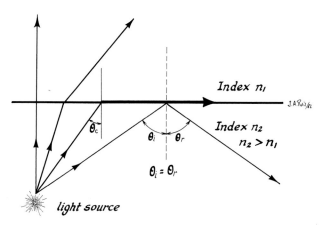

FIG 7–3.
Ray diagram showing the critical angle and total internal reflection.

This internal reflection is nearly total if the surface is microscopically smooth. The critical angle and total internal reflection are illustrated in Figure 7–3.

If a ray of light enters one end of a glass fiber in air at an angle such that the critical angle is exceeded at the cylindrical surface, the ray will be transmitted to the other end by a series of internal reflections, as shown in Figure 7–4. In a typical 10-μm diameter fiber, a ray

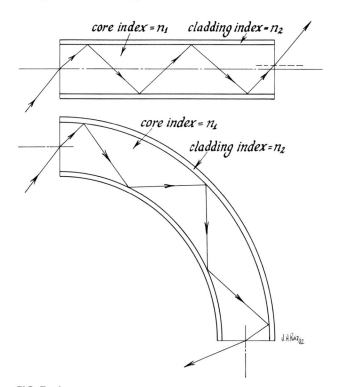

FIG 7–4.
Transmission of a light ray through a flexible fiber by total internal reflection.

reflects many thousands of times in traveling a 1-meter distance. Hence, it is necessary that the reflections be nearly perfect. If the surface of the fiber is not microscopically perfect or if any contaminant lies on the surface, the reflection coefficient will not be 100%, and some light will escape. For this reason, the transmitting fibers are clad with a lower index glass, as indicated in Figure 7–4. The coaxial fiber is produced by being drawn through a furnace so that the cladding is optically fused to the core.

Cladding the fiber changes the critical angle for total reflection from $\sin \theta_c = 1.00/n_1$. When the core is in air, the angle changes to $\sin \theta_c = n_2/n_1$ for the cladded case. Here n_2 is the refractive index of the cladding and n_1 is the refractive index of the core.

Numerical Aperture of a Fiber

Figure 7–5 shows a ray entering the end of a straight, cylindrical fiber core with an index of n_1, clad with a medium of index n_2 where $n_1 > n_2$. The ray is incident from a medium of index n_0 at an angle α to the fiber axis. The ray will be refracted at the end face of the fiber and will be totally reflected at the cylindrical fiber wall if the incident angle at the fiber wall is greater than the critical angle θ_c. The maximum value of the incident angle, α_m, for which the ray will be totally reflected at the fiber wall can be calculated using Snell's law $n_0 \sin \sigma_m = n_1 \sin \alpha_m' = n_1 \cos \theta_c = n_1 (1 - \sin^2\theta_c)^{1/2}$. $\sin \theta_c = n_2/n_1$. Hence, $n_0 \sin \sigma_m = (n_1^2 - n_2^2)^{1/2}$.

The numerical aperture *(NA)* of the fiber is defined as $n_0 \sin \sigma_m$. Hence, $NA = (n_1^2 - n_2^2)^{1/2}$. The numerical aperture is a measure of the light-gathering power of the fiber. A typical fiber core having a refractive index of $m_1 = 1.62$, and a typical cladding having a refractive index of $n_2 = 1.52$, would produce a numerical aperture of 0.56. If the ray is entering the fiber from an air medium, $n_0 = 1.00$, the acceptance half-angle would be 34°. Hence, the acceptance cone angle would be 68°. If the ray enters from water, $n_0 = 1.33$, and the acceptance cone angle is 50°.

In practice, a number of factors combine to produce a *NA* and an acceptance angle smaller than defined here. Attempts to increase the *NA* by increasing n_1, the refractive index of the core, will lead to a lower transmittance of the blue end of the visible spectrum. However, the selective transmittance is usually not a problem except for very long fibers or when ultraviolet light is being used for illumination.

Coherent Fiber Bundles

In order to transmit an optical image through a bundle of fibers, the fibers must have the same relative arrangement at the distal end as at the proximal end. Fiber bundles of this type are said to be coherent.

Light originating from an object and entering the distal end of a fiber, after a large number of internal reflections, emerges uniformly distributed over the exit face of the fiber, as illustrated in Figure 7–6. Any detailed distribution of light over a single fiber is lost after transmission through the fiber. This blurring of the light distribution by transmission through the fiber sets a limit to the ability of fiber bundles to resolve fine detail. For the case when the fiber bundle is stationary with respect to the object, the smallest detail of the light distribution on the distal face that can be resolved at the proximal end is approximately 2.5 *d,* where *d* is the diameter of a fiber.

To produce images for viewing, the fiberoptic coherent bundle makes use of an objective lens system and an eyepiece (Fig 7–7). The objective lens system focuses a real image of the object being viewed onto the distal fiber bundle face. The coherent bundle transmits this image to the proximal end face. Here the eyepiece views the transmitted image and forms a magnified virtual image at a distance of approximately 25 cm in front of the normal eye.

The overall magnification of the endoscope is given by the product of the magnification of the objective lens and the eyepiece. The eyepiece magnification is usually

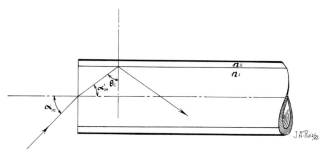

FIG 7–5.
Ray entering a straight fiber at an angle σ_m for which the incident angle on the fiber wall is θ_c.

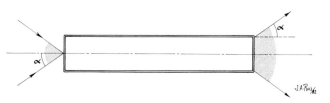

FIG 7–6.
Any distribution of light within the acceptance cone at the entry face of a fiber will be uniformly distributed over the exit face of the fiber.

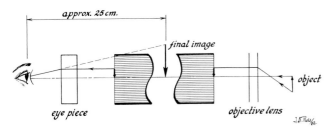

FIG 7–7.
Schematic of fiberoptic endoscope showing the object and image positions.

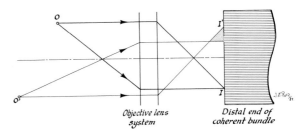

FIG 7–8.
The objective lens system focuses a sharp image of a source of light at O on the fiber face at I. Another object at O′, which is further from the objective lens than O, produces an out-of-focus image I′ on the fiber face.

limited to 10× because of the discrete nature of the fiber bundle. The magnification of the objective lens is less than 1 and is inversely proportional to the distance of the object from the lens. Hence, an exact magnification for a fiberoptic endoscope can be given only if the object distance is known.

In practice, objects to be viewed are located at different distances from the objective lens. Either some means of focusing must be built into the objective lens system, or sufficient depth of focus must be provided. For medical endoscopes, the latter approach is usually taken, since distal focusing presents mechanical as well as sterilizing difficulties.

Light focused on the distal fiber face is transmitted to the proximal end. If the distal image is poorly focused, the image on the proximal face will be of poor quality, and no refocusing of the eyepiece can bring the image to sharp focus. Figure 7–8 shows the schematic of an objective lens system and distal end of the coherent fiber bundle, set to produce a sharp focus on the fiber face of an object located at O. An object at O′ will produce an out-of-focus patch of light covering a number of fibers, resulting in a loss of image quality.

For a fixed-focus fiberoptic endoscope, the depth of focus can be increased by stopping down the objective lens with a small aperture. However, the image brightness is directly proportional to the square of the aperture radius. Therefore, any improvement in depth of focus achieved with an aperture is accompanied by a decrease in the image brightness.

The resolving power describes the ability of an optical instrument to distinguish between two point sources of light. The limit of resolution is usually given as the distance between two objects that can just be resolved. The limit of resolution of a fiberoptic bundle is set by the discrete structure of the coherent fiber bundle. Light from the object focused by the objective lens onto a single fiber appears at the proximal end, spread uniformly over the entire face of the fiber. When all factors are considered, the coherent bundle gives a limit of resolution of approximately $2.5\, d$, where d is the fiber

diameter. This limit refers only to the fiber bundle. If the objective magnification is m_o, the limit of resolution in the object is $2.5 d/m_o$. If d is taken to be 10 μm and m_o is taken as one-fifth, the smallest detail that can be resolved in the object is $2.5 d/m_o = 125$ μm.

The image focused on the distal fiber end is transmitted to the proximal face at unit magnification, and is viewed by the eyepiece under a magnification of m_e. Thus, the smallest resolvable separation in the final image is $2.5\, d \times m_e$. For $d = 10$ μm and $m_e = 10$, the resolution in the image is 250 μm. The limit of resolution due to diffraction by the limiting apertures at the objective lens and eyepiece is far smaller than that caused by the discrete structure of the coherent bundle.

Incoherent Illuminating Fiber Bundles

Nonimaging fiber bundles also carry light by total internal reflection, but in contrast to image carrying bundles, need not be coherent. Image resolving power is of no consequence for the illuminating bundle, hence fibers chosen are 25 μm in diameter and larger. Each fiber consists of a high refractive index core inside a low index cladding.

An important consideration for illuminating bundles is the spectrum of the transmitted light. The higher the refractive index of the core glass, the greater is the absorption of the blue end of the visible spectrum. Therefore, to maintain faithful color rendition for the viewer or camera, relatively low numerical aperture fibers of short length should be used.

The light sources for modern endoscopes are high pressure lamps having color temperatures as high as 5,500°K. The light from the lamps is focused through a heat filter or by a cold mirror onto a flexible fiber light guide, which is coupled to the incoherent fiber bundle of the endoscope, as shown in Figure 7–9. A higher color temperature is desirable to offset attenuation of the blue end of the spectrum by the fiberoptics and thus

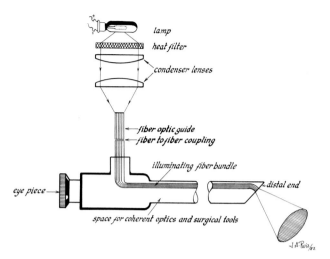

FIG 7–9.
Schematic diagram of an endoscope illuminating system.

produce a faithful color rendition of the tissue or organ under view. Reduced light transmission to the object may be due to reflection from air-glass surfaces of the heat filter, the condenser lenses, and the fiber end faces. Additional light losses arise because the core cross-sectional area occupies only about 70% of the bundle cross-section (Fig 7–10) and because of mismatches in the fiber-to-fiber coupling.

Rigid Endoscopes

The standard endoscope, which historically preceded the fiberoptic model, consists of an objective lens

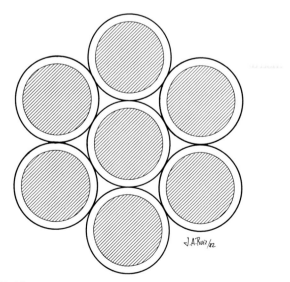

FIG 7–10.
Cross section of a bundle of fibers. Light passes only through the cores of the fibers.

system, an eyepiece, and a number of optical relay stages assembled and encased in a rigid, narrow tube. In early endoscopes of this type, the image relay optics consisted of a number of lenses separated by long air spaces (Fig 7–11,A), which allowed the image to be transmitted at unit magnification from the distal to the proximal end through a small-diameter tube without severely restricting the field of view. The light transmission of the lens relay system was greatly improved by the introduction of the rod-lens system, devised by H.H. Hopkins. The rod-lens system replaced the long air spaces and thin glass lenses with long glass rods and short air spaces (Fig 7–11,B).

The total amount of light transmitted by a lens relay endoscope is proportional to the square of the index of refraction of the medium between the relay lenses. If the medium is air, $n = 1$ and $n^2 = 1$. However, if the medium is glass, as in the Hopkins rod-lens system, and if $n = 1.52$, then $n^2 = 2.31$. Thus, filling the space between objective and eyepiece with glass rather than air more than doubles the transmission of light. In addition, the rod-lens endoscope allows a 1.4 times larger internal clear aperture radius for a given outer radius of the endoscope than the older lens-relay type. Light transmission through the endoscope tube is proportional to the fourth power of the radius. Thus, the combined increase in light transmission of the rod-lens over the thin lens relay amounts to approximately nine times.

The illumination of the object is provided by an incoherent fiber bundle arranged at the distal end to illuminate effectively the field of view of the endoscope.

Rigid endoscopes usually do not employ variable focus optics. To allow viewing of objects at different distances from the objective lens, the instrument must be provided with some depth of focus. The normal eye can create sharp images of objects which lie between optical infinity and 250 mm. Hence, the depth of focus for a rigid endoscope being used visually can be defined as the range of object distances which furnish images that fall within the range of the accommodation of the eye. Eye accommodation does not play a role in aiding the

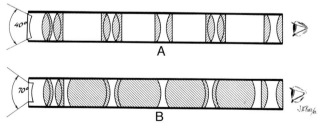

FIG 7–11.
A, conventional lens-relay rigid endoscope. **B,** the Hopkins rod-lens rigid endoscope.

depth of focus of a fiberoptic endoscope. If the image focused on the coherent fiber bundle is out of focus, it cannot be refocused by the eye.

The resolution of a lens-type endoscope is limited by the diffraction effects that are common to optical instruments employing lenses which limit the wavefront of the light emerging from the object under view. The image of a point on the object is a diffraction pattern consisting of alternating, concentric dark and light bands or rings. The overlap of these diffraction patterns sets a limit to the separation between points that can be judged by the viewer as being separate.

Unlike the fiberoptic endoscope, in which the diffraction limit of the resolution of the objective is not reached because of the discrete structure of the image-carrying fiber bundle, a high-quality rigid endoscope has a resolution near the limits set by diffraction theory.

The Contact Hysteroscope

The contact hysteroscope is a rigid endoscope that employs a rod-lens objective set for focus on an object plane at the distal surface of the lens (Fig 7–12). The objective lens, which is encased in a stainless steel sleeve, forms the image for the eyepiece, and also serves as the guide for the illuminating light. The visual field is limited to diameters slightly smaller than the outside diameter of the stainless steel casing, which is 6 mm and 8 mm for the two models available. The contact hysteroscope does not have the panoramic view of the conventional fiberoptic hysteroscope; however, there are a number of advantages in the use of this simple optical instrument for direct viewing of the uterine cavity.

The object to be viewed is illuminated by ambient light, which enters the body of the hysteroscope through a translucent collector. The light is transmitted down the rod-lens by total internal reflection and is concentrated at the object plane of the lens. Light is prevented from reflecting back into the eyepiece and decreasing contrast, by properly coated optics that enhance transmission down the light guide. A system of

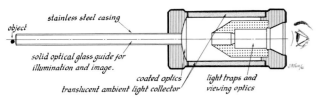

FIG 7–12.
Schematic diagram of a contact hysteroscope. This instrument, known under the trade name Hysteroser was designed by the Institute d'Optique de Paris and is manufactured in France.

light traps also helps prevent extraneous light from entering the eyepiece (see Fig 7–10).

The basic magnification of the Hysteroser is ×1.6. An adjustable magnifier, which attaches directly to the eyepiece, is also available. The use of this magnifier brings the magnification to ×3.2. The Hysteroser produces a high-quality image with a resolution of object of 20 µm. This far exceeds the resolution of the best fiberoptic system.

The color rendition of the image is excellent because the 20-cm glass stem, which carries both the image and the illuminating light, does not significantly attenuate the blue wave lengths.

Objects to be viewed are in clearest focus when in contact with the distal end of the objective lens. Contact of the lens with the object forces any liquid that may exist from between the lens and object. Consequently, clear images are produced in fields of opaque liquids, such as blood. Although the best focus is produced for objects in contact with the objective lens, structures at distances up to 5.0 mm can be brought into focus by the accommodation of the eye. This depth of focus allows sufficient visualization to direct grasping forceps for biopsies.

SOME ASPECTS OF IMAGE QUALITY

Endoscopes should present undistorted, bright images to the eye or camera. Consequently, setting aside the mechanical aspects of the scope and its convenience of operation, the most important aspect of an endoscope is the quality of its images under the various operating conditions. It is sometimes necessary in the manufacture and the use of an optical instrument to sacrifice one aspect of image quality to enhance another aspect of the instrument.

Magnification and Resolution of Detail

The term magnification is used in several ways when referring to optical instruments. Linear magnification is defined as the ratio of the image size to the object size. However, the apparent size of an object to an observer is determined by the size of the retinal image, which depends only on the angle subtended at the eye by the object of vision. Thus, as seen in Figure 7–13, the object closer to the eye is apparently larger than the more distance object because of the larger visual angle. Consequently, another magnification must be defined. Visual magnification or magnifying power is defined as the ratio of the angle subtended at the eye by the object to the angle subtended at the eye by the image when

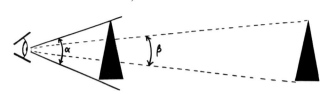

FIG 7–13.
Visual angles subtended at the eye by same size objects at different object distances.

the image is at the near point of the eye, which for the emmetropic eye is taken to be 250 mm. Actually, accommodation allows the eye to focus sharply for any object distance between infinity and the near point. Consequently, in panoramic endoscopes, such as a hysteroscope, the observer sees the near objects at different visual magnifications than those for more distance objects. The visual magnification of the scope is inversely proportional to the distal object distances.

Resolution refers to the ability of an optical instrument to separate fine detail in an object. The objective lens set essentially consititutes an aperture which, because of the wave nature of light, yields a circular diffraction pattern as an image. Thus, the images of two adjacent object points consist of two overlapping diffraction patterns, as seen in Figure 7–14. These images are defined as being resolved when this overlapping pattern can be identified as having originated from two points on the object. The effect of any optical aberrations, from any cause, such as poor alignment of optical components, will be to decrease the resolution, thereby increasing the size of the smallest detail resolved. Diffraction theory predicts that it is not possible to resolve detail smaller than about one half the wave length of the light being used.

The resolution of the human eye is determined by such factors as the pupil diameter, cone spacing on the retina, and various optical aberrations. The limit of res-

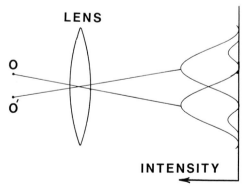

LENS

O

O´

INTENSITY

FIG 7–14.
Two overlapping diffraction patterns from objects O and O´ that are just resolved by the Rayleigh criterion.

olution of the eye is set at an angular separation of about 5×10^{-4} radians at best. Hence, at the near point of 250 mm, the eye can just resolve detail about 10^{-4} meters apart. This in turn limits the useful magnifications in optical instruments, as determined by resolution, to about $\times 500$. However, the necessity for large fields of view in endoscopes to examine gross detail and the instability of a hand-held optical instrument, dictate useful magnifications much smaller than $\times 500$. Generally, the most useful magnifications are about $\times 1$ to $\times 3$. However, some hysteroscopes made for panoramic as well as contact viewing have magnifications up to $\times 150$.

Contrast

A distinction should be made between detection of the presence of an object in the field of view and the ability to resolve its true shape and size. It is possible to detect the presence of objects that are smaller than the limit of resolution. The limit of detection depends to a large extent on contrast, assuming sufficient brightness of field. By contrast is meant the relative difference in intensity between the objects under view and its immediate surroundings or background. Contrast is affected by stray light, which produces a general haze over the image. Reflection from untreated lens surfaces, from the edges of lens, and, in the case of fiber bundles, the leakage of light into adjacent fibers due to broken fibers are frequent causes of stray light.

Depth of Focus and Depth Perception

Medical endoscopes are usually fixed-focus instruments, although some modern hysteroscopes have focusing eyepieces to allow panoramic as well as tissue contact operation. To view objects at different distances from the distal end of the endoscopes, a sufficient depth of focus, more properly called depth of field, is necessary. This depth of focus is greatly aided by the accommodation of the eye. For a panoramic endoscope it is important to clearly see detail near the distal end as well as detail at some distance without moving the instrument, because relative viewing angles and visual magnification change as the instrument is moved.

Depth perception in human vision is primarily a result of binocular vision (Fig 7–15). Objects at different distances produce different visual angles at the eye as well as images on different parts of the retina. The brain learns to interpret these differences in terms of distance from the eye. Endoscopes, being monocular instruments, provide little depth perception for the viewer. However, the interpretation of depth can be improved with practice.

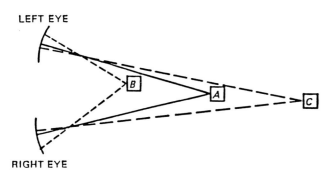

FIG 7–15.
A schematic diagram illustrating depth perception achieved as a result of binocular vision. Eyes are focused on object A.

Field of View

The field of view refers to the dimensions and area of the object that are seen in the image for a single setting of the endoscope. Generally speaking, the diameter of the field of view is dependent on the overall visual magnification of the endoscope but is more dependent on the objective than the eyepiece. The diameter of the field of view is one of the trade-offs that must be made with magnification, as it is inversely proportional to the visual magnification.

Color Rendition

The endoscopist uses size, shape, structure, and color as a basis of diagnosis. The color rendition of the object depends on the chromatic transmission of the imaging and illuminating optics as well as the spectral output of the illuminating lamp. Uniform representation of all wave lengths throughout the visible spectrum, shown in Plate 35, is needed for good color rendition. Generally, white light is desirable for eye viewing and color photography. Long glass fibers in flexible endoscopes selectively attenuate the blue end of the white light spectrum, producing images with a strong yellow hue.

Light sources may be classed according to their color temperature, which refers to the temperature necessary to achieve specifically defined spectral output. Modern light sources having color temperatures to 6,000°K, the approximate color temperature of the surface of the sun, are available for endoscopic use. These lamps provide a color temperature that approximates bright sunlight, and give excellent color rendition for viewing, photography, and video imaging.

BIBLIOGRAPHY

Driscoll WG, Vaughn W (eds): *Handbook of Optics.* New York, McGraw-Hill, 1987.

Gardner FM: Optical physics with emphasis on endoscopes, in Baggish MS (ed): *Clinical Obstetrics and Gynecology.* Philadelphia, Harper & Row, 1983, vol 26, p 213.

Hopkins HH: Optical principles of the endoscope, in Berci B (ed): *Endoscopy.* New York, Appleton-Century-Crofts, 1973.

Strong J: *Concepts of Classical Optics.* San Francisco, WH Freeman, 1958.

8

Instrumentation for Hysteroscopy

Michael S. Baggish, M.D.

Selection of the proper and most appropriate instruments is one of the keystones for the performance of a successful hysteroscopic examination. The prospective hysteroscopist is often overwhelmed by the variety of instruments available in the marketplace and may be confused when presented with the multitude of specialized endoscopes, sheaths, and accessories offered by instrument manufacturers and detail salespersons. The question "what best fits my needs and pocketbook" should be asked always before purchasing equipment. Obviously, a logical chronology of learning and experience should be followed in order to master any new technique. To jump headlong from no hysteroscopic experience into, for example, laser hysteroscopic surgery without intermediary steps is both foolish and reckless. Likewise, to attempt hysteroscopy and expect optimal results with jury-rigged equipment such as urethroscopes, cystoscopes, or laparoscopic insufflators is to court the unexpected. Purely and simply, fine, skilled procedures should be performed with precision instrumentation. Diagnostic skills and mastery in learning to orient oneself within the intrauterine milieu must always precede intrauterine operative intervention. In fact, every operative hysteroscopic procedure should be immediately preceded by a thorough diagnostic scan of the endometrial cavity.

For convenience, uterine endoscopes may be divided into two major categories: panoramic and specialty instruments.

PANORAMIC TELESCOPES

Modern panoramic telescopes are rigid instruments which consist of an optical (viewing) component and an illumination (lighting) mechanism (Fig 8–1). The resolution (small detail or point to point discrimination) of rigid instruments far exceeds that of fiberoptic, flexible instruments to such a degree that the latter will not be considered in the light of current technology to offer a reasonable alternative. The telescope can be subdivided into an eyepiece, a barrel, and a terminal lens (Fig 8–2). Most commonly the inner-barrel structures are encased in stainless steel. Within this steel cover are located groups of lenses or rods separated by air spaces. Surrounding the optical components are glass fiberoptic bundles that transmit cold light by way of a fiberoptic cable from a remote light generator. Generally speaking, the 4-mm outer diameter of the telescope is the narrowest diameter that can provide an optimally bright, clear, wide-angle view of an object together with a high-intensity light shower. Although telescopes of smaller diameters are marketed, they all suffer from shortcomings of low light capacities and/or suboptimal optics. Telescopes 2 to 3 mm in diameter will couple to small covering sheathes and permit easier entry into the cervical canal but clearly will suffer from the aforesaid deficiencies. Practically, therefore, a 4-mm telescope is the instrument of choice. The viewing angles most commonly available are either 0° (straight on) or 30° (offset) (Fig 8–3). Selection of these angles is pretty much a matter of personal preference. For the beginner, the 0° telescope is easier to use because orientation is similar to that of normal vision (Fig 8–4,A). The 30° telescope allows more rapid, dextrous evaluation of the anterior walls, posterior walls, and cornual recesses (Fig 8–4,B). Simply rotating the telescope slightly to the right or left permits the endoscopist to see the tubal ostia. In comparison, the same view with a 0° scope may only be possible by severely angulating the instrument to the left or right. One must remember that depth perception is limited substantially because the sighting is monocular

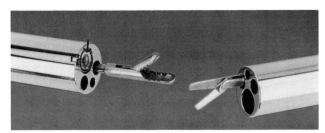

FIG 8–1.
Panoramic hysteroscope in the sheath. The *open arrow* points to the viewing component and the *solid arrow* to the illumination part of the telescope.

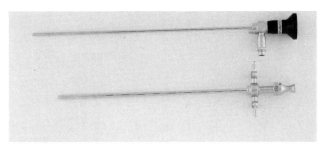

FIG 8–2.
Photograph showing the telescope (above) and diagnostic sheath. The most commonly used telescopes measure 4 mm outer diameter. The telescope consists of eyepiece, barrel, and objective (terminal) lens.

rather than binocular. Additionally, one should bear in mind, regardless of whether diagnostic or operative hysteroscopy is contemplated, that the telescope remains constant. This author prefers the 0° telescope for operative hysteroscopy, but again this is a matter of individual choice. Finally, these instruments are focused at infinity and therefore give an image that is smaller than actual size when positioned away from the object and, correspondingly, a magnified view when moved closer to the object. Therefore, it is impossible to determine accurate measurements without a frame of reference within the same viewing plane.

The quality of instruments may be judged by viewing a detailed object, for example, a piece of multicolored printing, and noting the brightness and clarity of the image viewed, the diameter of the field seen at various reference distances, and the intensity of illumination in a dark space, perhaps inside a double-thickness bag or opaque container.

Several varieties of focusing telescopes are available (Fig 8–5,A). These instruments differ from fixed-focus endoscopes in that they provide the ability to magnify the object by bringing the terminus of the telescope close to the object and/or even making light contact with the surface of the object. They function somewhat like a microscope and allow vision within the near range where a fixed-focus hysteroscope would prove unable

to provide a clear image. Therefore, these focusing instruments offer panoramic viewing as well as magnified close-up viewing (Fig 8–5,B). Generally, although the field is magnified (i.e., larger objects), these instruments suffer from a diminished peripheral field and less distant resolution than fixed-focus instruments. The focusing mechanism is usually located to one side of the telescopic eyepiece mounting within the housing where the barrel and eyepiece join (Fig 8–5,C). Focusing is accomplished by turning a small wheel. The gynecologist should be informed that a small movement of the wheel may take the instrument out of focus for panoramic hysteroscopy! Simply testing the focus may surprise the examiner who is fretting over why he or she can't see a clear image by suddenly bringing the field into excellent focus. The obvious advantage of these instruments is to provide precise viewing of mucosal patterns, vasculature, color, and to show detail of lesions within the cervical canal or uterine cavity. The microhysteroscopes allow switching to a lens system that magnifies up to ×150 when the endoscope is lightly in contact with the mucosa (i.e., producing an "in vivo" cytologic examination). This instrument operates similarly to an oil immersion lens of a microscope (Fig 8–6).

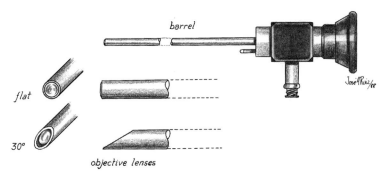

FIG 8–3.
The most common objectives are 0° (flat) and 30° (offset).

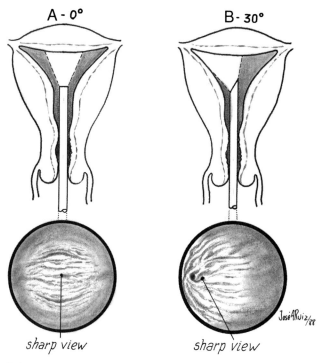

FIG 8–4.
Example of 0° view **(A)** and 30° view **(B).**

Sheaths

Before entering a body cavity such as the uterus, the telescope must be fitted to a sheath through which a distending medium can be infused into the uterine cavity, in order to provide necessary distention for panoramic viewing. To provide reasonable clearance for a 4-mm telescope, the smallest diagnostic sheath measures 5 mm in outer diameter (OD). Whether the sheath measures 300 mm in length or the 240 mm frequently used with microhysteroscopes, the diameter (5 mm) is the same, and the ease of entrance into the uterus is identical. The 5-mm diagnostic sheath is well suited for office hysteroscopy using gaseous distending media but makes instillation of liquid media difficult because of the small clearance space between the endoscope and the wall of the inner sheath (Fig 8–7). Entry into the interior cavity of the sheath is provided by a single stopcock with a luer-lock fitting. Although some diagnostic sheaths are equipped with two stopcocks, these offer no additional advantage and only add excess weight to the sheath.

Quality machining and construction should be evaluated. The terminus of the endoscope should fit flush with the end of the sheath. The stopcock should be constructed of heavy-duty stainless steel and should open and close smoothly (Figs 8–8,A and B). The ease or dif-

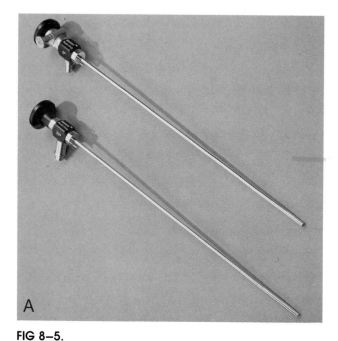

FIG 8–5.
A, focusing telescope combines panoramic and contact hysteroscopes into one instrument. The near point of the focusing telescope (top) is much closer to the object than the fixed focus instrument (bottom). **B** and **C,** detail of the focusing wheel of focusing telescope.

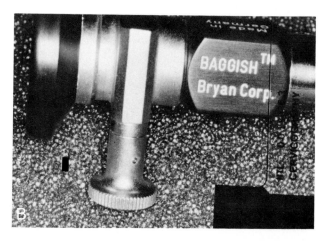

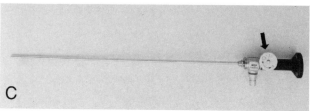

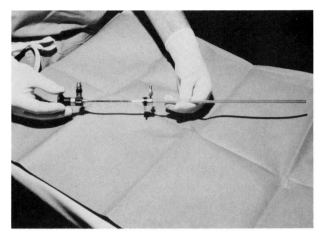

FIG 8-6.
Button *(arrow)* on microhysteroscope allows switching to a lens system that magnifies up to ×150.

ficulty of engaging and connecting the telescope to the sheath should be carefully evaluated. During an operative procedure, the hysteroscopist may wish to withdraw the telescope momentarily while leaving the sheath in situ. If the locking mechanism is difficult to open and close, the uterine cavity could be traumatized while the surgeon is fumbling to reassemble the sheath and telescope. The locking mechanism should also be checked under pressure injection of a liquid medium to determine whether leakage occurs at the telescope-sheath interface (Plate 36,A and B).

Operative sheaths come in several varieties depending on the manufacturer and range between 7 and 8 mm outer diameter. The most common design consists of a hollow tube, usually fitted with two stopcocks (right and left) for the instillation of the distending medium (Fig 8–9). An operating channel mounted on the posterior

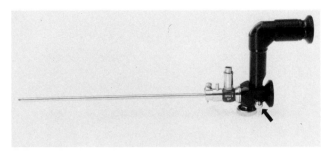

FIG 8-7.
Telescope inserted into a 5-mm diagnostic sheath.

surface and fitted with a stopcock feeds into the common channel. Opposite the operative channel is an interior groove where the telescope is seated. Since the distending medium is injected into a common channel (i.e., both instilling channels open into the same space), it is not feasible to flush the uterine cavity by injecting through one channel while leaving the opposite stopcock open. The operating channel must be fitted with a rubber nipple (gasket) to prevent the loss of medium and distention when operating instruments are introduced. One problem with this system is the tendency for the gaskets to slip off and/or leak when Hyskon is

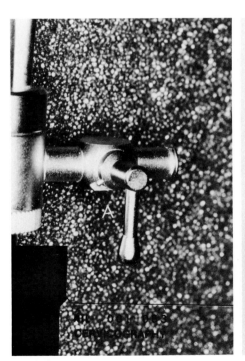

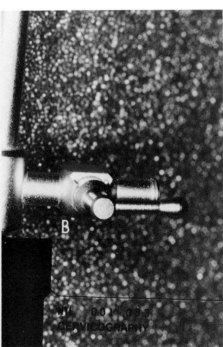

FIG 8-8.
Stopcock of diagnostic sheath in **(A)** closed position and **(B)** opened position.

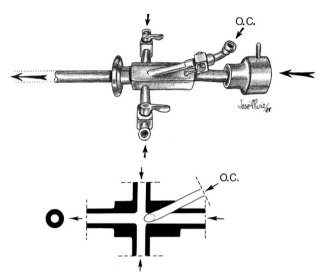

FIG 8–9.
An operating sheath with two stopcocks. The operating channel (O.C.) feeds into a common channel *(arrow)*. A rubber nipple prevents the loss of distending medium when an operating device is inserted.

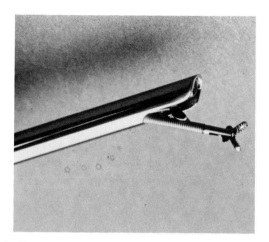

FIG 8–11.
Terminal deflector shown angulating flexible forceps.

the selected injection medium. A specialized sheath may be fitted with a terminal deflector that can be operated with two small wheels located just distal to the point where the sheath and telescope join (Fig 8–10). These special sheaths usually are constructed with an interposing bridge in order to allow selection with or without the deflector mechanism. The deflector may be utilized to angulate flexible instruments or fibers to one side by manipulating the wheel mechanism and has found greatest application for silicon plug–type hysteroscopic sterilization procedures (Fig 8–11).

One contemporary design in an operating sheath provides isolated channels for the telescope and medium installation, and incorporates two operating channels. With this system the uterine cavity can be flushed clear of debris. Additionally, the surgeon may operate and aspirate independently or simultaneously (Fig 8–12). New types of operating gaskets that are leakproof and lock onto the Luer-lock fittings of the operating channels provide substantial advantages compared with

the overfit types of nipples (Plate 37). Dual channel operating sheaths are clearly advantageous for control and clarity, especially during laser hysteroscopy employing a 300 to 600 μm quartz fiber to transmit the laser light to the target.

Light Sources

The quality and quantity of light delivered to the telescope depend equally on the type of the light generator and the transmitting fiberoptic cable. The sim-

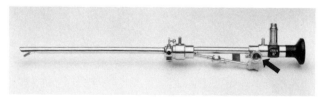

FIG 8–10.
Special operating sheath equipped with a terminal deflector (bridge), which is controlled by a wheel mechanism *(arrow)*.

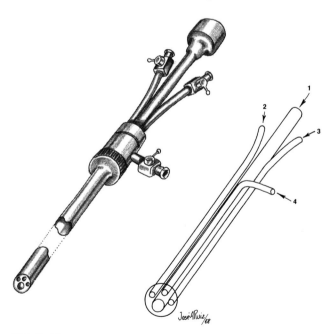

FIG 8–12.
Dual operating channel sheath permits aspiration and operating at the same time. The sheath consists of four isolated channels: *(1)* telescope, *(2)* operating, *(3)* operating, *(4)* medium instillation.

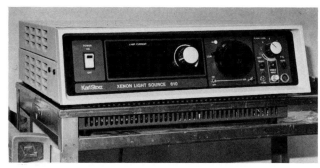

FIG 8–13.
Xenon light generator provides ample power for viewing as well as both still or television photography.

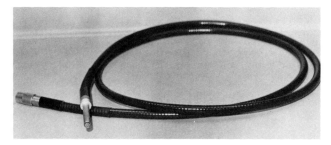

FIG 8–14.
The fiberoptic cable must be handled carefully since transmission of light from the generator to the telescope is as important as the light source itself.

plest light generator provides only 150 W of power, which suffices for direct view hysteroscopy when photography is not desired. These light sources may be purchased at a modest cost, and because of their compact design are ideal for office hysteroscopy. Very elaborate light sources are available which produce very high intensity light. The xenon generator provides 300 W of intense power with a current meter readout from 7 to 21 amp and is recommended for indirect video-control hysteroscopy as well as for photography (Fig 8–13). The variable illumination settings and special filters provide tailor-made light for a variety of situations. The metal-halide light sources produce a bluish coloration to the delivered light. Most of the less expensive tungsten type sources dominate in the orange-red wave lengths. Regardless of the type of light generated, whatever reaches the telescope depends on the quality and maintenance of the fiberoptic light cable. Generally, the liquid cables transmit the most effectively. These must be heavily clad to protect against explosion and rupture and are therefore less flexible than glass fiber cables. The surgeon should regularly check fiberoptic cables in a dark room to look for broken fibers, which are detected by noting illuminated spots along the cladding (Fig 8–14).

Sterilization

Most of the hysteroscopes described in this section may be sterilized by a variety of techniques. Unless one is endowed with several telescopes, gas sterilization with ethylene oxide is impractical. Liquid disinfection by soaking is the most frequently used method to "sterilize" these instruments. If the lens system is sealed, the entire telescope may be submerged for 20 minutes in Cidex (glutaraldehyde), then the instrument is thoroughly rinsed in sterile water. The sheaths can be steam autoclaved without damaging them or, alternatively, can be soaked in Cidex. The contact hysteroscope may be

totally covered with Cidex without risk of damage. The Hamou microhysteroscope cannot be submerged. Therefore, only the barrel (the portion entering the patient) is sterilized. Although several manufacturers purport that steam autoclaving is safe for their equipment, repeated exposure to the high heat damages the glue holding the lenses in place and can result in infiltration of water into the interior of the endoscope.

SPECIALTY INSTRUMENTS

Contact Hysteroscope

The contact hysteroscope differs in construction from the instruments previously described. First, this instrument does not require any distending medium; second, the hysteroscope is applicable for diagnostic purposes only and does not require a sheath; third, no fiberoptic illumination system is needed, since the instrument traps and collects directed as well as ambient light.

The contact hysteroscope is composed of three major parts. A solid core of optical mineral glass serves as both a light and optical guide that carries the image of an object to the examiner's eye. The glass core is supported and surrounded by an interior mirrored and exterior steel sheath (Fig 8–15). The outer diameter of the most popular model is 6 mm, and the core measures 350 mm in length (with magnifier). The second component is a cylindrical light trap onto which an external light source (e.g., the examination room light) is directed. A magnifying eye piece with focusing mechanism enlarges the image threefold. This endoscope provides discrimination to 20 μm. It is a portable instrument with a simple but ingenious optical system and is ideal for office and outpatient hysteroscopy. A special variant of this hysteroscope may be used for chronic biopsy. The latter endoscope is only 4 mm OD (a very small viewing field) and is fitted with a channel to transport a suction

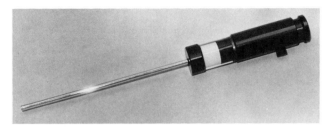

FIG 8–15.
The contact hysteroscope traps ambient light and conducts the light through a solid core of optical mineral glass.

cannula for chorion villus aspiration. Since the contact hysteroscope has a known diameter which is viewed as a ring, objects may be accurately sized.

The Autonomous Hysteroscope

A unique self-contained panoramic hysteroscopic system has been developed in Europe by Richard Wolf (Fig 8–16). The 4-mm foreoblique telescope and sheath are fit into a special cannula and mounting device. The handle of the autonomous system contains three cadmium-nickel rechargeable batteries and a short fiberoptic connecting cable. A second handle contains a CO_2 cartridge and delivery system. The end of the cannula is fitted with a cervical adapter to ensure a tight connection. The major disadvantages to the system are its weight and the fact that the instrument is useful for diagnostic purposes only. The obvious advantage is the portability and convenience of having the hysteroscope, light source, and distention system packaged in one compact bundle.

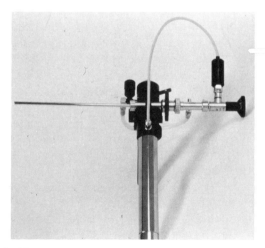

FIG 8–16.
Self-contained hysteroscope is powered by rechargeable batteries, and contains a CO_2 cartridge, a telescope, and sheath.

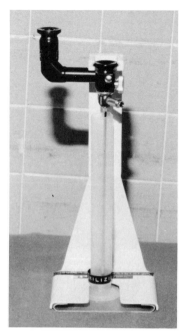

FIG 8–17.
Hamou microhysteroscope is soaked in a special container to prevent leakage into the lens system.

The Microhysteroscope

The microhysteroscope combines a 4×300 mm telescope, by the push of a button, with a $\times 80$ to $\times 150$ contact microscope (Fig 8–17). The instrument has an angulated distal end and foreoblique vision (30°). The diagnostic sheath measures 5.2 mm. Although an operating sheath is available, this system is rather clumsy for operative hysteroscopy. The unique feature of this endoscope lies in the ability for the gynecologist to perform microcolpohysteroscopy (i.e., examining in vivo the stained cells of the ectocervix and endocervix).

EQUIPMENT SELECTION

Panoramic hysteroscopy with standard instrumentation (i.e., nonspecialty endoscopes) is recommended for initiating a hysteroscopy program, whether for office, surgicenter, or operating room use. This choice offers the practitioner the greatest flexibility for use with any medium as well as a foundation for building a larger, more complex system. A 4-mm, fixed-focus telescope of standard length, 5-mm diagnostic sheath, and 150 W or more powerful light source will allow the new hysteroscopist to initiate diagnostic hysteroscopy with the least amount of money. When greater experience is gained, a focusing hysteroscope would be the next logical acquisition. Specialty endoscopes and operating hysteroscopes will subsequently be acquired for the performance of intrauterine surgery and will easily meld with the recommended first purchases.

BIBLIOGRAPHY

Baggish MS: Contact hysteroscopy: A new technique to explore the uterine cavity. *Obstet Gynecol* 1979; 54:350.

Baggish MS: New techniques for laser ablation of the endometrium in high risk patients. *Am J Obstet Gynecol* (in press).

Baggish MS: A new laser hysteroscope for nd-YAG endometrial ablation. *Lasers Surg Med* 1988; 8:248.

Edstrom K, Fernstrom I: The diagnostic possibilities of a modified hysteroscopic technique. *Acta Obstet Gynecol Scand* 1970; 49:327.

Gauss GJ: Hysteroskopie. *Arch Gynaek* 1928; 133:18.

Gribb JJ: Hysteroscopy an aid in gynecologic diagnosis. *Obstet Gynecol* 1960; 15:593.

Hamou, J: Microhysteroscopy. *Acta Endocrinol* 1980; 10:415.

Lindemann JH: The use of CO_2 in the uterine cavity for hysteroscopy. *Int J Fertil* 1972; 17(4):221.

Lindemann JH, Mohr J: CO_2 hysteroscopy, diagnosis and treatment. *Am J Obstet Gynecol* 1976; 124:129.

Lindemann JH: Pneumotra fur die hysteroskopie. *Geburtshilfe Frauenheilkd* 1973; 33:18.

Marleschki V: Hysterskopische feststellungen der spontanen perfusionsschwankungen am menschlichen endometrium. *Zbl Gynaek* 1968; 90:1094.

Norment WB: Hysteroscope in diagnosis of pathological conditions of uterine canal. *JAMA* 1952; 148:917.

Norment WB: The hysteroscope. *Am J Obstet Gynecol* 1956; 71:426.

Parent B, Toubas C, Doerler B: L'hysteroscopie de contact. *J Gynecol Obstet Biol Reprod* 1974; 3:511.

Porto R, Gaujoux J: Une nouvelle methode d'hysteroscopie instrumentation et technique. *J Gynecol Obstet Biol Reprod* 1972; 7:691.

Rubin IC: Uterine endoscopy, endometroscopy with the aid of uterine insufflation. *Am J Obstet Gynecol* 1925; 10:313.

Silander T: Hysteroscopy through a transparent rubber balloon. *Surg Gynecol Obstet* 1962; 114:125.

Wulfsohn NL: A hysteroscope. *J Obstet Gynecol Brit Emp* 1958; 65:657.

9

Accessory Instruments for Operative Hysteroscopy

Michael S. Baggish, M.D.

Rafael F. Valle, M.D.

A variety of instruments for hysteroscopic surgery have been designed in flexible, rigid, and semirigid forms. The flexible and semirigid instruments are of a 7 F caliber and can be slid through the hysteroscopic channel for intrauterine surgery. These include grasping forceps, biopsy forceps, scissors, and electrodes (Fig 9–1). The rigid or fixed instruments cannot be slid into the hysteroscopic channel but must be attached to the sheath itself; therefore, the attached telescope and sheath must negotiate the cervical canal as a unit.

Most manufacturing companies offer three different types of instruments, but the semirigid instruments are manufactured only by Storz Company, Richard Wolf Company, and Bryan Company. Generally speaking the flexible instruments are for light-duty procedures, since they are rather fragile (Fig 9–2,A). They do have the advantage of being positioned at varying angles by means of the deflecting sheath (Fig 9–2,B). Practically speaking, the need for this type of maneuver is infrequent. The semirigid instruments are preferred by most experienced hysteroscopists. These instruments are small enough to fit through standard operating channels (Figs 9–3,A and B). They may be manipulated for close-up work near the terminus of the telescope or slid out away from the telescope to permit panoramic surgery. Essentially the location of the operating instrument is relatively independent of the optical portion of the hysteroscopic system (Fig 9–4). Additionally, the semirigid instruments are manufactured to serve as heavier duty

equipment compared with the flexible instruments. For example, the semirigid scissors are reasonably well suited for cutting septa, synechia, and myomata, whereas flexible instruments are practical only for thin septa and fine adhesions. Although free intrauterine devices may be removed by either flexible or semirigid forceps, the former are totally unsuited for imbedded devices. Neither flexible nor semirigid biopsy instruments supply a very good specimen for the pathologist to evaluate. The jaws of these instruments are simply too small to obtain an adequate specimen for interpretation. When Hyskon is used as the distending medium, all accessory instruments must be immediately and thoroughly washed with hot water. If the Hyskon dries on the jaws of these accessories and an attempt is made to force them open by working the handles, it is likely that the instruments will break. These instruments may be steam autoclaved.

The rigid instruments are heavier and larger than either flexible or semirigid instruments (Fig 9–5,A and B). The size of these instruments necessitates that they be permanently incorporated into the construction of the specialized sheath. The telescope in effect looks through the interior of the rigid operating sheath (Fig 9–6). Thus the optical system provides a limited field of view and is permanently tied to the operating instrumentation at a fixed, unalterable distance (Plate 38). In fact, this distance is very close to the end of the telescope and produces a magnified close-up view with a small field. The size of these instruments permits cutting

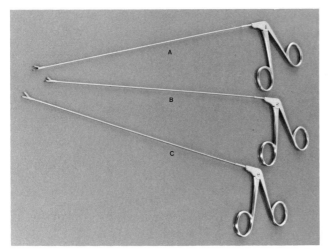

FIG 9–1.
Three types of semi rigid instruments which may be inserted through the operating channel of an 8 mm sheath: **(A)** grasping forceps, **(B)** biopsy forceps, **(C)** scissors.

large lesions and clearly allows great traction to be applied to imbedded intrauterine contraceptive devices. As noted, they must be slid through the cervix as an operating system, with the instruments protruding beyond the sheath. This makes for a more traumatic and difficult entry into the uterine cavity. Additionally, the cervical canal is not viewed during entry. These instruments can also be steam autoclaved.

ASPIRATION DEVICES

Plastic tubing is necessary to flush the uterine cavity to remove blood clots, mucus, and debris, and/or wash the fluid when it has become mixed with blood. These

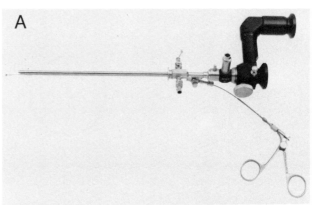

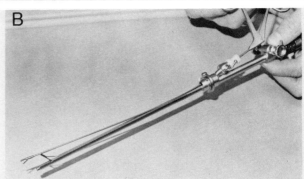

FIG 9–2.
A, flexible instruments, e.g., the grasping forceps pictured here, are of narrow caliber and tend to be fragile. **B,** deflector bridge with scissors.

catheters must be large enough to allow for this flushing effect and not become plugged with blood clots. The internal diameter of these catheters is 1.6 to 1.7 mm; the outer diameter, 2.0 to 2.4 mm (Fig 9–7,A). Several types of plastic tubing have been roughly adapted for use as aspiration cannulae but usually suffer from being too short and not having the proper fittings for syringes to

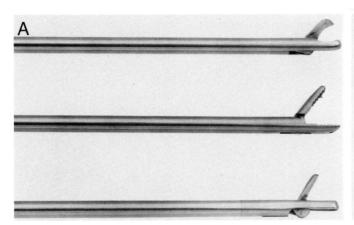

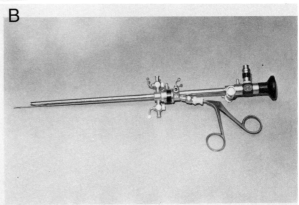

FIG 9–3.
A, semirigid instruments are stronger than their flexible counterparts. **B,** the instruments may be adjusted to any working distance from a position relative to the telescope.

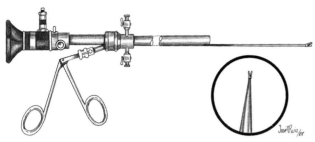

FIG 9–4.
View through telescope using semirigid scissors.

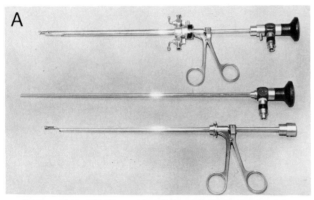

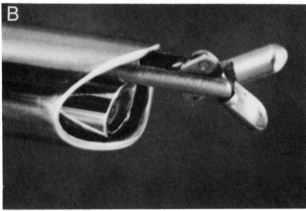

FIG 9–5.
A, the rigid operating instruments are constructed in two components: an operating sheath through which a telescope is inserted, and the operative tool, which forms a portion of the sheath. **B,** the rigid forceps is fixed and protrudes slightly beyond the specialized sheath.

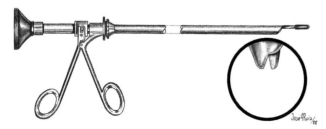

FIG 9–6.
View through rigid scissor sheath.

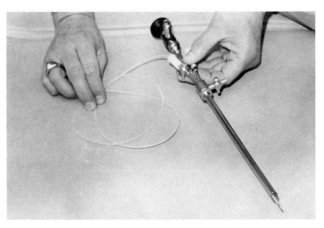

FIG 9–7.
A (above), aspiration cannula engaged into one channel of dual channel operating sheath. **B** (see Plate 39), terminus of aspirating cannula. Bands at the end of the cannula are 1 mm apart and may also serve as a measuring device.

be attached. Recently the Cook Corporation has distributed specially designed cannulae for hysteroscopic aspiration. These are banded with terminal 1-mm-spaced markings for purposes of measurement and, additionally, have terminal and side aspiration ports (Plate 39). These are available in lengths ranging from 35 cm to 100 cm and are constructed with Luer-lock type fittings for easy leak-proof syringe attachment. These aspiration cannulae are invaluable for suctioning debris out of the uterine cavity. Liquid media may be injected through the cannulae in order to flush the uterine cavity. Since they may be moved back and forth, they are independent of the optical system. Most experienced hysteroscopists utilize aspiration cannulae freely and frequently. To attempt operative hysteroscopy maneuvers with less than optimal vision is fraught with unnecessary hazards. Simply aspirating debris transforms a cloudy field to one

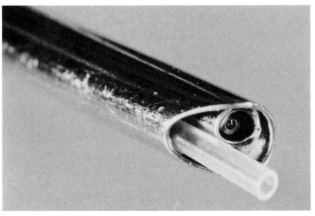

FIG 9–8.
Detail of aspirating cannula exiting through the operative sheath. The telescope is above and to the left.

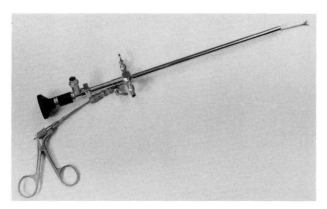

FIG 9–9.
Most operating sheaths are equipped with a single access channel.

that is sharply clear and is well worth the modicum of time expended (Fig 9–8).

OPERATING PLUGS

Most operating sheaths are equipped with a single access channel (Fig 9–9). The Baggish hysteroscopic system provides dual operating channels side by side; Storz provides a dual channel system with an over-and-under design (Fig 9–10; Plate 40). The operating channel(s) is equipped with a stopcock which can be switched to an open or closed position in order to prevent leakage of the distending medium. When a flexible instrument, semirigid instrument, laser fiber, or aspiration cannula is engaged into the channel, a gasket or nipple must be applied to the fitting of the channel to suppress leakage. Until recently, adaptations of urologic rubber nipples have been utilized (Plate 41,A). Some of these nipples have oversized openings, which results in leakage of media when narrow-gauge instruments are inserted.

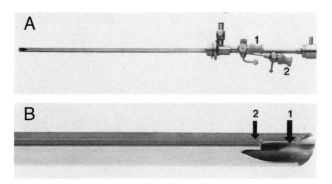

FIG 9–10.
A, Storz over and under dual channel operating sheath. **B,** detail of terminus of operating sheath shown in **A. C** (see Plate 40), Baggish dual operating sheath.

Those nipples with pinpoint openings are best suited for operative hysteroscopy (Plate 41,B). Another problem with these urology nipples is their tendency to slip off the channel when Hyskon is used as the distending medium, particularly when lateral traction is placed on the operating instrument or aspiration cannula. Recently, Baggish has developed a new operating gasket that attaches to the sheath channel by means of a Luer-lock connection (Plate 42,A and B). This plug precludes slippage. Additionally, the fine-leaf construction of the gasket provides very close clearance for the narrow-gauge laser fibers and thereby reduces leakage of media with even extreme side-traction.

EXTENSION CANNULAE

Hyskon can be injected into the operating sheath by attaching a 30- or 50-cc syringe directly to the Luer-lock fitting of the medium instillation port of the hysteroscopic sheath (Fig 9–11). This method has several drawbacks. First, the angle for injection is awkward and does not allow adequate pressure to be applied, especially when the diagnostic sheath is used. Second, attachment and detachment of syringes are awkward. Third, not infrequently the syringe angulates to the side and becomes detached; the operator is then sprayed with Hyskon. It is more advantageous and convenient to inject Hyskon by the incorporation of an intermediary, large-diameter connecting tube (Fig 9–12). This should be approximately 12 cm in length, with a 4-mm outer diameter. This tube must be constructed with Luer-lock fittings to couple securely to the hysteroscope sheath and to allow very secure attachment of the 50-cc injection syringe.

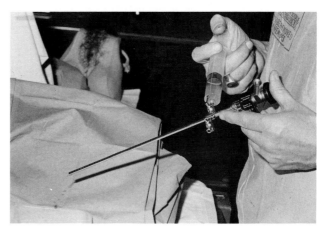

FIG 9–11.
A syringe is attached directly to inflow port of the hysteroscope. This is unwieldy and may result in difficulty injecting Hyskon.

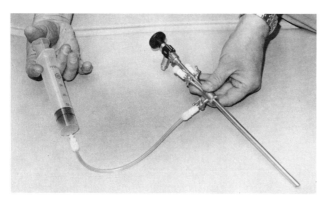

FIG 9–12.
Large-bore connecting tube is interposed between 50-ml syringe and intake port of the hysteroscope. The person injecting Hyskon can now be relatively remote in relation to the immediate operating field.

RESECTOSCOPES

The urologic resectoscope can be adapted to hysteroscopy for the resection of intrauterine lesions and/or ablation of the endometrium by modifying the urologic instrument and techniques to better fit the anatomy and size of the uterine cavity. These resectoscopes are available from Storz and Richard Wolf companies (Fig 9–13,A and B).

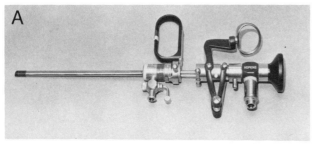

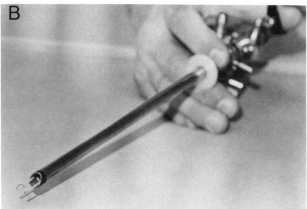

FIG 9–13.
A, the cystoscopic-resectoscope is identical to the instrument used for prostatectomy. **B,** a fine loop activated by electric current serves as a cutting/shaving tool.

STILL PHOTOGRAPHY EQUIPMENT

Because hysteroscopy relies on visualization of the different aspects of the uterus, documentation by photography is important, particularly for record keeping and reevaluation of planned surgery and follow-up. Many small cameras are available for this purpose. We have utilized successfully the Olympus-OM2 camera because of its light weight and capability of electronically controlling the light required, without additional flash generators (Plate 43). Other cameras may require strobes or electronic flash generators, which indeed provide the best pictures in hysteroscopy. Such units are available from Richard Wolf, Storz, Olympus, and other companies (Fig 9–14). An easy way to obtain pictures immediately for documentation and charting is by using Polaroid systems, with special films and camera attachments.

VIDEO CAMERAS

Any endoscopic examination is essentially a dynamic process, and one of the best ways to document the technique for teaching, instruction, and review is by utilizing video cameras. This is particularly helpful when other ancillary persons are present, such as students, nurses, or a patient who wishes to view her own examination. To obtain this documentation, it is important to have a light camera of small size in order to perform the examination with minimal impedance. In general, two types of video cameras are available on the market: the chip mode and the tube camera. Both are small, lightweight, and can be used for documentation interchangeably. Many of these cameras have been manufactured to be disinfected by soaking, should this be required (Fig 9–15). In order to obtain excellent pictures with these cameras, a potent light is required (i.e., a 300 W metal halide or the more powerful xenon lamp).

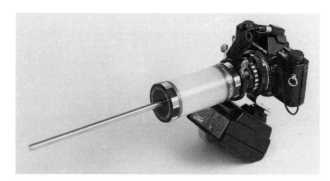

FIG 9–14.
Olympus camera adapted with bayonet mount and special flash bracket for the contact hysteroscope.

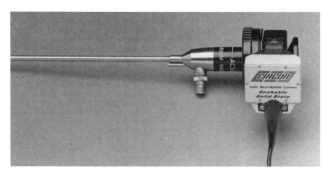

FIG 9–15.
New model endoscopic video camera with beam splitter attached to the endoscope's eyepiece.

These light sources provide appropriate, intensive light. Other cine fountains are available from most manufacturers.

The best resolution and widest field video pictures are obtained with microchip cameras attached directly to the eyepiece of the hysteroscope (Fig 9–16). Under the circumstance described, the hysteroscopist must see and operate by viewing the video monitor screen in a manner analogous to that used by orthopedic surgeons performing arthroscopy (Plate 44). This technique obviously requires practice and great skill, since the field is viewed in two dimensions only. A great advantage to working directly from the video monitor screen is that this technique allows the endoscopist to sit upright rather than hunched over thereby reducing operator fatigue. By using video camera adapters with lenses of different focal lengths, one may obtain a variety of views and visual fields.

CINEMATOGRAPHY EQUIPMENT

For specific documentation and production of movies, a special endoscopic camera is required. Of these, the most commonly known and used is the Beaulieu camera (Fig 9–17).

LASERS

Specific lasers have proved to be especially useful for intrauterine surgery. The criteria for a laser in this location include the following: the beam must be conducted and delivered to the operative site by a flexible, fine quartz fiber; the laser must produce relatively high power (e.g., 40 to 100 W); and the characteristics of the light must penetrate liquid media efficiently. Clearly, the best laser for use in hysteroscopy to date is the Nd-YAG

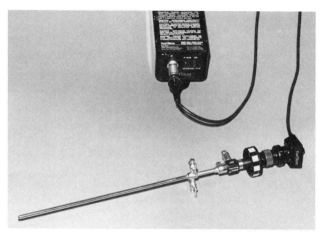

FIG 9–16.
Microchip endoscope television camera provides high-resolution video pictures during hysteroscopy.

laser (Fig 9–18). This laser is particularly useful because it has the properties of front scatter and excellent coagulation capabilities. The fact that this wave length, 1,064 nm, is effectively transmitted by 300 to 600 μm quartz fibers is highly advantageous since the fiber easily passes through the operating sheath of standard hysteroscopic systems. Carbon dioxide lasers are unsuited for hysteroscopic surgery. Both argon and KTP 532 lasers may be useful for hysteroscopic surgery, but suffer from insufficient power.

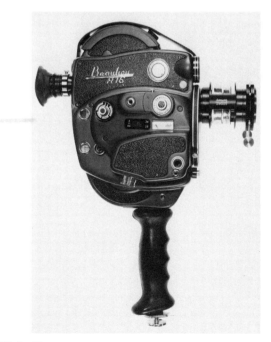

FIG 9–17.
High-quality films are obtained with the endoscopically adapted movie camera.

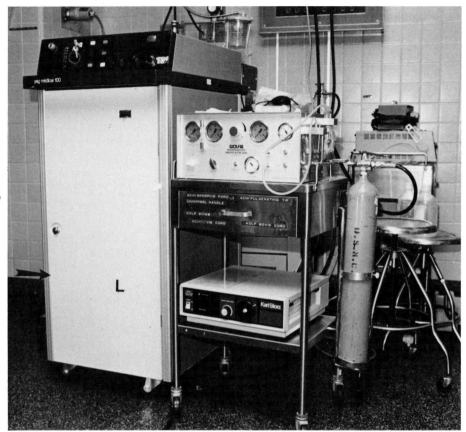

FIG 9–18.
The laser most often utilized *(L)* is the Nd-YAG laser. This laser provides high power, penetrates liquid media, and is delivered to the operative site by fine quartz fibers.

The laser is an ideal operating accessory since it can deliver ablative power to the surgical site without the necessity of touching the tissue and also allows surgery to be performed with the added bonus of simultaneous hemostasis (Plate 45,A and B). Further, the laser, unlike the cautery, is not conducted through the tissues or fluid and surpasses electrocoagulation in its ability to enable precision operations.

A new development in the use of the Nd-YAG laser is the sapphire tip (Plate 46). This tip attaches to the end of the quartz fiber and allows the laser beam to be focused to a fine point over a very short focal distance. This in turn permits very high power densities to accrue at the target.

BALLOONS

Not infrequently, sustained bleeding ensues following operative hysteroscopy, especially when the pressure of the distending medium on the uterine walls has been relieved. Under these circumstances insertion of a balloon into the uterine cavity is the most practical method for controlling the uterine hemorrhage. In the past these balloons were jury-rigged 10- to 30-cc Foley catheters. These catheters were inserted into the uterus, then the catheter balloons were inflated with sterile water or saline. The pressure of the balloon on the uterine wall allowed clotting to occur, and the bleeding stopped. The catheter should be left inflated for an hour or two, then partially deflated while observing for bleeding. We have in fact left such devices in place for up to 48 hours.

Recently, the Mentor Company (Goleta, Calif.) has marketed specifically designed intrauterine balloons (Plate 47). Three sizes are available: 150 cc, 500 to 1,000 cc, and 1,000 to 4,000 cc. The 150-cc size is appropriate for use after hysteroscopy. The balloon can be filled with 6 to 150 cc of water or saline, and a manometer may be attached to measure the actual intrauterine pressure. The advantage of these balloons is that they conform to the shape of the uterine cavity and exert uniform pressure on the uterine walls. Obviously, as the intraluminal pressure increases, the veins will be closed first; then, as pressure approaches 90 to 100 mm Hg, the arteries within the endometrium and superficial myometrium will be compressed (Fig 9–19).

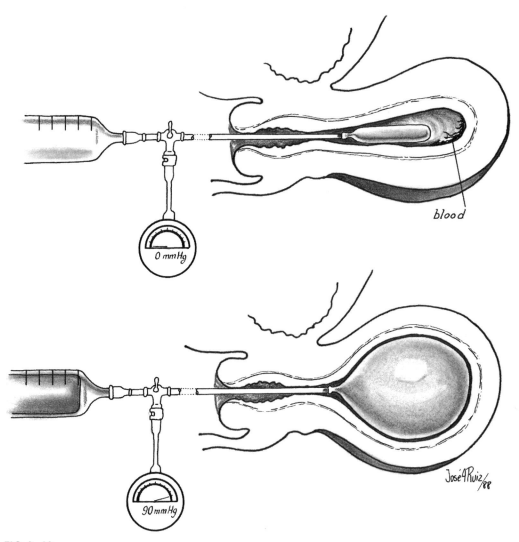

FIG 9–19.
Schematic diagram of balloon inserted in the uterine cavity and exerting hemostatic pressure on the uterine walls.

BIBLIOGRAPHY

Amin RF: Hysteroscopy for gynecologic diagnosis. *Clin Obstet Gynecol* 1983; 26:253.

Baggish MS: A new laser hysteroscope for Nd-YAG endometrial ablation. *Lasers Surg Med* (in press).

DeCherney A, Polan ML: Hysteroscopic management of intrauterine lesions and intractable uterine bleeding. *Obstet Gynecol* 1983; 61:392.

Deutschmann C, Lueken RP: Hysteroscope findings in postmenopausal bleeding, in Siegler AM, Lindemann HJ (eds): *Hysteroscopy Principles and Practice.* Philadelphia, Lippincott, 1984, p 132.

Edstrom KGB: Intrauterine surgical procedures during hysteroscopy. *Encoscopy* 1974; 6:175.

Gallinat A: Hysteroscopy as a diagnostic and therapeutic procedure in sterility, in Siegler AM, and Lindemann HJ (eds): *Hysteroscopy Principles and Practice.* Philadelphia, Lippincott, 1984, p 180.

March CM, Israel R: Hysteroscopic management of recurrent abortion caused by septate uterus. *Am J Obstet Gynecol* 1987; 156:834.

Neuwirth RS: Hysteroscopic management of symptomatic submucous fibroids. *Obstet Gynecol* 1983; 62:509.

Neuwirth RS: A new way to manage submucous fibroids. *Contemp Obstet Gynecol* 1978; 12:101.

Parent B, Guedi H, Barbot J, et al: Hysteroscopie panoramique. Paris, Maloine, 1985.

Siegler AM, Kemmann E: Hysteroscopy. *Obstet Gynecol Surv* 1975; 30:567.

Valle RF: Hysteroscopy for gynecologic diagnosis. *Clin Obstet Gynecol* 1983; 26:253.

10

Care and Maintenance of Hysteroscopes and Nursing Procedures

Janice Luke, R.N., B.S.N.

Doris Laurey, R.N.

Beverly Mayette, R.N.

The prime purpose for the proper handling and care of hysteroscopic instruments is to keep the equipment in top working order and to protect patients from cross contamination. Poorly cared for instruments will make the procedure more difficult if not impossible to perform.

Some cardinal rules for reasonable maintenance are:

1. Always handle telescopes at the eyepiece end and not by the shaft or objective end because the instrument can be bent, fractured, or easily dropped (Fig 10–1).

2. Never force a frozen stopcock or working part, since it can be easily broken off.

3. Never place heavy instruments on top of delicate endoscopes because the latter may become distorted and subsequently fit improperly into the sheath.

4. If a piece of equipment is inadvertently dropped, inspect it immediately for damage by looking through the eyepiece at an object and by attaching the fiberoptic cable to illuminate the telescope.

PREOPERATIVE PREPARATION OF EQUIPMENT

When setting up the table for a hysteroscopic procedure, all heavy instruments should be placed to one side of the table and the sheaths on the other side (Fig 10–2). Delicate equipment that has a tendency to roll about, for example, the telescopes, should be placed near the center of the table so that they will not fall off the table when it is moved into position for use at the surgical field (Table 10–1). All working parts such as stopcocks, working elements of the catheterizing bridge, forceps, or scissors should be checked to be sure they are functioning properly (Table 10–2). Hyskon is a favorite medium for viewing during panoramic, operative hysteroscopy and is very difficult to remove during cleaning. The slightest residue left on the scopes will result in the working parts and stopcocks becoming frozen. If this happens, flash autoclaving all metal pieces for 3 minutes or soaking nonmetal pieces in boiling water will liquefy the Hyskon and allow the working pieces to move freely.

INTRAOPERATIVE MANAGEMENT

During use, some hysteroscope pieces will be used for a short period of time and then exchanged for others. The scrub nurse should be supplied with a basin of very hot sterile water and syringes so that thorough rinsing can take place immediately to help prevent the Hyskon from setting. This will make the cleaning process at the end of the procedure easier.

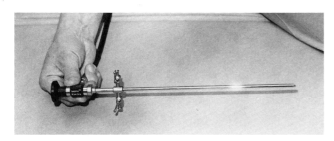

FIG 10–1.
Telescopes should be securely handled by the eyepiece end.

POSTOPERATIVE CARE

When the operative procedure is finished, the equipment should be rinsed immediately in hot water. All equipment including telescopes should then be washed in hot, soapy water, and all stopcocks should be taken apart and thoroughly cleaned.

The following cleaning supplies are needed:

- Water pistol.
- Long pipe cleaners.
- 4 × 4 sponges.

- Duraglit silver polish wadding (Reckitt Household Products).
- Blitz (3-M Company) surgical instrument cleaner and lubricant.
- Cotton-tipped swabs (such as Q-tips).
- Bioclean (Stanbio Laboratories), a phosphate-free biodegradable cleaner.

A water pistol is a wonderful tool to use when cleaning hysteroscopic equipment. It can be easily attached to a sink faucet by hospital plumbers and can save much time in the cleaning process. The pistol has tips of various sizes. There is one that will fit every sized hole in the sheath. The pistol is better than simple running water from the faucet because more pressure can be generated by the pistol, resulting in more adequate cleaning. Each individual piece of the apparatus is then dried and lubricated separately.

Telescopes

The telescope can be damaged very easily by improper handling. As previously mentioned, it should always be held by the eyepiece. It should be cleaned with

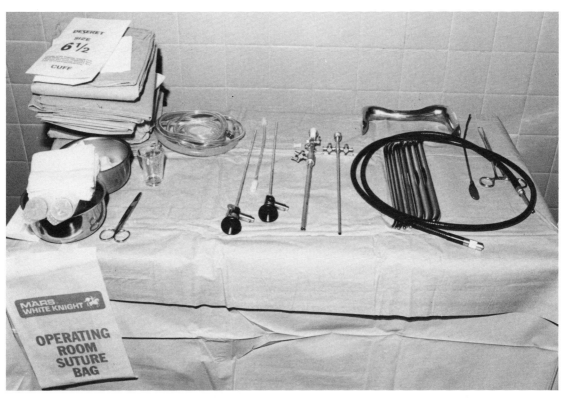

FIG 10–2.
Setup table for hysteroscopy. The heavier instruments are placed on either end of the table. The fragile equipment (e.g., telescopes) is placed in the center.

TABLE 10–1.

Contents of Hysteroscope Tray

Standard items
   1 Double-ended Sims speculum
   1 Uterine sound
   1 Single-toothed straight tenaculum
   1 Solution bowl
   4 50-cc syringes
   1 Set Pratt dilators
   1 Length of 1 in. silicone tubing fitted
     with one male connector and one
     female connector
   1 30° telescope
   1 0° telescope
   1 Sheath and obturator, diagnostic
   1 Sheath and obturator, operative
   1 Short bridge
   1 Catheterizing bridge
   1 Aspirating cannula
Other items that may be used
   Rigid or semirigid scissors
   Rigid or flexible biopsy forceps
   Rigid or flexible grasping forceps
   Fulgurating tip with high-frequency cord

either the water pistol or with a 4×4 sponge that has been soaked in water and Bioclean. It should be rinsed well with warm water and carefully dried. Careful attention must be directed to the optics. Cotton-tipped swabs or lens paper should be used to dry these delicate areas. If proper care is not taken, the objective lens may be scratched. After the telescope has been thoroughly cleaned and dried, it should be inspected. This can easily be done by looking through the eyepiece while holding it up to the light. By rotating the lens, small spots at the edges of the lens can be detected. This inspection will also uncover damage to the telescope itself. If small spots do appear, clean the lens again as previously described. Persistent spots after repeated cleaning can mean that the sealed ends are leaking and the instru-

TABLE 10–2.

Complete Setup for Hysteroscopy

The hysteroscopic tray
A small table
A light source
A drape pack, consisting of under-the-buttocks
   drape, leggings, and abdominal sheet
Hyskon or a CO_2 hysteroscopic insufflator with sterile
   tubing
Stirrups and straps with Clark sockets
4×8 radiopaque sponges, which should be counted
A prep set
A 16 F red rubber catheter
An unsterile prep pad

ment must be sent for repair. To remove "fogging" residue, a drop of 90% alcohol may be applied with a cotton-tipped swab. If this does not relieve the problem, the lens seal has probably been broken and fluid has leaked into the system, necessitating repair. A "half moon" appearance to the view usually means that there is a dent in the shaft of the telescope as a result of improper handling or dropping of the instrument.

Fiberoptic Cable

The light cable should be cleaned with Bioclean and water utilizing 4×4 sponges. It should be thoroughly rinsed. After drying, wadding silver polish can be applied to the ends of the cable to remove any debris. The polish is then removed with a dry 4×4 sponge, leaving a clean, shiny surface.

Inspection of the cable should then be done. As with the telescope, the overhead lights may be utilized. By holding one end of the cable to the light and directly viewing the other, broken fibers will be seen as numerous black dots. A new cable will have no black dots and will appear very shiny. Liquid cables are cleaned and inspected in a similar manner.

Stopcocks

Stopcocks should be completely disassembled after each use. The holes in the stopcocks must be cleaned particularly of Hyskon residue. The water pistol is invaluable here. The force of the water from the pistol can dislodge stubborn Hyskon residue. If a pistol is not available, a long pipe cleaner may be used to thoroughly clean and dry stopcock holes. After drying, Blitz spray can be used to remove any residue. After application, the excess should be removed with a dry 4×4 sponge. The stopcocks are then reassembled and tested for ease of movement. Mineral oil can serve as a substitute lubricant if the Blitz is not available; because the oil spreads easily, very little is needed (Fig 10–3).

Sheath and Obturator

Stopcocks on the sheath are cared for as previously discussed. The sheath itself is quite easily cleaned using the pistol or long pipe cleaners. The external surface is cleaned and dried using 4×4 sponges. After the thorough cleaning and drying, wadding silver polish is used to remove debris from the outside of the sheath. Frequent soaking in Cidex can result in discoloration of the sheath and obturator. The polish quickly eliminates this tarnish and restores the instrument to a "like-new" appearance. Removal of debris and soap residue also ren-

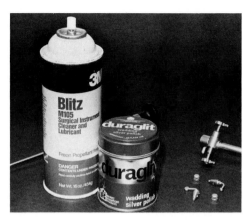

FIG 10–3.
Stopcocks, moving parts, and operative instruments are lubricated with Blitz. Telescopes, sheaths, and obturators are cleaned then polished with wadding silver polish.

ders the surface of the sheath smoother, making insertion during the procedure easier.

Catheterizing Bridge and Biopsy Forceps/Scissors

Both of these pieces of equipment have hinges and joints that cannot be taken apart; therefore, thorough cleaning, rinsing, and drying are necessary before lubricating. Again, the water pistol is invaluable, allowing water under pressure to remove any debris from the tiny hinges and the hollow interior. Long pipe cleaners can be used for both washing and drying when the water pistol is not available. Because the jaws of the biopsy forceps are required to exert force sufficient to enable an adequate biopsy specimen to be taken, Blitz lubrication of their working parts is necessary. Mineral oil is an inexpensive lubricating agent that can be applied with a medicine dropper or syringe to the deflecting mechanism of the bridge and the jaws of the biopsy forceps or scissors.

Fulgurating Tip and High-Frequency Cord

It is best not to immerse the fulgurating tip and HF cord when cleaning. The outside can simply be washed with Bioclean and water, then rinsed, with specific attention being given to the tip of the fulgurating electrode. A small toothbrush can be used to help remove any char that has adhered to the tip. If immersion is necessary, as with chemical disinfection, all connections must be thoroughly dried before being connected to the electrosurgical generator. Wet connections can cause arcing of current and damage to the equipment as well as injury to the surgeon or patient.

STERILIZATION

The three sterilization methods that will be discussed are steam sterilization, gas sterilization with ethylene oxide, and soaking with chemical disinfectants.

Steam Sterilization

All pure metal parts can be flash autoclaved at 270° for 3 minutes at a pressure of 30 lb/in.[2] Stopcock valves must be either in the open position or disassembled. Some manufacturers claim that their lenses can be steam autoclaved provided that certain conditions are met. They must be placed in a perforated metal container and wrapped loosely with open-weave gauze. Spontaneous cooling must take place to help prevent shrinking of the telescope's metal sheath, which could cause rupture of the seals between the sheath and the lens cover. This type of sterilization may therefore be impractical and possibly dangerous or damaging to the lens if all considerations are not met. For this reason, autoclaving is not recommended. Some manufacturers state that their fiberoptic cables can be flash autoclaved without damage to the cable as long as care is taken to keep the cable in large loops to prevent strain on the fiber bundles.

Gas or Ethylene Oxide Sterilization

Gas or ethylene oxide sterilization is the method of choice for all endoscopes (Fig 10–4). Trays are designed specifically for housing hysteroscope sets and can usually be purchased from vendors who manufacture endoscopes. The trays are perforated and contain padding

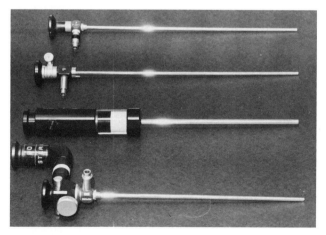

FIG 10–4.
All telescopes may be sterilized with ethylene oxide gas, depending on the construction material. They must be aerated from 4 to 30 hours.

for protection of the instruments. There are specific steps that must be followed prior to gas sterilization:

1. After use, instruments must be disassembled, thoroughly cleaned and rinsed, and each and every item thoroughly dried, to allow adequate penetration by the gas.

2. After reassembling equipment, all stopcocks must be left in the open position to allow the gas to flow through them.

3. After repackaging the hysteroscope set, it should be wrapped in paper or muslin.

Aeration is a critical issue. Metal pieces require no aeration time because the metal does not hold the ethylene oxide. However, material that is used to protect the individual pieces and the wrappings themselves will hold the gas. Therefore, a minimum of 4 hours is recommended to allow removal of the potentially harmful gas from these items. If the hysteroscope set contains rubber, the aeration time must be increased. The same is true for plastics, whether they be rubberized or constructed of polyvinyl chloride (PVC). Such materials tend to retain the ethylene oxide for a longer time period. Eight hours' aeration is recommended by the Occupational Safety and Health Administration for rubber or plastics (which do not contain PVC) that will not come into direct contact with the patient.

Non-PVC rubber or plastic items that will directly touch the patient, for example, the flexible cautery tip or the coating on the flexible forceps, should be aerated for 12 hours. Plastic items containing PVC must be aerated for 30 hours. If the nurse is unsure of equipment composition or aeration time, the manufacturer should be contacted. It may be advantageous to autoclave certain items separately when they are used infrequently. The aeration time of the more frequently used equipment can be decreased without these items.

This technique is also a satisfactory method for sterilization of fiberoptic cables.

Soaking or Chemical Disinfection

Cidex, a long-life activated aldehyde solution (Surgikos), is perhaps the most widely used chemical disinfectant. Cidex is generally used between patients, when gas sterilization is impractical. Before disinfection with Cidex, all equipment must have been thoroughly cleaned and rinsed. The instruments are then submerged in the solution, care being taken that all hollow parts are completely filled with the solution (a syringe filled with Cidex can be used to accomplish this). Obviously, all stopcocks must be in the open position or disassembled.

New fluid-filled light cables now on the market cannot be safely steam or gas autoclaved and must be chemically disinfected.

The minimum time for soaking instruments is 10 minutes. All organisms with the exception of spores will be destroyed. To eliminate spores, the instruments would have to be immersed for 10 hours. This would severely damage if not totally destroy most instruments. The 10-minute soak time should not be exceeded by more than 30 minutes, as Cidex is very corrosive to the seals between the lens covers and the metal sheaths.

When the soaking period has been completed, the instruments are thoroughly rinsed with distilled, sterile water to prevent any residue from coming into contact with either the patient or the eye of the surgeon, as Cidex is very irritating to tissues (Fig 10–5). Gloves should be worn by the nurse or technician charged with the soaking and rinsing procedure.

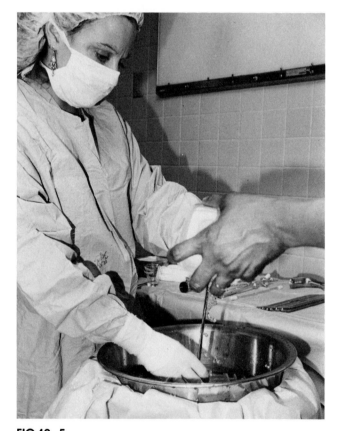

FIG 10–5.
Instruments disinfected with Cidex must be thoroughly rinsed in sterile water. One nurse is pouring sterile water while the other (sterile gloved) is holding the instrument.

Proper care, handling, and attention to detail when cleaning and sterilization hysteroscopes will add additional years to the lifetime of the equipment.

POSTSTERILIZATION CARE

After the hysteroscope and accessories have been wrapped in either muslin or paper, sterilized with ethylene oxide, and aerated for the appropriate time, storage now becomes the issue. One month is the recommended time limit for those items which are wrapped. If a longer shelf life is desired, overwrapping with a plastic dust cover will add another 5 months to the expiration date.

The instruments should be kept in storage either in a closed cupboard or in a cart that has doors or drawers. These measures will help to prevent accidental splashes of contaminants from contact with the wrapped set. If open storage is the only means available, all sets should have the additional protection of a plastic outerwrap.

INTEROPERATIVE NURSING CARE

Admission of the Patient to the Operating Room

The hospital or surgicenter operating room policy and procedure manual should contain authoritative statements that define necessary actions and detailed explanations for carrying out specified activities. The admission procedure should include the following:

- Proper identification of the patient.
- Surgical consent forms.
- Proper testing and completion of these tests.
- Reaffirmation of the completion of the appropriate items on the preoperation check list.
- Patient safety and comfort.

Proper identification of the patient should include checking her identification bracelet prior to bringing her into the operating room. Ask the patient her name and the name of her surgeon. Reconfirm the operative site whenever possible. Surgical consent forms should be checked for the patient's signature and that of the witness. The form should contain the name of the operation in a language that is easily understood. If the laser will be used, this should be stated on the permit. If any investigational lasers or fibers are anticipated, a special permit with detailed explanations should be signed. The consent signatures should be appropriately

dated. Each institution has different requirements for preoperative tests; the usual requirements are a complete blood count, urine analysis, and, depending on the age of the patient, an electrocardiogram and chest radiograph. These all should be available on the chart and should be reviewed by the anesthesiologist and surgeon.

Reaffirming the preoperative check list completed by the floor nursing staff will prevent oversights and omissions. Any allergies and reactions to blood transfusions or anesthetics should be noted.

The patient should never be left alone after admission to the operating room. Side rails and safety straps should be applied. The patient's privacy should be respected at all times. The demeanor of the operating room staff must be at all times reassuring, pleasant, and professional.

Nursing Interactions

Once the patient is admitted to the operating room suite, there are several nursing interactions with which the operating room nurse has to be concerned. These include:

- Moving the patient to the operating room (OR) table.
- Anesthesia (general versus regional, plus nursing responsibilities).
- Patient positioning (lithotomy; safety).
- Prepping the patient for a hysteroscopy.
- Draping the patient for a hysteroscopy.
- Reversing anesthesia.
- Transferring the patient from the OR table to the stretcher.
- Instrumentation (care and maintenance of the hysteroscopic equipment).

Transferring the patient to the OR table will require a nursing assessment to determine if any special equipment or additional personnel will be required. The patient should remain covered; efforts should be made to maintain her privacy and dignity. All team members should be ready for the transfer. The anesthesiologist should remain at the patient's head, making sure all lines and monitoring equipment are unencumbered. One team member should be on each side of the table. The patient is made as comfortable as possible. The OR nurse should not leave the patient unattended and should ensure that the safety strap is secured.

Anesthesia is selected based on the patient's age, medical history, physical status, patient preference, surgeon preference, anesthesiologist preference, and previous anesthesia experience of the patient. There are two basic types of anesthesia: general and regional. General anesthesia depresses the central nervous system and results in a loss of consciousness. Regional or local anesthesia blocks the conduction of pain impulses from a specific part of the body. Nursing responsibilities for either type of anesthesia are the same. The operating theater should be as ready as possible prior to the patient's admission in order that the circulating nurse can be available to assist the anesthesiologist. The room should also be kept as quiet as possible.

Nursing interventions should focus on providing emotional support to the patient, ensuring her safety, and assisting with the induction of general anesthesia or administering the regional or local block. These interventions would include calming the patient, explaining everything that is happening to her, limiting the amount of unnecessary exposure, and keeping the noise level to a minimum. Proper positioning during induction is important; therefore, the nurse will check the patient for correct body alignment, making sure the legs are not crossed and there are no pressure areas. Suction should be available, and the circulating nurse should be at the side of the patient. During the administration of a regional or local anesthetic block, the nurse should be available to set up the trays and medications. She may assist with positioning the patient for the block, while speaking to the patient in a calm, reassuring manner. After the patient has been anesthetized, the circulating nurse should assist with positioning the patient in a lithotomy position.

The lithotomy position is used to gain surgical access to the pelvic organs. The patient is supine with her legs elevated and abducted. Various stirrups are used, but principles of proper body alignment and protection are the same. The buttocks must be even with the lower break in the table. The stirrups must be level to prevent pressure at the knee and the lumbar spine. When raising the legs, two team members are needed to elevate the legs at the same time. They are raised and lowered evenly and slowly to prevent hip dislocation. Knee support stirrups should be well padded to prevent injury to the peroneal or saphenous nerve. The lower part of the leg should be free from pressure against the metal bars to prevent pressure on the common peroneal nerve. Pressure against the soft tissues of the leg may predispose the patient to venous thrombosis. The patient's arms should be secured on padded armboards or crossed loosely on her chest and secured with a sheet, making sure not to restrict respiration. When the arms are extended on the table the fingers will extend below

the foot extension and are in danger of injury when the foot extension is raised. When the procedure is completed the legs must be lowered by two team members slowly and simultaneously to prevent sudden hypotension and lumbosacral muscle strain.

Next, the preoperative preparation is done according to individual hospital policy, taking into consideration the allergies of the patient and whether or not the laser may be used. No alcohol or flammable prep solution should be used if the laser is being considered; this could cause serious burns to the patient and personnel in close proximity.

The patient is now draped with leggings and a fenestrated drape to expose the perineum. A sheet is placed across the abdomen. If the Nd-YAG laser may be used, four wet towels should outline the perineum. Even though water is not a barrier for the Nd-YAG laser, if a stray beam were to pass through the wet towels and heat the sheets below, the water would cool it down or extinguish a flame.

Hysteroscopic operations performed with the use of a high-resolution endoscopic television camera offer a great advantage to the understanding of the hysteroscopy technique and associated operative procedures. Nursing personnel essentially have the same view of the operative field as the surgeon and can provide more effective help during the operation. Frequently, nurses will operate video recording equipment, adjust light generators, and monitor Nd-YAG laser equipment intraoperatively. During laser operations, nurses are usually responsible for supervising laser safety measures (Fig 10–6).

When the procedure is finished the circulating nurse must be available to again aid the anesthesiologist during reversal of the anesthesia. The safety strap should be reapplied after the patient is placed in a supine position. Suction should be readily available. When the anesthesiologist is ready, the patient may be transferred back to her stretcher, with the assistance of at least three team members, depending on the condition of the patient. The anesthesiologist will remain at the head to support the patient. If the patient has been given a regional block, her legs must be supported, and a team member must be at either side to transfer her. The patient is covered to maintain her body temperature and privacy and is transferred to the recovery room.

Orientation for New Operating Room Personnel

Perioperative nurses must have knowledge of the policies and procedures of the OR. A manual should have detailed explanations for carrying out specific ac-

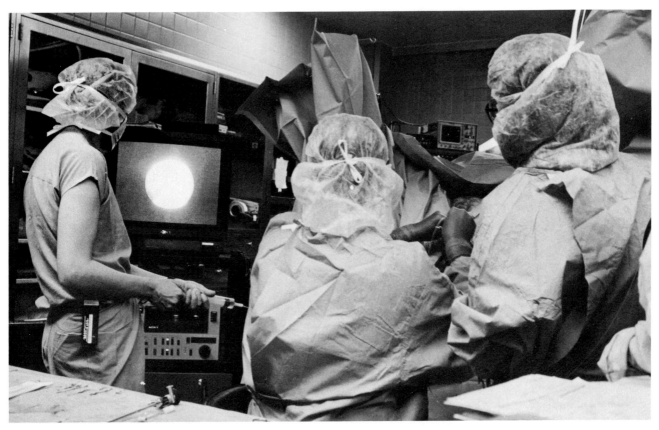

FIG 10–6.
When surgery is performed under guidance of an endoscopic television camera, nurses and assistants see the same field as the surgeon.

tivities. The nurse must have an understanding of the hysteroscopy procedure and why it is being done. This will help in making future judgments about what is needed for a particular case. The nurse must understand proper positioning techniques, to ensure the patient's safety. She/he should know what hazards exist and how to prevent them. The perioperative nurse should have knowledge of surgical asepsis, instrument care, and maintenance. At Crouse-Irving Memorial Hospital, nursing care/teaching plans are written for every procedure performed in the operating suite. These detail the procedure, anatomy involved, instrumentation needed, equipment required, operation and care of the equipment, and surgeon preferences. These plans are incorporated into a detailed orientation program for use of both new and experienced nurses. All new employees can be directly supervised by an experienced nurse until she/he is ready to circulate comfortably alone.

BIBLIOGRAPHY

Groah LK: *Operating Room Nursing, The Perioperative Role.* Reston, Va, Prentice Hall Co, 1983.

Gruendemann BJ, Meeker, MH (eds): *Alexander's Care of the Patient in Surgery,* ed 8. St Louis, CV Mosby Co, 1987.

Lach J: *OR Nursing: Preoperative Care and Draping Technique.* Chicago, Kendall Co, 1974.

Perkins J: *Principles and Methods of Sterilization in Health Sciences.* 1978; pp 327, 501.

Spry C: *Essentials of Perioperative Nursing,* Rockville, Md, Aspen Publications, 1988.

Storz C: *Gynecology Instruments: Care and Maintenance of Telescopes and Instruments,* 1985.

11

How to Learn Hysteroscopy

Michael S. Baggish, M.D.

Rafael F. Valle, M.D.

Visual examination of the uterine cavity to detect disease dates back to the first known demonstration of hysteroscopy by Pantaleoni in 1869. Gynecologists generally have preferred blind methods of examination: tactile appraisal, exploration with forceps or curettes, and radiographic studies with radiopaque material to demonstrate any filling defects in the uterine cavity. These blind methods have limitations however, and, since the early 1970s when hysteroscopy became a practical method for intrauterine visualization, precision-oriented gynecologists have preferred to evaluate the uterine cavity hysteroscopically, with the degree of success depending on the endoscopist's skill.

Lack of familiarity with intrauterine visualization and difficulty in obtaining satisfactory uterine distention have frustrated gynecologists in attempting to use hysteroscopy in their practice. Skillful use of hysteroscopy requires thorough training, dedication, and experience. In the past, gynecologists learned the technique by self-teaching and solved their own problems without guidelines or tutors to help them. We believe that there is a more effective and more appropriate method for learning hysteroscopy.

WORKSHOPS, SEMINARS, AND LECTURES

Lectures and workshops on hysteroscopy have multiplied during the past few years and are now offered almost monthly at various institutions. Most of these seminars are didactic and theoretical, looking at methods, results, complications, practical applications, indications, and contraindications.

The selection of the best seminar to attend should be based on the number and expertise of the faculty and the course content. For example, basic physics, basic methodology, distending media, instrumentation, panoramic hysteroscopy, contact hysteroscopy, operative hysteroscopy, and laser hysteroscopy should be detailed as well as expansive. The best courses include a "hands-on" component.

This "hands-on" experience should allow the physician to assemble a number of instruments and use uterine models to become familiar with the direct and foreoblique views. Such exercises permit a wide variety of equipment to be used in a concentrated time period. Additionally, a substantial number of experienced hysteroscopists should be available to answer questions and demonstrate techniques.

TUTORIALS

Ideally, the technique is best learned by performing endoscopy under the guidance of an expert who can correct mistakes and encourage success. Tutorial training is available in most major hospitals, where usually at least one physician is an experienced hysteroscopist. Tutorials are more difficult to conduct effectively at workshops or seminars with large numbers of participants, owing to the lack of time and volunteer patients. Under circumstances where no local hysteroscopy expertise is available, course directors may suggest programs offering visiting hysteroscopy preceptorships.

WHERE TO BEGIN

Familiarization with instruments is a key factor in learning any new technique. Examine objects of known

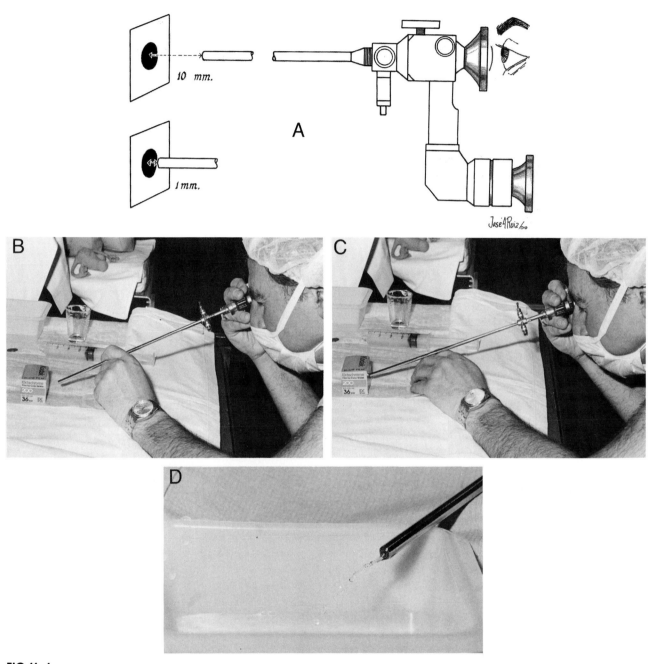

FIG 11–1.
A, objects of known sizes are examined at various distances from the terminus of the endoscope. **B,** the fine print on a box of film is viewed with a focusing telescope in the panoramic mode. **C,** next, the objective lens is brought close to the box's surface for a highly magnified view of the details. **D,** examination with a 0° telescope. Water is flushed through the sheath.

sizes and shapes at distances from 3 in. to 1 to 2 mm from the terminus of the endoscope (Fig 11–1,A–C). Do this examination with both 30° and 0° telescopes (Fig 11–1,D). Next, repeat the examination in a glass container—first using air, then water, then Hyskon. Drop a coin into the glass (Fig 11–2,A and B) and examine the detailed etchings and inscriptions on the coin after at-

taching the fiberoptic light cable to the hysteroscope and connecting it in turn to the light generator. Settings should be made with different powers ranging from low- to high-intensity illuminations. Next, attempt these examinations first with a diagnostic sheath then with various operating sheaths.

The most valuable and practical model on which to

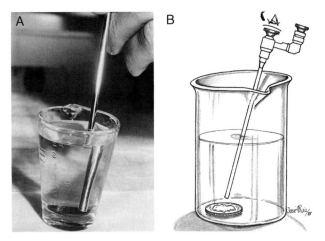

FIG 11–2.
A, the effects of different media on the quality of view may be seen by examining objects in air, water, and Hyskon. Note the effect of diffraction on the hysteroscope at the air-liquid interface. **B,** a coin may be examined at the bottom of a beaker and the detailed inscriptions read by bringing the hysteroscope close to its surface.

practice diagnostic and operative panoramic hysteroscopy is an extirpated uterus (Fig 11–3). The best uterus to examine is a normal uterus; these are readily available following surgery (vaginal or abdominal hysterectomy) for the correction of pelvic relaxation and/or stress incontinence. The specimen should be placed in saline and secured in a timely fashion following the operative procedure. Obviously, removal of the specimen should be coordinated with the Department of Pathology beforehand. Additionally, in the present climate of sexually transmitted diseases, a negative serologic report

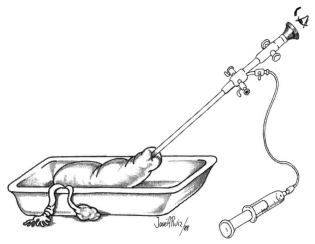

FIG 11–3.
An extirpated human uterus is an ideal specimen for the beginner to practice various hysteroscopy techniques. The uterus is usually distended with water or Hyskon.

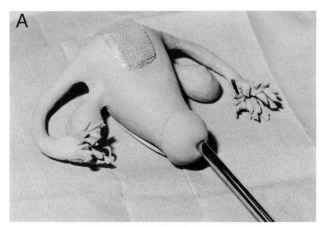

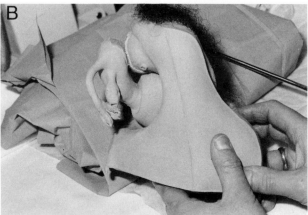

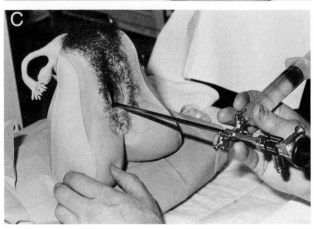

FIG 11–4.
A, this latex rubber life-size model of a human uterus is useful in practicing endoscopic observation and orientation. **B,** the uterus model in **A** may be attached to a latex vagina and hemisected pelvis. **C,** now the hysteroscopic examination may be performed under lifelike conditions using water to distend the uterus.

for syphilis and human immune deficiency virus is recommended. In fact, because of AIDS risk, the practice of using human specimens for exercises during hysteroscopy didactic courses has largely been abandoned (Fig 11–4,A–C). Once a specimen has been obtained, exam-

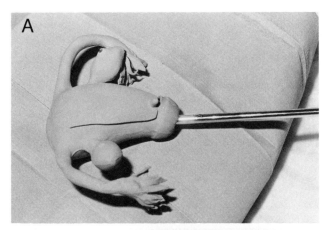

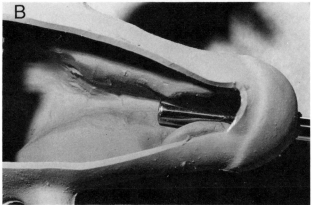

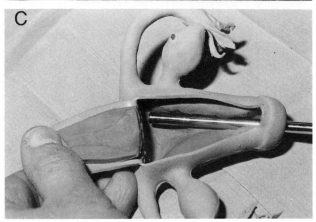

FIG 11–5.
A, the hysteroscope is engaged at the external os of the cervix. **B,** the internal cervical os is negotiated, and the endoscope enters the lower part of the corpus. **C,** the hysteroscope is angulated to the right and left to view the cornual recesses.

ination should be performed with the hysteroscope fitted with a 5-mm diagnostic sheath. Sterile water or saline is used to distend the uterus and is delivered to the sheath through a 50-cc syringe. The endoscope should be engaged at the external cervical opening so as to afford a good view of the endocervical canal (Fig 11–5,A),

and then follow the canal up to the level of the internal os. If possible, the endometrial cavity should be entered without dilatation (Fig 11–5,B). When the os is too tight to allow unfettered passage of the endoscope then careful dilatation should be performed with Pratt dilators. Just enough dilatation should be obtained to allow passage of the 5-mm sheath. The cavity is distended fully and examined from below upward, obtaining a wide-angle, panoramic view of the entire cavity. By pulling the instrument back into the upper endocervical canal and carefully entering the endometrial cavity again, an excellent view can be assured. Next, each cornua is inspected by angulating the instrument first to the right then to the left (Fig 11–5,C). The endoscope is pulled back to midcavity level and swung from the right to the left cornua in order to observe the central point where the Müllerian ducts fused to form the uterus. Then, while one is continuously viewing, the instrument is withdrawn from the cavity and back into the cervical canal.

After several "in vitro" hysteroscopic examinations, the gynecologist is ready to begin examining uteri "in vivo." We feel this is best done at the time of dilation and curettage (D&C). In fact, we believe there is little justification for the performance of blind D&C in this day and age. The operation of choice to investigate the uterine cavity for whatever reason is hysteroscopy, followed by directed endometrial sampling.

For the beginner, the preferred medium with which to begin "in vivo" hysteroscopic examinations is Hyskon, which is injected into the uterus through a 50-cc syringe attached to the hysteroscopic sheath with the intermediary of a large bore connecting tube similar to the one pictured in Plate 48. Again, the examination technique is similar to that described earlier for the extirpated uterus. The major differences in the examination of the "in vivo" uterus compared with the "in vitro" specimen are position differences, color differences, and mucosal bleeding. We strongly suggest the following procedure:

1. It is wise to set a limit on the time allowed for the examination (e.g., a maximum of 15 minutes).
2. The quantity of Hyskon should be limited to less than 200 cc.
3. Before initiating any endoscopic examination, a thorough pelvic examination must be performed and the position of the uterus accurately determined.

This type of exercise is valuable not only to familiarize the gynecologist with the hysteroscopic technique and the intrauterine milieu, but also because it orients the surgeon as well as the nursing personnel to the instru-

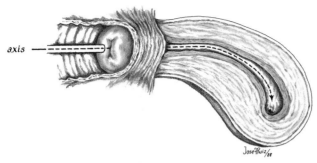

FIG 11–6.
Maintaining the hysteroscope coincident with the axis of the cervical canal and uterine cavity is a key factor in avoiding trauma to the sensitive mucosa.

mentation and to the necessary mechanics for initiating a successful examination.

The most important aspect of the "in vivo" examination is to maintain the hysteroscope in line with the axis of the uterus and its cervical extension (Fig 11–6). The operator must position himself/herself accordingly; for example, in the anteflexed circumstance, the endoscopist should be low in relation to the patient (Fig 11–7). The endoscope should be engaged into the external os while maintaining traction on the uterus by means of a single-toothed tenaculum placed on the anterior cervical lip. Exposure is provided either by a single-hinged speculum or with a Sims retractor placed in the posterior vagina. It is preferred to prepare the cervix and vagina with a cleansing solution of povidone-iodine (Betadine) (if the patient is not allergic to iodine). When the hysteroscope is inserted into the cervix it should be tried without dilatation, using the 5-mm sheath and with the Hyskon flow initiated. The interior of the cervix is examined with a constant flow of Hyskon and slow,

steady movement of the endoscope upward, steering the instrument through the center of the endocervical canal. The internal os, which is viewed as a constricted opening at the top of the canal, is easily identified by witnessing the Hyskon current accelerate as the flow enters the expanded space of the uterine cavity. In fact at this point of entry into the uterine cavity an extra Hyskon push is advised. The cavity is next examined in the fashion described for the "in vitro" examination. The tubal openings may be readily identified by watching the Hyskon flow and seeing small flecks of blood exit the cavity through these ostia. Frequently the tubal ostia have a light-bluish tint (Fig 11–8). When a systematic examination of the cavity has been completed, the instruments are withdrawn under direct vision. If it is required, dilation of the internal os may be accomplished by the use of Pratt dilators lubricated with Hyskon (Plate 49). Again, this must be done carefully and sparingly in order to avoid overdilatation, with resulting loss of medium. At the completion of hysteroscopy a more intelligent curettage (i.e., directed sampling) can be performed. We recommend that approximately 25 "in vivo" learning examinations be performed to attain sufficient diagnostic skill to allow subsequent competent diagnostic hysteroscopic examinations. We likewise believe that approximately 50 diagnostic hysteroscopies be done before attempting operative hysteroscopy. During this latter period it is worthwhile to learn to use other media, particularly CO_2, to perform diagnostic endoscopy.

To prepare for operative hysteroscopy, the novice endoscopist should again repeat the steps suggested to learn diagnostic hysteroscopy but incorporating the 7- to 8-mm operating sheath. This sheath frequently requires dilatation of the cervix. Again, the overriding principle should be to dilate only enough to allow pas-

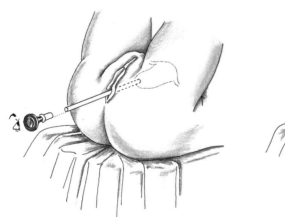
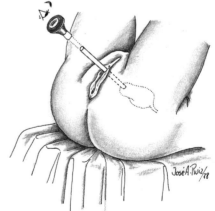

FIG 11–7.
Proper positioning of the endoscopist in relation to the patient's uterine position is essential for a successful examination and is complementary to the axis alignment shown in Figure 11–6.

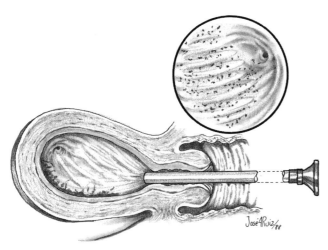

FIG 11–8.
The tubal ostia may be identified by watching small blood particles exit the tubal ostia by way of the Hyskon flow. As the hysteroscope reaches the internal os, an extra push of Hyskon is recommended.

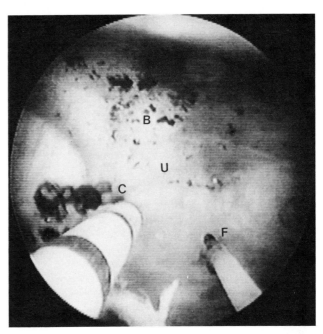

FIG 11–9.
Hysteroscopic view of an aspirating cannula *(C)*, which is inserted through one operating channel, and a quartz fiber *(F)*, which has been passed through a second channel. Flecks of blood *(B)* are suspended in the Hyskon within the uterine cavity *(U)*.

sage of the sheath while maintaining very close clearance relative to the cervical tissues. This close proximation will diminish retrograde leakage of the distending medium.

Next, nipples or gaskets (Plate 50) should be placed over the operating channel fittings. After turning the stopcock to the opened position, one inserts various operating instruments (e.g., forceps, biopsy scissors) through the channel viewed, and manipulates them within the cavity. Although several varieties of operating instruments are available (flexible, semirigid, rigid), the authors prefer to use semirigid instruments, as these fit easily through the sheath's operating channel and also have enough strength to permit a number of maneuvers to be performed with reasonable alacrity. Additionally, the semirigid instruments are sturdy enough to allow relatively heavy-duty work to be performed. As the instruments are positioned closer to the objective lens of the telescope they appear larger, and as they are moved away from the lens they appear smaller than actual size (Plate 51). It is important to learn to appreciate depth with monocular vision by touching the surface of the endometrium. It is also important to estimate the thickness of the endometrium by putting pressure on the uterine wall with the endoscopic sheath and then elevating the instrument and pulling it back toward the endocervix to view the induced groove (Plate 52). The novice should also insert an aspirating cannula through the second channel of the operating sheath to clear debris from the uterine cavity while at the same time instilling additional distension medium (Fig 11–9). Again, gently touch the surface of the endometrium with the cannula. Finally, rotate the endoscope to view the

cornua, and insert the cannula into the cornua and aspirate. Next, pull the cannula back into the sheath and bring the endoscope close to the tubal ostium while injecting distending medium (Plate 53).

Once these techniques are well understood, hysteroscopy may be undertaken while the patient is under local anesthesia or has had systematic analgesia.

When the gynecologist has mastered hysteroscopic examination and manipulated operative hysteroscopic instruments, therapeutic hysteroscopy may begin. Training should begin with easy cases, such as biopsies or removal of intrauterine contraceptive devices, to learn the manipulations required to operate under hysteroscopy, then include more difficult operations, such as the removal of small submucous leiomyomas and division of intrauterine adhesions and uterine septa.

Photographic equipment is helpful in documenting progress in training. A camera should always be ready for use during examinations or operations, and the operator should be familiar with its use. Patient charts utilizing simple diagrams are another important means of documenting and explaining findings to the patient.

A systematic training process will help the gynecologist learn effective intrauterine visualization, make the transition from the asymptomatic patient to the symptomatic one, and understand the disease processes. With a training plan, the transition from diagnostic to operative hysteroscopy will also be easier.

Flexible or rigid teaching devices or microvideo cameras that allow the student to see what the hysteroscopist sees are especially helpful. Videotape machines and closed-circuit television are an excellent method for viewing the dynamic character of hysteroscopy and clearly demonstrating normal and pathologic findings.

Hysteroscopy should be used within a framework of specific clinical indications; a technique or an instrument cannot replace sound clinical medical judgment. Experimental methods or techniques should not be undertaken as the first step in hysteroscopy; they should be reserved for those investigating newer techniques who have access to great numbers of patients and resources.

These guidelines should increase the ease and effectiveness of training in the use of hysteroscopy, thereby increasing its safety and efficiency.

BIBLIOGRAPHY

Baggish MS: Gynecologic endoscopy and instrumentation. *Clin Obstet Gynecol* 1983; 26:211–376.

Baggish MS: Use of hysteroscopy in gynecology, in Nelson J, Taymor M (eds): *Progress in Gynecology VII.* Grune & Stratton, New York, 1983, p 67.

Neuwirth RS: Hysteroscopy, in *Major Problems in Obstetrics and Gynecology.* Philadelphia, WB Saunders Co, 1975, vol 8.

Siegler AM: Learning and teaching hysteroscopic tubal sterilization, in Sciarra JJ, Butler JC, Speidel JJ (eds): *Hysteroscopic Sterilization.* New York, Intercontinental Medical Book Corp, 1974, pp 133–143.

Valle RF, Sciarra JJ: Hysteroscopy, in Sciarra JJ (ed): *Gynecology and Obstetrics.* Hagerstown, Md, Harper & Row, 1974, chap 19.

Valle RF: Hysteroscopy: Basic principles and clinical applications. *J Continuing Educ Obstet Gynecol* 1977; 19:19–28.

12

Distending Media for Panoramic Hysteroscopy

Michael S. Baggish, M.D.

Because of the substantial thickness of the uterine walls, the potential rather than true nature of the uterine cavity, and the tendency of the endometrial mucosal lining to bleed on contact, distention is necessary to view objects within the uterus when using the panoramic mode. Three general types of media have undergone sufficient clinical trials to qualify them for the status of standard techniques.

HYSKON

Thirty-two percent dextran with a molecular weight of 70,000 is a crystal-clear, viscid fluid (Plate 54). This branched polysaccharide, which is electrolyte-free, has the consistency of honey in the liquid state and assumes the characteristics of airplane glue when dried. The advantages of this material as a medium to distend the uterus are multiple. It is the easiest material with which the beginner can learn panoramic hysteroscopy, since it consistently and promptly dilates the cervical canal and uterine cavity. The thickness of Hyskon diminishes the likelihood of massive retrograde leakage characteristic of other liquid media (Plate 55). Hyskon mixes poorly with blood and remains reasonably and optically clear during the procedure. Because of its clarity, Hyskon is the best material to use in performing operative hysteroscopy, since debris can be easily aspirated and if required the cavity may be flushed with fresh material. By observing the flow of fragments of blood and cellular material suspended in the Hyskon, the endoscopist can rapidly and accurately identify the tubal ostia. Finally, Hyskon is an excellent lubricant and may be employed to facilitate dilatation of the cervix by dipping the dila-

tors in the material before engaging them in the external os. However, this same benefit may also create a hazard when the Hyskon spills onto the floor of the operating room, since it can cause personnel to slip and fall. Uncommonly, a patient may experience an anaphylactic reaction to Hyskon. This is far less likely, however, than a similar idiosyncratic reaction to the injection of local anesthesia. Hyskon is not easy to instill through the narrow (5-mm) diagnostic sheaths, and it does require some degree of force to instill it even through the larger diameter operative sheaths. The volume of instilled Hyskon must be carefully monitored, since prolongation of bleeding time has been reported with volumes of 500 cc or more. Additionally, when the uterine wall is damaged (e.g., during endometrial ablation), large volumes of Hyskon may be absorbed into the vascular space and, because of its high osmotic pressure, pulmonary edema may be precipitated. Upon completion of hysteroscopy, all instruments and channels must be repeatedly flushed with very hot water to prevent solidification of the Hyskon (see Chapter 10). If this is not done, the dried material will assume the consistency of cement within these small channels. Nevertheless, with exposure to heat, the material liquefies and can be flushed out of the instruments. When everything is said, Hyskon is probably the overall most popular medium used for hysteroscopic distension in the United States. It gives very reproducible results.

CARBON DIOXIDE

Carbon dioxide (CO_2) has essentially the same index of refraction as air and provides a very clear view

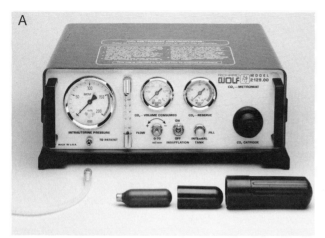

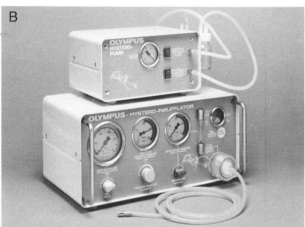

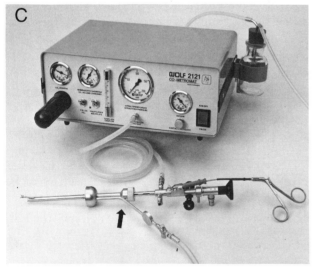

of the endometrium. Since it is a gas it is very easy to infuse and the least messy of all intrauterine distension media. CO_2 is the medium of choice when small diagnostic sheaths are employed, even if clearance around the telescope is limited. It is ideal for office panoramic hysteroscopy. Likewise, there is no problem in so far as cleansing of instruments postoperatively as is the case with Hyskon. CO_2 is also the medium of choice for panoramic hysteroscopic investigation of the endocervix. CO_2 must be insufflated by means of a specialized apparatus designed for hysteroscopy and flowing in the order of cubic centimeters per minute (Fig 12–1,A). Under no circumstances should laparoscopic insufflation equipment, which allows gas to flow at a rate of liters/minute, be utilized for hysteroscopy. Deaths have been reported when CO_2 has been infused without proper flow and pressure regulation. The most common mistake for inexperienced endoscopists is to instill CO_2 at too high a flow rate, which produces obstructive bubbles of gas. It has been recommended that a flow rate of 30 cc/min is best to dilate and view the cervix; increasing to a 40 to 50 cc/min flow for viewing the uterine cavity; the maximal flow rate should not exceed 100 cc/min (Fig 12–1,B). The key to success with CO_2 is a tight fit of the endoscope to the cervix and prevention of mucosal contact, which produces bleeding. In the presence of bleeding, CO_2 hysteroscopy may have to be abandoned because of a foaming interaction between blood and gas. Although some CO_2 insufflators have pressure gauges exceeding 200 mm Hg, the upward pressure limit during CO_2 endoscopy should rarely exceed 100 to 150 mm Hg (Fig 12–1,C). Although most hysteroscopy equipment sets include suction collars to be applied to the cervix to prevent the loss of CO_2, the practicality of these devices is questionable and they not infrequently provoke bleeding, which makes the hysteroscopic examination technically impossible. It is preferable to guide the endoscope through the cervix and gingerly slip "just through" the internal os. CO_2 media is the least advantageous for operative hysteroscopy, but a combination of CO_2 for small sheath diagnostic hysteroscopy followed by Hyskon for the operative portion of the case is a highly satisfactory approach (Plate 56). Some of the newer insufflators can be automatically adjusted not to exceed an intrauterine pressure of 150 mm Hg and to also maintain continuous flow, which keeps

FIG 12–1.
A, hysteroscopic CO_2 insufflator flows at the rate of cc/minute and should not be confused with laparoscopic CO_2 machines which deliver gas at the rate of liters/minute. **B,** intrauterine pressure should rarely exceed 150 mm Hg, and flow rate should not exceed 100 cc/min. **C,** frequently, hysteroscopic equipment is supplied with CO_2 cervical suction collars. Although these devices have some theoretical advantages, in practice they are not useful. **D** (see Plate 56), CO_2 medium is clearly advantageous for diagnostic hysteroscopy using the 5-mm diagnostic sheath.

the uterine walls reliably separated. Gallinat has described experiments on dogs that received direct femoral vein insufflation of CO_2. At flow rates of 200 cc/min, minimal variations in pulse rate and breathing were observed. Toxic effects occurred at flow rates of 400 cc/min, and the animals died within 1 minute when 1,000 cc/min was insufflated.

WATER/SALINE

Five percent dextrose in water (D_5W) or 5% dextrose in saline (D_5S) have the great advantage of always being available in the operating suite or surgical day care center (Plate 57). These solutions are packaged conveniently in plastic infusion bags in 500- or 1,000-cc units. They may be delivered to the intake stopcock of the hysteroscope by a 50-cc syringe, by simple gravity flow from an intravenous infusion pole, or by a pneumatically inflated pressure bag. In fact, the most effective method of administration is by means of a specially designed aneroid pressure cuff, which can be inflated by pumping a rubber bulb (Fig 12–2). The pressure gauge should be inflated to approximately 100 to 110 mm Hg to enable constant delivery and to ensure consistent uterine distension. A bonus advantage to instilling D_5W is its excellence as a lavage solution to wash out clots from within the uterine cavity. After the cavity has been "cleansed," an alternative distension medium may be selected (e.g., CO_2 or Hyskon).

On the negative side, both D_5W and D_5S tend to create a mess as a consequence of leakage and are clearly not recommended for office use. Additionally, these low-viscosity liquids readily flow through the tubal ostia, carrying cellular debris, bacteria, and other flotsam into the oviducts and out into the peritoneal cavity, where they are readily absorbed. Likewise, they tend to

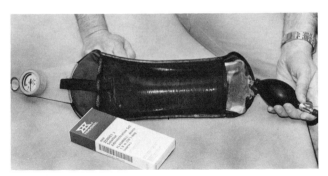

FIG 12–2.
The most convenient method for delivery of D_5W, D_5S, or glycine is by pressure bag, which can be inflated to a desired pressure by means of a pneumatic bulb.

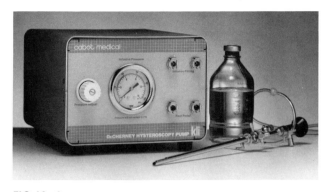

FIG 12–3.
A modification of the Quinones pump is shown here. This refined pump has the advantage of foot switch control and may be used to instill Hyskon.

leak retrograde from the uterus through the cervix into the vagina. Large quantities of D_5W can be absorbed during prolonged operative hysteroscopy, exposing the patient to the risk of water intoxication. Because of the latter consequence, many gynecologists who perform laser ablation of the endometrium prefer D_5S, which results in clouding of the operative field as the case progresses. Since surgery is impossible to perform safely when vision is poor, frequent flushing may be required. If leakage between the hysteroscope sheath and a floppy cervix is excessive, the uterine walls may collapse around the hysteroscope, obtunding the slightest modicum of vision and causing extensive endometrial bleeding. This set of circumstances may preclude reinitiating the procedure, even after extensive lavage. Recently Quinones described a compact regulating-compression apparatus that facilitates the flow of D_5W and reduces the possibility of loss of uterine distension (Fig 12–3).

Although both D_5W and D_5S have their adherents, they are the least popular infusion media for hysteroscopy. They are, however, extremely useful, cheap media for novice hysteroscopists to practice diagnostic and operative hysteroscopy on extirpated uteri. For that matter, simple tap water also suffices for such endeavors.

Regardless of the medium selected, it is wise for the hysteroscopist to become adept with the use of one medium for diagnostic work and probably two for operative techniques. Obviously, the user must be thoroughly informed about possible untoward actions from whatever medium he or she chooses. The delivery of the medium to the hysteroscopy sheath is as important as the choice of medium. Simply attaching a 50-cc syringe loaded with a distending medium is not a very satisfactory method for delivery, since leakage may be prevalent if the force of injection is applied at an angle other than the perpendicular to the hysteroscope sheath (Fig

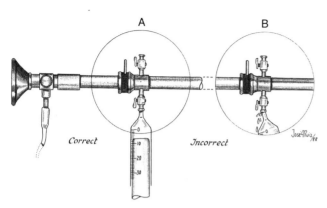

FIG 12–4.
A, attaching a 50-ml syringe to the intake valve of the hysteroscopy sheath is unsatisfactory, since pressure must be delivered perpendicularly to the valve. **B,** when pressure and motion cause the syringe to become angulated, leakage eventuates.

12–4). An extension tube constructed with male and female Luer-lock fittings and of at least 4- to 5-mm bore is best suited for remote attachment of a syringe filled with distention medium (Fig 12–5). Although several "Hyskon pumps" have appeared in the marketplace, none of these has performed more satisfactorily than a 50-cc syringe pushed by hand (Plate 58). The key to continuous distention of the uterus by any medium relies on the tightness of fit between the hysteroscope and the cervix. The operator should always try to negotiate the cervix without dilating, since the ability to enter the endometrial cavity sans dilatation will usually guarantee minimal medium leakage. Other benefits also accrue, for example, less chance of bleeding, no distortion of the endometrial cavity, and little discomfort for the patient. When the cervix is so patulous (usually secondary to obstetric

lacerations) that substantial clearance exists between the diagnostic sheath (5 mm) and the surrounding tissue, the operator may at his or her discretion: (1) utilize a larger sheath (e.g., a 7- to 8-mm operating sheath) or (2) apply a shallow purse-string suture around the cervix and tighten it appropriately to ensure a tight fit to the endoscope (Fig 12–6,A and B). Recently Baggish has described a banding device which can routinely be applied to the cervix during hysteroscopic procedures even in the office setting. When dilation is required—this is frequently necessary when operative hysteroscopy is done—finely tapered dilators are preferred (Pratt dilators) and should be lubricated with Hyskon. Slow, careful dilation will avoid cervical and uterine trauma. Attempts to pass the hysteroscope sheath should be tried frequently in order to avoid passing the optimal tight fit mark between cervix and hysteroscope. As stated

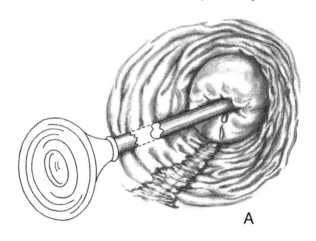

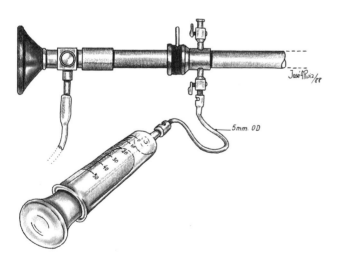

FIG 12–5.
Hyskon is delivered to the sheath by a wide-bore extension tube constructed with mole and female antislip Luer-lock fittings.

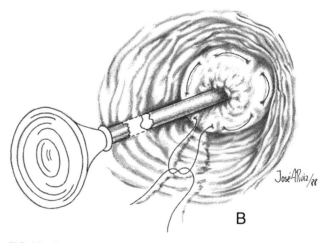

FIG 12–6.
A, the cervical canal is of greater diameter than the hysteroscope and sheath. Leakage and resulting loss of distention are inevitable. **B,** a purse-string suture is placed in the cervix and tightened around the hysteroscope sheath.

TABLE 12–1.

Comparison of Distension Media

Factor(s)	Hyskon	D_5W/D_5S	CO_2
Facility for beginner	Best	Intermediate	Worst
Complexity of equipment	Best	Intermediate	Worst
Ease of instillation	Intermediate	Intermediate	Best
Availability	Intermediate	Best	Intermediate
Maintenance of distention	Best	Worst	Intermediate
Messiness	Worst	Intermediate	Best
Office use	Worst	Worst	Best
Optimal clarity	Best	Worst	Best
Miscibility with blood	Best	Intermediate	Worst
Ability to aspirate	Best	Intermediate	Worst
Flushing capability	Intermediate	Best	Worst
Operative capability	Best	Intermediate	Worst
Complications	Intermediate*	Low†	Low‡

*Rate = *Worst* if >700 cc is utilized after estimating losses.
†Rate = *intermediate* when water is used for operative endoscopy.
‡Rate = *Worst* if operator does *not* use specifically designed hysteroscopic insufflation equipment.

earlier, the operator is obliged to keep careful track of the volume of liquid medium instilled into the uterus. Equally important is judging the amount of these liquids that are lost through retrograde leakage. In a study performed by the author in Syracuse, NY, such losses utilizing Hyskon as the medium were reasonably estimated to range from 20% to 30% of the insufflated volume. Approximately 5% of the instilled Hyskon was found in the peritoneal cavity when a simultaneous or immediately subsequent laparoscopy was performed. When D_5W or D_5S is utilized, a plastic or rubber drape should be placed under the patient's buttocks and led into a bucket in order to collect as much leaked liquid as possible. Obviously, soaked drapes will have to be estimated in calculating the amount of fluid absorbed. The critical figure to know or reasonably estimate is the difference between the total volume instilled minus the volume lost.

Experience with the medium used is the most valuable asset for the hysteroscopist (Table 12–1). Only with time and use can fine tuning be appreciated. Such little things as warming the Hyskon, introducing the CO_2 at a 30 cc/min flow rate, and keeping the hysteroscope in midchannel of the medium-distended uterus come only with experience.

BIBLIOGRAPHY

Edstrom K, Fernstrom I: The diagnostic possibilities of a modified hysteroscopic technique. *Acta Obstet Gynecol Scand* 1970; 49(4)327.

Hamou JE: Microhysteroscopy. *Clin Obstet Gynecol* 1983; 26:285.

Lindemann HJ: The use of CO_2 in the uterine cavity for hysteroscopy. *Int J Fertil* 1972; 17:221.

Lindemann HJ: Pneumometra fur die hysteroskopie. *Geburtshilfe Frauenheilkd* 1973; 33:18.

Lindemann HJ, Mohr J, Gallinat A, et al: Der einfluss Von CO_2-Gas wahrend der hysteroskopie. *Geburtshilfe Frauenheilkd* 1976; 36:153.

Neuwirth RS, Levine RV: Evaluation of a method of hysteroscopy with the use of 30% dextron. *Am J Obstet Gynec* 1972; 114:696.

Porto R, Gaujoux J: Une nouvelle methode d'hysteroscopie, instrumentation et technique. *J Gynecol Obstet Biol Reprod (Paris)* 1972; 1(7):691.

Porto R: La pneumo-hysteroscopie. *Acta Endoscopica* 1973; 3–4:86.

Quinones RG: Hysteroscopy with a new fluid technique, in Siegler AM, Lindemann HJ, (eds): *Hysteroscopy: Principles and Practice.* Philadelphia, Lippincott, 1984, p 41.

Siegler AM, Kemmann EK: Hysteroscopy, a review. *Obstet Gynecol Surv* 1975; 30:567.

Siegler AM, Kemmann EK, Getile GP: Hysteroscopic procedures in 257 patients. *Fertil Steril* 1976; 27:1267.

Valle RF: Hysteroscopy for gynecologic diagnosis. *Clin Obstet Gynecol* 1983; 26:253.

13

Technique of Panoramic Hysteroscopy

Rafael F. Valle, M.D.

The uterus is an organ with thick, muscular walls in apposition with a central virtual cavity lined with an epithelium that bleeds cyclically and whose surface changes constantly during the menstrual cycle (Fig 13–1). To convert this virtual cavity to an actual volumetric space for panoramic visualization, positive pressures of a distending medium are required. Because the endometrial lining varies in thickness and friability, distension of the uterine cavity is easier at some periods rather than others during these cyclic changes (Fig 13–2,A–E).

These anatomic and physiologic reasons help explain why use of hysteroscopy did not keep pace with cystoscopy, despite their common initial origin. The bladder requires gravity pressure for its distension rather than positive pressure, since a thin muscle can achieve distension easily. Furthermore, its transitional epithelium does not bleed cyclically and seldom bleeds on contact (Table 13–1). This explains why cystoscopy was a practical technique since the introduction of the original cystoscope by Desormeaux in 1865. Rubin noted these differences in the 1930s when he began distending the uterine cavity with CO_2 gas to perform hysteroscopy and, therefore, adapted the positive pressures to the uterus to maintain uterine wall separation while visualization was taking place.

MODERN METHODS OF UTERINE DISTENSION FOR HYSTEROSCOPY

Since the early 1970s when hysteroscopy became a practical method for uterine visualization, the media used most commonly for uterine distension to perform panoramic hysteroscopy are dextran 32% weight/volume (W/V) in dextrose 10%, CO_2 gas insufflation, and dextrose 5% in water (Fig 13–3).

Dextran in Dextrose

Dextran 32% W/V (Hyskon) is an optically clear, viscous solution with a high refractory index and high viscosity of 225 centipoise at 37°C. It has a molecular weight of 70,000 and does not mix easily with blood. It offers excellent, clear vision in panoramic hysteroscopy, requiring only about 50 ml of solution for each examination. Spillage during the examination is minimal. During the hysteroscopic examination an assistant delivers the Hyskon by means of a syringe through connective tubing attached to the inflow channel of the hysteroscope.

Carbon Dioxide Gas Insufflation

CO_2 gas insufflation permits excellent visualization of the uterine cavity; it provides good uterine distension and keeps the instruments and the operative field relatively clean. Delivery of the gas to the uterine cavity requires special hysterosufflators that monitor the intrauterine pressure and flow rate to the uterine cavity electronically (Table 13–2).

Because of possible intravasation of CO_2 during hysteroscopy, electrocardiographic monitoring of the patient is recommended, particularly when operative hys-

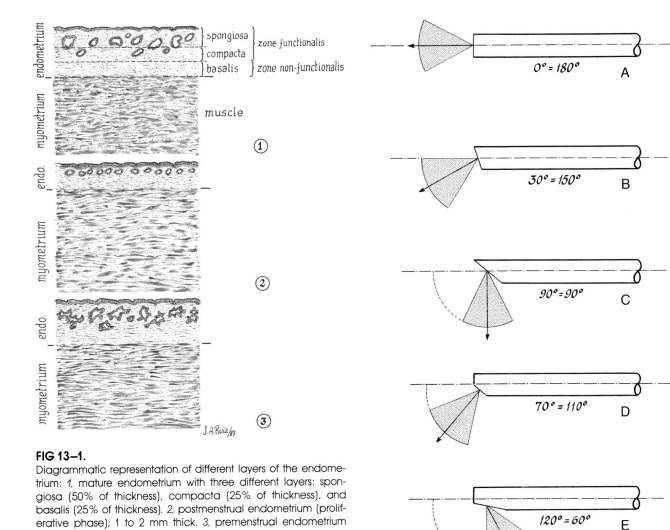

FIG 13–1.
Diagrammatic representation of different layers of the endometrium: *1,* mature endometrium with three different layers: spongiosa (50% of thickness), compacta (25% of thickness), and basalis (25% of thickness). *2,* postmenstrual endometrium (proliferative phase); 1 to 2 mm thick. *3,* premenstrual endometrium (secretory phase); 3 to 8 mm thick.

FIG 13–2.
Directions of view and angular notations of different endoscopes. Shaded area shows visual field. Direct or straight view **(A),** fore-oblique view **(B),** right angle view **(C),** lateral view **(D)** retrospective view **(E).**

teroscopy is being performed and the procedure exceeds the usual time for diagnostic hysteroscopy (usually about 5 to 7 minutes). Monitoring will detect possible arrhythmias secondary to hypercarbia and acidosis. An intravenous line is, therefore, desirable should medications be required.

Dextrose in Water

The most commonly used low-viscosity medium is 5% dextrose in water (D_5W). It mixes less readily with blood than normal saline, owing to the sugar's flocculation of the erythrocytes. This medium offers an advantage of washing the uterine cavity prior to uterine distention, or when debris, mucus, or clots are encountered with manipulation, particularly after operative procedures. This washing procedure is performed through a polyethylene catheter introduced through the operating channel of the hysteroscope to obtain a true inflow and outflow system under a low gravity pressure. When the returning fluid becomes clear, the polyethylene catheter is occluded, and adequate distention begins.

This medium clears the endometrial cavity from debris, mucus, or blood clots and aids in the assessment of tubal patency when hysteroscopy is concomitant with laparoscopy.

In general, no one of these three methods is better

TABLE 13–1.

Factors Related to Panoramic Endoscopy of the Uterus and Urinary Bladder

Uterus	Urinary Bladder
Virtual cavity has thick muscle walls	Has thin muscle walls, easily distensible
Positive pressure needed for distension	Requires gravity pressure
Bleeds at monthly cycles	Does not bleed
Has columnar epithelium with glands	Has transitional epithelium
Epithelium changes during cycle	No cyclic changes
Communicates with the peritoneal cavity through the fallopian tubes	No communication with peritoneal cavity
Has individual embryology, anatomy, physiology, and pathology	Has different embryology, anatomy, physiology, and pathology

TABLE 13–2.

Flow Rates and Intrauterine Pressure for CO_2 Hysteroscopy

	Flow rate (ml/min)	Intrauterine Pressure (mm Hg)
Conventional panoramic hysteroscopy	40–60	100–150 (maximum)
Microhysteroscopy	30	90 (maximum)
Salpingoscopy	10	40–50 (intratubal pressure)

than the others; with each, examination and hysteroscopic interventions can be performed adequately when the specific technique is well known and the operator is familiar with the properties, peculiarities, and possible side effects of each specific method. When the operator has experience with all of them, they can be interchanged and combined during an examination. Nonetheless, gas insufflation remains the method of choice for office hysteroscopy (Fig 13–4).

TECHNIQUE

Selection of patients is based on appropriate indications, a complete medical history, and physical examination—including a pelvic examination, a recent Papanicolaou smear, cervical vaginal smears, and cultures and pregnancy tests when appropriate.

Although specific indications for performing panoramic hysteroscopy may vary according to a patient's needs and the skill of the endoscopist, the contraindications to this technique should be ruled out.

CONTRAINDICATIONS

There are few absolute contraindications to hysteroscopy. They are pregnancy, cervical infection, profuse uterine bleeding, and known cervical malignancy.

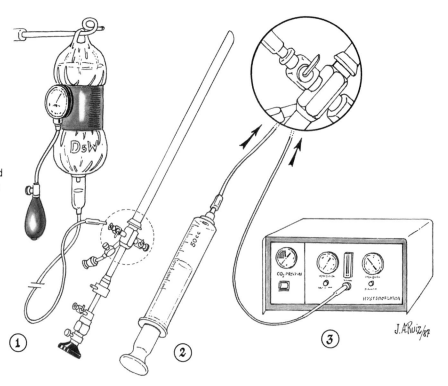

FIG 13–3.

Setup for uterine distension with different methods: *1,* a blood pressure cuff around a plastic bag containing dextrose 5% in water kept under pressure; *2,* plastic 50-cc syringe for delivering the Hyskon; *3,* CO_2 insufflator for controlled delivery of the gas.

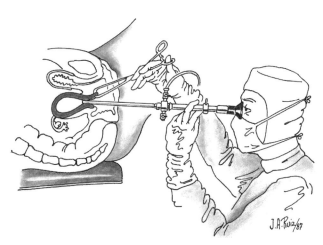

FIG 13–4.
Schematic representation of the hysteroscopic examination.

Pregnancy

Because hysteroscopy invades the uterine cavity, pregnancy is a contraindication owing to the dangers of introducing infection to the early conceptus or interrupting a desired pregnancy. Hysteroscopy may be modified as an amnioscopic examination in selected patients under strict criteria and specific technique.

Recent or Existing Uterine or Cervical Infection

The danger of spreading infection from the lower genital tract into the peritoneal cavity by way of the fallopian tubes or the systemic circulation dictates avoidance of hysteroscopy when infection is suspected.

Profuse Uterine Bleeding

In the presence of excessive uterine bleeding or menstruation, hysteroscopy cannot be performed satisfactorily, regardless of the distending medium, and should therefore be avoided.

Known Cervical Malignancy

The presence of invasive cervical malignancy is another absolute contraindication to hysteroscopy, not only because hysteroscopy is of doubtful value but also because cervical manipulation may spread the malignant cells.

Relative contraindications to hysteroscopy are known carcinoma or adenocarcinoma of the endometrium when a practitioner is not familiar with this disease, marked cervical stenosis not resolved by usual dilatation, and operator unfamiliarity with the instru-

mentation and technique used, particularly, unfamiliarity with the delivery of the distending medium used.

CLINICAL INDICATIONS FOR HYSTEROSCOPY

Clinical studies are now demonstrating the value of hysteroscopy in the diagnosis and treatment of patients afflicted with a variety of gynecologic problems. The present indications for hysteroscopy are the following:

1. Abnormal premenopausal and postmenopausal uterine bleeding (Plates 59 and 60).
2. Diagnosis and possible transcervical removal of submucous leiomyomas or endometrial polyps (Plates 61 through 63).
3. Location and retrieval of "lost" intrauterine devices or other foreign bodies.
4. Evaluation of infertile patients with abnormal hysterograms (Fig 13–5 and Plate 64).
5. Diagnosis and surgical treatment of intrauterine lesions.
6. Diagnosis and division of uterine septa (Plates 65 through 67).
7. Exploration of the endocervical canal and uterine cavity in patients with repeated pregnancy losses.

As experience and simplification of instrumentation increase, new applications will be evaluated, and indications will undoubtedly increase. At present, the most common indications for hysteroscopy are the evaluation of persistent or recurrent abnormal uterine bleeding, the evaluation of abnormal hysterograms, the surgical treatment of intrauterine adhesions, the treatment of uterine septa, and the location and removal of misplaced intrauterine foreign bodies.

Despite the multiple application and indications of hysteroscopy, the method is no panacea, and should be used as a helpful adjunct to other techniques and as an excellent alternative in the diagnosis and treatment of intrauterine lesions.

TECHNIQUE OF PANORAMIC HYSTEROSCOPY

With this background of clinical indications, absence of contraindications, and appropriate selection of patients, the technique of hysteroscopy will provide a safe, simple, and efficient examination of the endocervical canal and uterine cavity.

With the patient in a dorsal lithotomy position, the

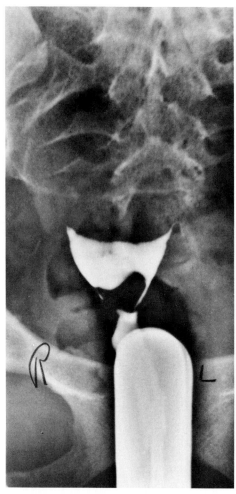

FIG 13—5.
Hysterosalpingogram shows a large filling defect, essentially dividing the uterus into two chambers. This picture is highly suggestive of uterine synechiae.

vulvar area and vagina are cleansed with an appropriate antiseptic solution.

Office hysteroscopy requires less manipulation and no cervical dilatation, as the instruments are less than 4 mm in diameter and can be introduced easily under direct vision through the endocervical canal. Nonetheless, the vaginal and cervical area should be cleansed with an appropriate antiseptic solution. Although no surgical drapings are required, the usual no-touch sterile technique should be respected. A local anesthetic is optional, although useful in small amounts, particularly when a patient is somewhat apprehensive. The cervix is visualized with the aid of a vaginal speculum, and a paracervical block is performed. Five milliliters of chloroprocaine hydrochloride 1% (Nesacaine) is injected superficially on each side of the cervix.

A small dot of anesthestic is also placed at the ante-

rior cervical lip where the tenaculum will be placed; this minimizes any feeling that the patient may have during initiation of the procedure. The cervix is grasped with a tenaculum, and the instrument and hysteroscope are attached to its light source. Insufflation flowing directly through the hysteroscope is introduced at the external cervical os. By gentle manipulation, the endoscope is advanced slowly, following the small cavity seen in front of the hysteroscope which the gas has created. When vision is impaired, the instrument is gently withdrawn and a new attempt is initiated, allowing the gas to distend the cavity. The cervical canal is visualized in its totality and once the junction between the cervix and uterus is passed, the uterine cavity is observed, first in its totality, and then systematically in each portion of the anterior wall, posterior wall, and uterine cornua (Fig 13–6).

When larger instruments or operative hysteroscopes are used under local anesthesia, the paracervical block is performed in the same manner, but 5 to 8 ml of the anesthetic may be required on each side of the utero-

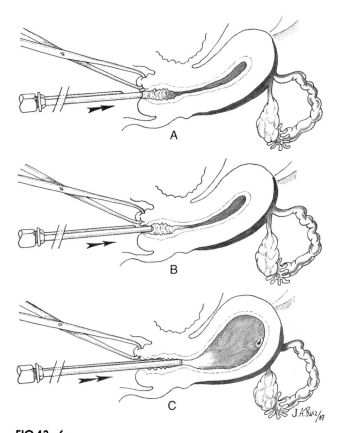

FIG 13—6.
Hysteroscopy with diagnostic endoscopes (<4 mm OD). Examination begins at external cervical os without previous cervical dilatation **(A)**; The endoscope is advanced under direct vision **(B)**; After the endoscope crosses the internal cervical os, the uterine cavity is systematically examined **(C)**.

sacral ligaments. The cervical canal is then gradually dilated to 6, 7, or 8 mm of diameter, depending on the endoscope used. The endoscope is introduced to the level of the internal cervical os. If the instrument has an obturator, this is replaced with a telescope at this point. Visualization of the uterine cavity is performed; at the conclusion of the systematic observation of the uterine cavity, while this instrument is being withdrawn, the cervical canal is explored (Fig 13–7).

When operative hysteroscopes with low-viscosity fluids are being used, before uterine distension is achieved, a polyethylene catheter is introduced through the operating channel up to the distal tip of the hysteroscope, and the uterine cavity is irrigated with D_5W until the returning fluid is clear; then the polyethylene catheter is occluded and uterine distention begins (Fig 13–8).

Although the technique of operative hysteroscopy is specific to each operative procedure planned, several common principles apply to all hysteroscopic operative procedures. First, an appropriate operative hysteroscope at least 7 mm in diameter should be available, and the

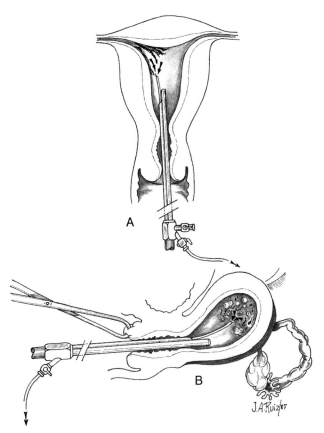

FIG 13–8.
Polyethylene tube is inserted through hysteroscopic operating channel for aspiration of debris, blood clots, mucus, and air bubbles, when using liquid media. **A,** anteroposterior view; **B,** lateral view.

accessory instruments ready in good working condition. These include biopsy forceps, grasping forceps, scissors, calibrated probes, and polyethylene tubes for aspiration. Additional instruments may be required; flexible, semirigid, and rigid instruments should be available. When extensive intrauterine surgery is planned, laparoscopy may be necessary. (See Chapters 20 and 21.)

Hysteroscopy is best performed after the patient has completed menstruation, when the endometrial lining is thin and the uterine cavity is relatively free of blood or debris. Intrauterine surgery must be performed at this time. In patients with infertility problems, when hysteroscopy is performed in the midcycle or in the secretory phase of the menstrual cycle, care should be taken not to distort the endometrial lining with undue manipulation and not to abrade the endometrial lining, causing impaired visualization or undue bleeding. Hysteroscopy should not be performed on a menstruating patient. The patient should be placed at a level comfortable to the operator's view. Therefore, it is important to have a special stool that can be lowered at will to allow for the

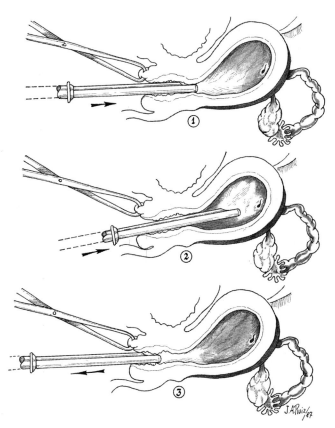

FIG 13–7.
Hysteroscopy with operative endoscopes (> 6.5 mm OD). *1,* the endoscope is introduced at the level of the internal cervical os: *2,* the hysteroscope is advanced under direct vision to complete the examination. *3,* the endocervical canal is examined during withdrawal of the endoscope.

operator's comfort without impairing his or her direct view through the endoscope.

POSSIBLE COMPLICATIONS OF HYSTEROSCOPY

Careful selection of patients may obviate most complications; nonetheless, because some blind manipulations are required (particularly when operative hysteroscopes are used, such as sounding the uterine cavity or dilating the endocervical canal), uterine perforations may occur, as is the case in the use of dilatation and curettage. Patients should be screened for possible cervical, uterine, or pelvic infections. Injury to the uterine walls is possible, particularly for significant uterine surgery. The most significant complications arising from the hysteroscopic technique are uterine perforation, infection, and significant bleeding.

Uterine Perforation

Because hysteroscopy is performed under direct vision, no perforation is possible with a hysteroscope unless the instrument is forcefully pressed against the uterine wall without panoramic vision. Perforation of the uterus may occur during sounding of the uterine cavity or during cervical dilatation; because with smaller diagnostic instruments these manipulations are not required, uterine perforation cannot occur if the instrument is advanced gently, with delicacy, and always under direct vision (Plate 68).

Infection

Infection seldom has been encountered subsequent to hysteroscopy; nonetheless, the instrument is passed from the vaginal area and cervical canal to the sterile endometrial lining. To avoid infection, the procedure is performed under strict and meticulous protocols.

Bleeding

Although minor spotting may occur after hysteroscopy, excessive bleeding is unusual, except in cases of extensive manipulations under operative hysteroscopy. Minor spotting may occur following intrauterine examination but generally subsides spontaneously within a few hours.

Other possible complications are those related to the medium utilized for uterine distension and those related to intrauterine operations.

Medium-Related Complications

Complications from media used during the procedure include an anaphylactic reaction to dextran, pulmonary edema secondary to fluid overload, and bleeding disorders (e.g., disseminated intravascular coagulation) secondary to excessive infusion of dextran. Problems related to the controlled CO_2 gas insufflation are rare. Nonetheless, when improper delivery gas sources are used, massive intravasation of CO_2 gas with secondary hypercarbia and acidosis may occur. Cardiac arrhythmias may also occur, but are unlikely when appropriate instrumentation for the CO_2 gas is used. With inappropriate perfusion of large quantities of D_5W, water overload and electrolyte imbalance may occur. This problem is easily avoided by controlling and limiting the quantity of the fluid used and by expediting the procedure.

Complications Related to Intrauterine Operations

When intrauterine dissections are performed—such as lysis of intrauterine adhesions; removal of pedunculated submucous leiomyomas or polyps; division of uterine septa; multiple biopsies of lesions, particularly when electrocautery or coagulation is used; and tubal cannulation—uterine perforations may occur, especially at the uterotubal junctions. Concomitant laparoscopy is useful when intrauterine dissections are extensive, particularly for the lysis of thick and extensive intrauterine adhesions, the division of uterine septa, the use of electrocoagulation, and the removal of submucous leiomyomas. The use of laparoscopy permits monitoring of the uterine walls during the hysteroscopic operation and alerts the hysteroscopist of imminent damage. Concomitant laparoscopy, should, nonetheless, be individualized.

ANESTHESIA

For office hysteroscopy with a hysteroscope less than 4 mm in diameter, the instrument can be inserted into the endocervical canal and uterine cavity safely and painlessly without anesthesia. Should the patient request anesthesia, paracervical block is sufficient with small amounts (less than 5 ml of anesthetic) in each uterosacral ligament. For operative hysteroscopes with diameters of 7 mm, some anesthesia or analgesia is required, most commonly, a paracervical block or general anesthesia. Occasionally, systemic analgesia is sufficient. Systemic analgesia may be sufficient when smaller instruments are used for diagnostic purposes, when the patient is somewhat apprehensive, and when no cervical dilatation is required.

Perhaps the best means of analgesia is a thorough explanation to the patient by a physician who reassures, instructs, and explains the procedure and its goals and benefits.

As with any other surgical techniques, the keys to success with panoramic hysteroscopy are knowledge of the instrumentation; use of appropriate instruments; gentle, sequential performance of each step in the technique; and cognizance of the limitations, indications, contraindications, and possible complications. Attention to all of these factors will undoubtedly result in a successful examination.

BIBLIOGRAPHY

Desormeaux AJ: *De L'Endoscope et de ses Applications au Diagnostic et au Traitement des Affections de L'Urethre et de la Vessie.* Paris, Bailliere, 1865.

Gallinat A: The effect of carbon dioxide during hysteroscopy, in Van Der Pas H, von Herendael B, van Lith D, et al (eds): *Hysteroscopy* Hingham, Mass, MTP Press Limited. 1983, pp 19–27.

Hamou J: Microhysteroscopy. A new procedure and its original applications in gynecology. *J Reprod Med* 1981; 26:375–382.

Lindemann HJ: The use of CO_2 in the uterine cavity for hysteroscopy. *Int J Fertil* 1972; 17:221–224.

Rubin IC: Uterine endoscopy, endometroscopy with the aid of uterine insufflation. *Am J Obstet Gynecol* 1925; 10:313–327.

Siegler AM: Adverse effects from hysteroscopy, in Siegler AM, Lindemann HJ (Eds): *Hysteroscopy: Principles and Practice.* Philadelphia, JB Lippincott Co, 1984; pp 108–111.

Siegler AM: Panoramic CO_2 hysteroscopy. *Clin Obstet Gynecol* 1983; 26:242–252.

Valle RF: Indications for hysteroscopy, in Siegler AM, Lindemann HJ (eds): *Hysteroscopy: Principles and Practice.* Philadelphia, JB Lippincott Co, 1986. pp 21–24.

Valle RF: Hysteroscopy for gynecologic diagnosis. *Clin Obstet Gynecol* 1983; 26:253–276.

Valle RF: Hysteroscopy: Diagnostic and therapeutic applications. *J Reprod Med* 1978; 20:115–118.

Valle RF: Hysteroscopy, Obstet Gynecol Annu 1978; 7:245–382.

Valle RF: Hysteroscopy: Basic principles and clinical applications. *J Continuing Ed Obstet Gynecol* 1977; 19:19–28.

Valle RF, Sciarra JJ: Hysteroscopy, in Sciarra JJ (ed): *Obstetrics and Gynecology.* Hagerstown, Md. Harper & Row, 1986, vol 1, chap 36.

Valle RF, Sciarra JJ: Current status of hysteroscopy in gynecologic practice. *Fertil Steril* 1979; 32:619–632.

14

Contact Hysteroscopy

Michael S. Baggish, M.D.

The first endoscopes were simple hollow tubes which, upon coming into contact with the highly vascular surface of the endometrium, produced bleeding. When Charles David sealed the distal end of his hysteroscope with a piece of glass, contact with the mucosa forced out the blood, allowing clear vision to become possible. Thus the endoscopic examination performed was a typical contact hysteroscopy. The modern contact hysteroscope is a highly refined, precise instrument compared with its primitive ancestor and provides the endoscopist with the simplest and most portable hysteroscopic system available. The quality of the image obtained with the contact optical system is excellent and can discriminate between two points which are as close together as 20 μm (Plate 69). The basis for contact hysteroscopy is completely different from that of panoramic hysteroscopy, since the endoscope lies within the tissue itself; whereas in panoramic hysteroscopy, the tissue is viewed from above or from a distance (Plate 70). Additionally accurate interpretation of the object under scrutiny depends on an intact vascular supply to allow proper color differentiation. Since the uterine cavity is not distended, the endometrium is viewed in its most natural state, that is, with the anterior and posterior endometrial walls in apposition. Contour as well as color is critical in differentiating one lesion from another. In a manner analogous to colposcopy, patterns seen by the hysteroscope are then interpreted. Additionally, the endoscopist can appreciate spatial relationships and actually feel the lesion. Much in the manner of a computer, all this information is fed into the endoscopist's brain, interfaced, analyzed, and a resulting diagnosis is revealed. In contrast to panoramic hysteroscopes the focal field of the contact instrument provides an accessible, accurate spatial relationship and permits accurate measurement of lesions (Plate 71). Since the principles of contact endoscopy depend on interpretation of color, contour, vascular patterns, and touch, clinical-pathologic correlations based on previously learned patterns are vital for the technique and must be learned. Although the setup and actual use of the instrument are simple, the interpretation of patterns is difficult and requires diligent practice and patience to learn.

Another difficulty encountered when first starting contact hysteroscopy is the very small field of view and an optical field totally foreign to an observer who has been familiar since birth with panoramic vision. Magnification is therefore always required. There are certain areas in which contact endoscopy is useful and advantageous compared with other methods of hysteroscopy. These categories include detailed evaluation of (1) the endocervix, (2) endometrial carcinoma, (3) the female urethra and bladder, (4) the vaginas of infants and children, and (5) the uterus of the pregnant woman. The contact hysteroscope is not an advantageous selection for evaluation of space-occupying lesions, for uterine synechiae, for septa, and for operative hysteroscopy. Finally, contact hysteroscopy is a diagnostic technique only.

INSTRUMENTATION

No distending media are required for contact hysteroscopy. The contact endoscope is composed of three principal parts: (1) an optical guide; (2) a cylindrical chamber which collects and traps ambient light; and (3) a magnifying eyepiece (Plate 72). A magnifying telescopic attachment is built into the eyepiece of the endoscope and can be focused in a manner similar to an eyepiece of a microscope. This extra magnification equipment is clearly a necessity which permits examination in detail. The optical guide consists of a solid piece of high-grade mineral glass measuring 200 mm in

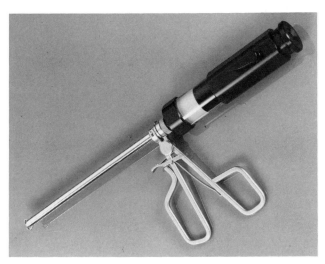

FIG 14–1.
The newest version of the contact hysteroscope has a built-in magnifying device. The focusing lever is noted just forward of the eyepiece.

length and 6 mm in diameter (Fig 14–1). The glass is protected by a mirrored, stainless steel jacket. At each extremity, a tight silver ring maintains an air space between the metal and the glass, which ensures total light reflection. The cylindrical chamber collects directed or ambient light and concentrates that light into the optical guide. It additionally eliminates annoying reflections. The outer surface of the hollow cylinder is glossy, whereas the inner surface is unpolished. This component measures 120 mm in length and 50 mm in diameter and contains two light-trapping devices: a black, polished concave mirror, and a conical, metallic diaphragm (see Plate 72). These respective optical and mechanical light traps are so arranged that only the light coming from the optical guide can pass through the cylinder to reach the observer's eye. Ambient light entering the cyl-

inder from the outside is reflected onto the concave mirror and captured by the metallic diaphragm. The instrument is watertight and can be sterilized by soaking in a Cidex solution for 15 minutes. A telephoto, bayonet adapter is available for taking photographs. A single-lens reflex camera with a specially adapted clear focusing screen is fitted to the endoscope with a special flash bracket. The flash unit is directed onto the light-collecting chamber to provide an effusive flood of light. The telephoto lens clamps onto the eyepiece, that is, it replaces the adifoser (magnifying option) (Fig 14–2; Plate 73).

METHOD OF EXAMINATION

Grasping the Instrument

The contact endoscope must be held in such a manner as not to obstruct the light-collecting chamber. The focusing and magnifying eyepiece is usually perfocused on a piece of gauze. Utilizing the index finger and thumb of the opposite hand allows the operator to focus the eyepiece as the endoscope is introduced into the cervix (Fig 14–3).

Preparation

The preoperative preparation for contact hysteroscopy is very simple and consists of a single-toothed tenaculum, a single hinged speculum opened on one side, and Pratt dilators or rubber bougies.

Light Source

The light source may consist of the operating room light, an examining room lamp, or a special high-intensity halogen lamp (Burton-Cavitron). The authors prefer the latter when photography is anticipated. Because of the simple setup and the availability of a variety of light sources, contact endoscopy can be carried out in virtually any setting (e.g., office, outpatient clinic, emergency room, hospital examining room, labor room, delivery room, or operating suite) (Fig 14–4).

Anesthesia

In many multiparous women the cervix is patulous enough to allow the insertion of the 6-mm contact hysteroscope without the need for dilation. Similarly, many mulligravid cervixes are sufficiently opened, especially at midcycle, to allow inspection without anesthesia. In every case, insertion should be attempted without re-

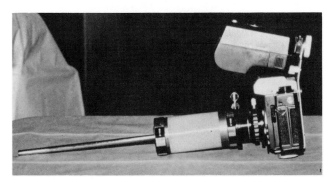

FIG 14–2.
A 35-mm camera attaches to the eyepiece of the contact hysteroscope by a bayonet mount. The flash is tipped so as to flood the light-collecting chamber of the hysteroscope.

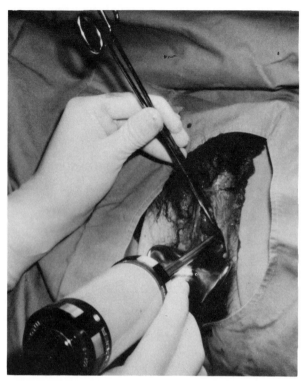

FIG 14–3.
The endoscope is introduced into the cervix without obstructing the light-collecting chamber.

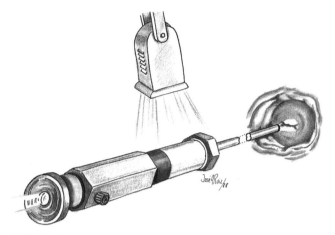

FIG 14–4.
Distribution of light. First the light is collected in the light trap, then distributed to illuminate the object, and finally carried back to the examiner's eye.

sorting to dilatation. Frequently, simple pressure on the cervical tissue is all that is required to stretch the tissue sufficiently to allow the smooth barrel of the endoscope to pass through the cervix into the uterine cavity.

Dilatation

Pratt dilators lubricated with Hyskon or water-soluble jelly offer gentle, atraumatic means for dilating the internal os of the cervix. This may be necessary when dealing with the narrowed, atrophic endocervical canal encountered when examining postmenopausal women. Obviously, dilatation is painful and should be preceded by the injection of 6 to 8 cc of 1% lidocaine (Xylocaine) directly into the cervix at the 12, 3, 6, and 9 o'clock positions. A 3-cc syringe equipped with a 25- or 27-gauge needle is preferred to carry out this maneuver.

When the contact endoscope is used, a gentle touch and very light contact with the structure to be viewed is important. The distance between the object and the extremity of the endoscope must be zero or nearly zero to obtain a clear image. Incident light from the room or other directed sources penetrates into the guide by the proximal extremity and exits at the distal end into the uterine cavity, where it illuminates the object under

scrutiny. The reflected light brings the image back to the observer's eye through the same guide. The loss of light is minimal, about 15%, due to its propagation by total reflection. Since the angles of entry and exit of the light rays are identical, the image is transmitted without distortion. The quality of the image obtained with the contact optical system is excellent. The distally coated convexity of the system is in direct contact with the mucosa, which is always covered by a thin film of liquid and acts as its own immersion lens (Fig 14–5). This means better

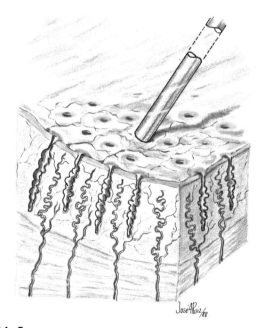

FIG 14–5.
As the distal convexity of the hysteroscope comes into light contact with the liquid film covering the mucosa, an oil-immersion lens is produced.

transparency, a suppression of the light diffusion on the surface of the mucosa, and an "inside" view of the tissue with particularly good detail of vascular networks. Contact vision does not mean a total absence of relief, space, or volume. The depth of field of the current system is approximately 5 mm to surface, and the vision in this field is perfectly clear; the background beyond this range becomes gradually more and more blurred. The most decisive advantage of the contact system is that the intrauterine milieu plays no part in the vision or obstruction thereof because it does not exist between the endoscope and the area to be viewed (i.e., blood or other body fluids have been forced out by light tissue contact).

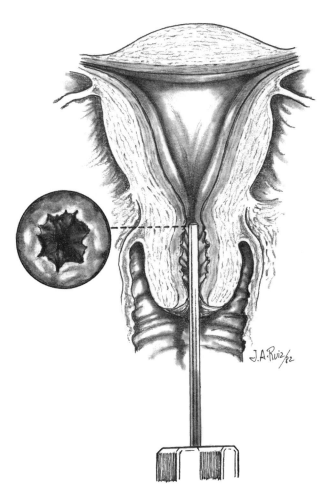

FIG 14–7.
Slight pressure is placed on the hysteroscope as its barrel passes the narrow isthmus.

TECHNIQUE

The vagina is prepared with povidone-iodine (Betadine), or a similar antiseptic solution, utilizing a large cotton swab. The cervix is then exposed with the single hinged speculum. The anterior lip of the cervix is next grasped with a single-toothed tenaculum. Under direct vision, the endoscope is engaged at the external os, and the cervical canal is inspected (Fig 14–6, A). Care should be taken to make very light contact with the mucosa. Too little contact will result in the intrusion of blood, and too much pressure will result in compression of the tissue to such an extent that only white is seen. With the correct technique, the arborescent aspects or columns of the plicae palmitae will be seen (Fig 14–6,B). It is preferred to inspect the posterior aspect of the canal up to the internal os, then pull the scope back to the external os and reinsert it and examine the anterior wall. Likewise, the instrument may be reinserted after a sam-

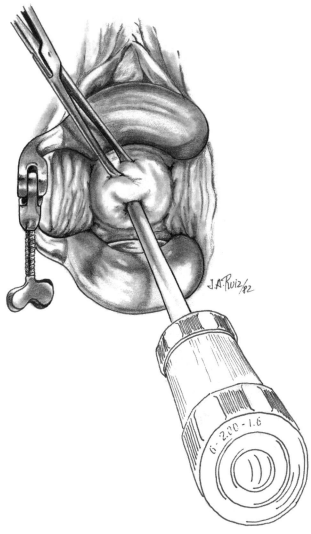

FIG 14–6.
A (above), the contact hysteroscope is gently engaged at the external os. **B** (see Plate 73), details of the endocervical mucosa are observed. Mucosal (pink) papillae are separated by clefts or tunnels.

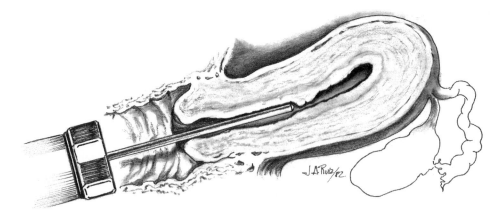

FIG 14—8.
The anterior wall of the uterus is examined maintaining light contact with the mucosa.

pling biopsy to determine whether the appropriate pathologic sample has been removed. For an ante-verted uterus, the endoscope must be angulated upward and anteriorly. To accomplish this maneuver the operator must sit very low in relation to the patient. Four percent acetic acid may be applied by inserting a wet, cotton-tipped applicator gently into the endocervical canal prior to the examination. The hysteroscope is then passed into the endometrial cavity. At the level of the isthmus it may be necessary to exert slight pressure on the instrument to make it enter the expanded uterine cavity. A definite plan or pattern should be followed in order to visualize the entire cavity. This necessitates moving the endoscope in and out of the cavity from the cervix (lower boundary) to the fundus (upper boundary). Our plan investigates the left wall, the anterior surface, posterior surface, right side-wall, and finishes with a back and forth sweep across the fundus (Figs 14–7 through 14–12). Inspection may be performed with this rigid instrument by proper angulation for each segment of the examination. Observation of the tubal ostia is best performed during the early proliferative phase of the cycle. Examination, however, may be done during any phase of the cycle, including the menstrual phase.

Since the viewing circle measures 6 mm in diameter, objects viewed within this circle may be sized. For example, a lesion occupying half this area may be approximated to measure 3 mm; one occupying three fourths of the space could be said to be 4 to 5 mm, and one filling the space would measure 6 mm. The objects seen outside the circle represent reflections from the interior mirrored, stainless steel sheath (Plate 74).

Appearance of Normal Endometrium

Proliferative phase endometrium is relatively flat, pink in color, and lacks any specific vascular pattern. If

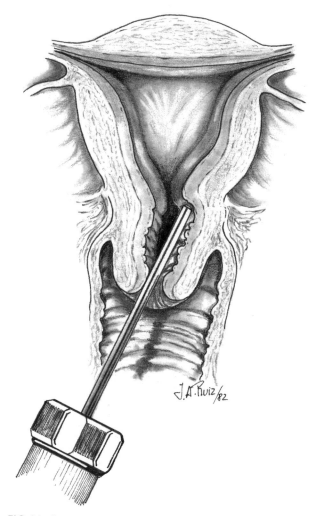

FIG 14—9.
The left side of the uterus is viewed from below upward.

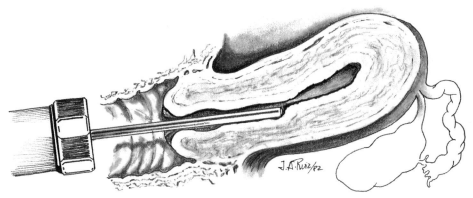

FIG 14–10.
The posterior wall is examined.

the end of the hysteroscope is held back from the surface 2 to 3 mm, small depressions or craters representing gland openings may be identified. Secretory endometrium is thick, polypoid, and appears deep red in color (Plate 75). As the endoscope moves across the endometrial surface, the mucosa does not peel away. Additionally, the relative thickness of the tissue may be determined by applying pressure with the barrel of the endoscope on the uterine surface and gauging the groove or depression that the instrument creates.

Atrophic endometrium and the tissue of women using contraceptive pills is flat, white, and generally devoid of vessels (Plate 76). On the other hand decidua is thick and white, with an occasional large, coiled vessel. As the endoscope is swept from side to side from one cornua to the other, the tubal ostia may be seen if the phase of the cycle is correct. The ostia are only seen

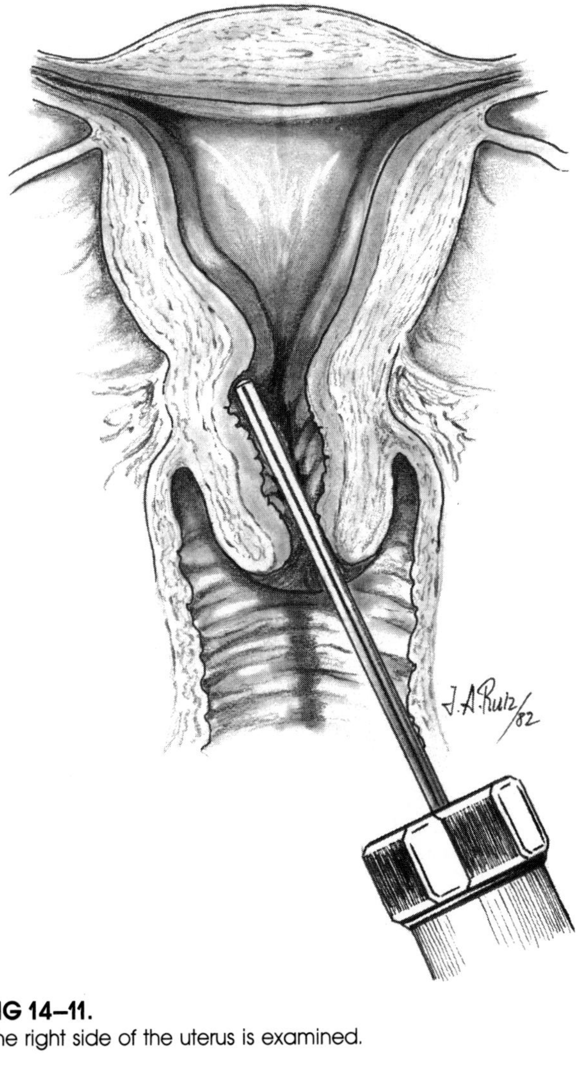

FIG 14–11.
The right side of the uterus is examined.

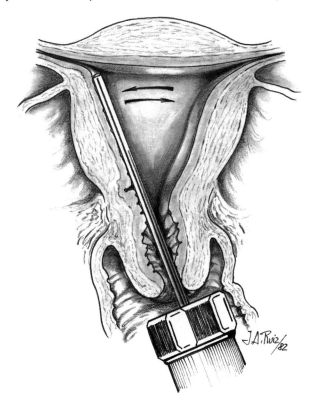

FIG 14–12.
The examination is completed with a fundal sweep.

during the early proliferative phase or when an atrophic mucosa pattern is present (Plate 77). The best results can be expected when the endoscope is guided carefully between the two opposing anterior and posterior uterine walls. When this can be accomplished bleeding is minimal, and the examination can be more easily done.

Evaluation of the Endocervical Canal

The normal endocervical canal is lined by mucous-secreting and tall columnar epithelium. In order to accommodate the large number of cells, a substantial surface area must be created; therefore, this surface is thrown into numerous folds and multiple branchings. The pattern of the folds may be described as polypoid or cobblestoned. At the bottom of these folds are the crypts (frequently misnamed "glands") or tunnels, which are especially prominent during pregnancy (Plate 78). A detailed view of the midportion of the canal shows the pink-white color of the epithelium and the relief of the folds. The instrument may come into contact with white, round protrusions or iridescent, pearl-like structures. These are cysts that result after the obliteration of the crypt orifices. The small cysts are equivalent to nabothian cysts seen on the endocervix (Plate 79). Because these formations are seen very frequently, they should not be considered pathologic. At the top of the endocervix, the lower portion of the uterine cavity can be seen.

One of the most frequent lesions seen by contact hysteroscopy is the endocervical polyp. This protrusion generally has a long, thin pedicle and is very mobile. One can precisely see the origin of the pedicle on a branch of the arbor vitae. These polyps are typical because they are covered with a very rich, netlike vascular pattern (Plate 80). The hairy, shaggy aspect of the vascular network is very different from the endometrial polyp. Sometimes the endocervical polyp is visible at the external os of the cervix, but most often, they are incidental findings seen during routine endoscopic evaluation of the canal. The contact hysteroscope is very useful in controlling the complete removal of the polyp, since knowledge of the exact location of the pedicle facilitates seizure of the polyp with forceps. Blind manipulations with the curette or forceps often leave the pedicle behind and may even cause a second or third polyp to be overlooked.

Cervical myomas projecting into the canal are rarely seen. The hysterogram demonstrates a round filling defect that can be seen protruding into the enlarged cervical canal (Fig 14–13). The hysteroscopic view of the defect is a white-yellow fibrous formation bulging into

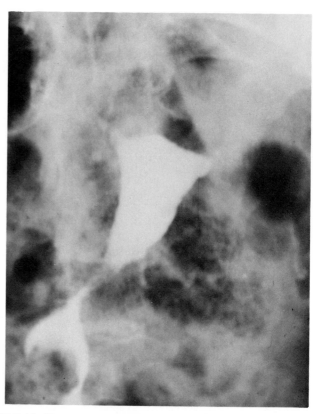

FIG 14–13.
A round filling defect protruding into the cervical canal can be seen in this hysterogram.

the canal. By touch, the lesion is firm and immobile. The diagnosis is therefore cervical myoma. Another relatively rare cervical lesion is endometriosis. This appears as blue-black spots that are visible on the walls of the endocervical canal. Hysteroscopy is frequently the only method by which to make a diagnosis because the lesions are rarely visible by hysterography (Plate 81).

Cervical intraepithelial neoplasia (CIN) is the most common neoplastic lesion of the cervix. When atypical epithelium extends into the cervical canal beyond the view of the colposcope, the 6-mm contact hysteroscope has been helpful to determine the extent and severity of the lesion as well as to direct biopsy equipment to the site of the lesion (Plate 82). Over 66 women who had endocervical extension of CIN were examined by the contact endoscope (Baggish and Dorsey, 1982). Essentially one is performing colposcopy in the canal. Since the diameter of the hysteroscope is fixed and known, the extension of the white epithelium may be accurately measured and related to a specific reference point (Plate 83). Examination by endoscopy is very useful during pregnancy, when endocervical curettage and/or conization may be hazardous. The instrument may be reinserted after sampling to be certain that the correct le-

TABLE 14–1.

Evaluation of 66 Women With Cervical Neoplasia Extending Into the Endocervical Canal

Colposcopic Biopsy	ECC*		Contact Endoscopy†			Excisional Cone (when done)		
	Negative	Positive	Less‡	Same	Worse	Less‡	Same	Worse
CIN I (11)	11	0	9	2	0	—	2	—
CIN II (17)	16	1	14	2	1	—	1	2
CIN III (33)	29	4	1	28	4	2	10	2
Invasive (3)	1	2	0	3	0	—	1	—
Negative (2)	1	1	0	0	2	—	1	1

*ECG = Endocervical curettage.
†Includes directed sampling
‡Compared with colposcopic biopsy.

sion has undergone biopsy. For lesions extending less than 6 mm into the canal (measuring from the external os), conservative techniques, for example, laser vaporization, may be done. When lesions are more than 6 mm from the external os, conization is done following hysteroscopy. The atypical epithelium is usually white and will frequently show atypical vascular patterns (e.g., punctuation or mosaic). Table 14–1 provides a list of the correlative findings relative to colposcopically directed biopsy, endocervical curettage, contact endoscopy with directed curettage, and conization. In the study done by Baggish and Dorsey, blind endocervical curettage resulted in eight positive diagnoses of CIN. Contact endoscopy plus directed curettage revealed 42 instances of CIN within the canal. Several of those cases extended only 6 mm or less from the level of the external os and were treated by laser vaporization (Table 14–2). In this same series, six cases of invasive carcinoma were diagnosed by endocervical endoscopy, two of which were primary adenocarcinomas of the endocervix (Plates 84 and 85). The latter were identified as stark white, waxy lesions that protruded into the canal. Although the recognized standard for determining the status of the endocervical canal is conization biopsy, this frequently requires general anesthesia and an operating room setting. Additionally, a sharp cone may be associated with cervical scar formation and sterility. Contact endoscopy is simpler and certainly less traumatic and therefore should be used prior to conization. There are virtually no complications associated with endoscopy.

Invasive epidermoid carcinoma of the cervix shows patterns similar to invasive adenocarcinoma of the endometrium by contact hysteroscopy (Plate 86). The tissue appears flocculent and gray with luminescent particles (Plate 87). Prior to sharp conization, the endocervical canal is thoroughly doused with 4% acetic

TABLE 14–2.

Treatment Regimen for 66 Women Following Endocervical Contact Hysteroscopy

Diagnosis*	Laser Excision Cone	Laser Vaporization	Radiation Therapy	Radical Surgery	Simple Hysterectomy
CIN I	2	9	0	0	0
CIN II	3	14	0	0	0
CIN III	14*	19	0	0	2†
Invasive epidermoid	0	0	1	0	2
Invasive adenocarcinoma	0	0	2†	2†	0
Total	19	42	3	3	4

*Two patients had cone excision, then hysterectomy.
†Two patients were treated by combination of radiation and radical hysterectomy.

acid by means of a small cotton-tipped applicator. Careful endoscopy may then be performed to approximate extension of epidermoid neoplasia into the canal. By using the diameter of the viewing circle of the endoscope, the height of the cone can be estimated preoperatively.

CONTACT CYSTOURETHROSCOPY

The urethra, bladder neck, and trigone are easily inspected with the patient in the dorsal lithotomy position. The vast majority of women require no anesthesia for the procedure. Use of the 6-mm contact endoscope seldom requires any dilatation of the meatus for easy acceptance, and, with very gentle dilatation, most patients will accept the 8-mm instrument with only minimal discomfort. The patient voids prior to the procedure, and the urethral meatus is then cleansed with a povidone-iodine solution and swabbed with 2% Xylocaine jelly (Plate 88).

The urethra is visualized throughout its length as the scope is inserted and again as it is withdrawn (Plate 89). The vesical neck is observed to open and close as the probe passes from urethra to bladder and back again. It is possible to gain some information about the sphincter mechanism if the patient is asked to attempt to void and then to cut off the urinary stream while the vesical neck is carefully observed from the urethral side (Plate 90). Usually the trigone and ureteral orifices are easily visualized, although it may be helpful to elevate the trigone by means of a finger placed in the vagina if the patient has a significant cystocele. The ureteral orifices and trigone are thereby manipulated into view of the scope (Plate 91).

The contact endoscope will usually afford a complete view of the bladder, although the use of a straight, direct view scope for bladder inspection may require some repositioning of the patient. Historically, in the early days of cystourethroscopy before the advent of "indirect" cystoscopy, air cystoscopy was performed with the patient in the knee-chest position. This position may allow easier access to the posterior bladder wall, as the force of gravity actually brings the trigone into contact with the air cystoscope. The knee-chest position may also be used in contact cystoscopy if difficulty is encountered in viewing the entire bladder. Upward pressure on the anterior abdominal wall will enable the anterior portions of the bladder to be seen more completely. In general, however, direct view endoscopy lends itself to inspection of urethra and trigone area, and cystoscopy is more easily accomplished with an angled scope.

BENIGN AND NEOPLASTIC LESIONS OF THE ENDOMETRIUM

Perhaps the most important application of the contact hysterscope is for the diagnosis of endometrial hyperplasia and carcinoma. Since this technique may be carried out with minimal preparation in virtually any setting (e.g., physician's office, emergency room, clinic, or operating room), it is ideally suited for investigative oncology.

Three general presentations of endometrial polyps may be identified by contact hysteroscopy. The histologic appearance of the polyp mirrors its appearance under the scrutiny of the contact hysteroscope. The lesion appears lighter or whiter than the surrounding normal endometrium and is characterized by thick-walled vascular channels (Plate 92). Polypoid endometrium presents as diffuse micropolyps covering a large area of the endometrial surface rather than a solitary discrete lesion. These small projections measure approximately 2 to 3 mm in height and 1 to 1.5 mm in width. Larger polyps are either pedunculated or sessile, depending on the characteristics and mobility of the pedicle (Plate 93). As the end of the contact hysteroscope encounters the lesion, the polyp swings or rotates away in a manner analogous to pushing a teabag with the index finger of one hand, while suspending the bag by its string with the other hand. The combination of the observed pattern of color, vasculature, encounter motion, and touch allow an accurate diagnosis of polyp. By careful manipulation, the polyp may be positioned to show the site of pedicle attachment and aid in its removal. Similarly, after inserting the polyp forceps and extricating the lesion, the operator may wish to reinsert the contact hysteroscope to ensure that no part of the polyp remains behind. The surface pattern of the polyp may vary in appearance, depending on whether the lesion is functioning or nonfunctioning: for example, cystic atrophy may appear as small bluish cysts, whereas a secretory polyp appears to be deep red, not dissimilar to the surrounding endometrium. The characteristics of the enlarged vasculature may be best appreciated by alternatively increasing and decreasing the pressure of the hysteroscope on the pedicle and observing the flow of blood through the vessels. Benign endometrial hyperplasia (benign cystic hyperplasia) presents a characteristic picture during contact endoscopy. The endometrium is thick and easily "grooves" with pressure produced by the hysteroscope. The endometrium is white to gray in color and shows multiple grayish cysts and craters mirroring the dilated glands so typical of "swiss cheese" hyperplasia (Plate 94). No atypical vessels are seen. Occasionally the cystic pattern is seen in conjunction with the diffuse polypoid changes noted earlier. Hertig and Sommers described a number of intrauterine pathologic conditions which they considered precursors to endometrial cancer. These consisted of endometrial polyps, endometrial hyperplasia, and adenomatous hyperplasia. Progression to malignancy is most frequent and occurs in the shortest time interval with atypical (adenomatous) hyperplasia. In 82% of endometrial hyperplasia cases which have been evaluated by contact hysteroscopy, bleeding was the major factor which led women to seek medical attention. The patterns of hyperplasia seen by contact endoscopy allow the gynecologist to make a presumptive diagnosis at the time of hysteroscopic examination; however, as with colposcopy (for cervical disease), the final diagnosis must await pathologic confirmation. Contact hysteroscopic observation lies between panoramic vision and microscopic views. The examiner's vision is within the tissue.

Plate 95 is a view of atypical hyperplasia as seen by contact hysteroscopy. As the degree of glandular proliferation and complexity increases, the epithelium appears whiter and raised; atypical vessels may also be observed. Some of the channels are long and thin; others are short and dilated. The latter changes are seen with severe degrees of atypical hyperplasia, but may also be observed in adenocarcinoma. In some instances, as is true with microscopic evaluation, the differentiation between severe atypical hyperplasia (Hertig's carcinoma in situ) and adenocarcinoma may be difficult or impossible. One of the major difficulties in the differential diagnosis of endometrial neoplasia when compared with cervical neoplasia is the fact that well-differentiated adenocarcinoma of the endometrium as well as its precursors appear to have a diploid chromosome pattern as compared with cervical carcinoma, which is aneuploid.

In a report published in *Gynecologic Oncology* in 1980, a tumor pattern that subsequently was characteristic of a mixed mesodermal sarcoma was thought to be a bleblike polypoid hyperplasia. Since that time, this pattern has been associated not only with uterine sarcomas but also with poorly differentiated adenocarcinomas. In the same series, atypical hyperplasia was misdiagnosed by contact hysteroscopy in 6% of the cases; these cases subsequently were revealed to be adenocarcinoma.

Adenocarcinoma presents characteristic patterns when viewed by the contact hysteroscope; therefore, the diagnosis and localization of tumors are easy. Figure 14–14 shows an irregular filling defect on hysterography. The defect extends from the right wall of the corpus to the isthmus. Panoramic CO_2 hysteroscopy examination of the same patient showed a polypoid process with a gray-white uneven surface extending onto the posterior

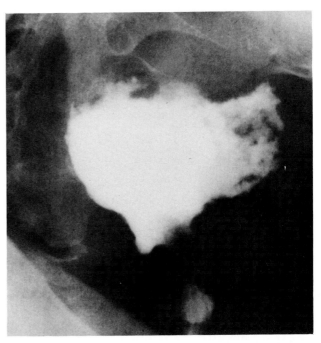

FIG 14–14.
A hysterogram suggests endometrial carcinoma. The study shows a ragged, irregular filling defect.

and right walls of the uterine cavity toward the isthmus. Contact hysteroscopy performed immediately after panoramic hysteroscopy showed white, irregular vegetations projecting from the mucosal surface and appearing in the field of the endoscope (Plate 96).

The question may be asked whether it is possible to classify endometrial carcinoma according to its gross appearance. Without hysterectomy this is only possible by examination of the hysterectomy specimen. Unfortunately this type of observation is substantially different from viewing dynamic, living tissue. Even previous curettage may substantially alter the original appearance of the tumor.

Sugimoto has proposed a classification according to the appearance of the tumor by panoramic hysteroscopy using a liquid distending medium. He describes four patterns: polypoid, nodular, papillary, and ulcerated. He was able to correlate hysteroscopic and histologic findings based on these types. Similarly, tumors can be identified by certain predominant patterns by contact hysteroscopy. However, one must recognize that most adenocarcinomas show more than one of these patterns and frequently show a full spectrum of changes. We could identify four major subcategories. (1) a vegetative lesion, gray in color, resembling cumulus clouds just before a summer thunderstorm with exuberant outgrowths ranging forth in many directions; (2) a cerebroid type, which is smooth and white, with a brainlike

TABLE 14–3.

Contact Hysteroscopic Patterns of
Adenocarcinoma

1. White epithelium, raised in relief
2. Gray, flocculant
3. Luminescence
4. Brain-like vessels
5. Abnormal vascular patterns

vascular pattern and small micropapillary projections whose convolutions are reminiscent of cerebral gyri (Plate 97); this pattern has been a consistent finding associated with well-differentiated adenocarcinoma and markedly atypical hyperplasia; (3) a luminescent or phosphorescent glow (which appears as zones of irregular staining, streaks, or spikes) to the cancerous tissue has been observed in almost every patient (Plate 98); (4) bleb formation associated with atypical vessels has been observed with poorly differentiated tumors (grade 3) as well as mixed mesodermal tumors. Atypical vessels may appear on a background of a smooth, waxy surface. In general, as the tumor becomes more dedifferentiated, very bizarre vascular changes are noted in a fashion analogous to the colposcopic patterns seen with invasive epidermodoid cancers of the cervix (Plate 99 and Table 14–3).

In a combined series of cases from Paris, France, and Syracuse, N.Y. (Table 14–4), 75 patients with endometrial carcinoma have been evaluated by contact hysteroscopy (42, France; 33, United States). Three women had endocervical tumors; the rest had primary adenocarcinoma of the endometrium. The ages of the patients in this combined series ranged from 37 years to 75 years of age, with the mode falling into the 59.5 range (61%). In every case in which endometrial cancer was discovered, the indication for contact hysteroscopy was abnormal bleeding. Ten patients (France) were referred by other physicians with a hysterogram suggestive of carcinoma. In the remaining 65 cases, no hysterography was performed. Endometrial sampling was always carried out to obtain material for pathologic diagnosis. A comparison between hysteroscopic and pathologic diagnoses indicated total agreement in 69 of the 75 cases (92%). In six cases, diagnosis of atypical hyperplasia was made by contact hysteroscopy. Therefore, the correlation between contact hysteroscopic and pathologic findings was excellent. No confusion occurred between benign cystic hyperplasia and adenocarcinoma. However, atypical hyperplasia may occasionally be confused with adenocarcinoma since delicate transitions are difficult to differentiate. The major advantage of contact hysteroscopy other than discovering the presence of tumor was to evaluate extension, particularly with respect to the isthmus. In spite of the fact that we had to deal with relatively older people, general anesthesia was unnecessary in half the cases. The use of contact hysteroscopy complemented by directed biopsy of the tumor can obtain the diagnosis, determine the extent of the tumor, and identify histologic type and pathologic grade. All information necessary for proper treatment is obtained without performing a fractional curettage. Thus, the potential danger of forcing cancer cells into the blood or lymphatic circulation or into the peritoneal cavity is minimized. This outpatient technique has been particularly helpful for following the progress of patients receiving estrogen replacement therapy as well as reassuring these women that they have no cancer.

THE CONTACT VAGINASCOPE

The differential diagnoses for vaginal bleeding in female infants and children include trauma, tumors, and

TABLE 14–4.

Comparison of Hysteroscopy and Pathologic Diagnoses in 75 Women
With Endometrial Endocervical Malignancies

Method of Diagnosis			
Hysteroscopy	Pathology	No.	%
Polypoid endometrium and hyperplasia	Mixed mesodermal tumor	1	1
Atypical hyperplasia	Adenocarcinoma, endometrium	6	8
Adenocarcinoma, endometrium	Adenocarcinoma, endometrium	65	87
Adenocarcinoma, endocervix	Endocervical adenocarcinoma	3	4
		75	100

infections. Even today rather poor, makeshift instruments are available with which to examine these children's vaginas, for example, the nasal specula. The contact hysteroscope has obvious advantages over current instrumentation. The smooth 6-mm hysteroscope can be inserted into the vagina of a newborn infant without trauma. The entire vagina including the fornices as well as the cervix may be viewed in detail (Plate 100). Foreign bodies may be felt as well as seen; swabs may be directed precisely under direct vision to a site of infection; tumors or other suspicious lesions may be sampled. When children are examined under awake but sedated conditions the lateral decubitus position or knee-chest position are the most conducive to good viewing, since the introitus is better exposed and the air distends the vagina.

BIBLIOGRAPHY

Baggish MS: The evaluation of the amniotic fluid by means of the contact endoscope. *Obstet Gynecol* (in press).

Baggish, MS: New instruments and techniques for hysteroscopy. *Contemp Obstet Gynecol* 1984; 22.

Baggish MS: Evaluation and staging of endometrial and endocervical adenocarcinoma by contact hysteroscopy. *Gynecol Oncol* 1980; 9:182.

Baggish MS: Contact hysteroscopy: A new technique to explore the uterine cavity. *Obstet Gynecol* 1979; 54:350.

Baggish MS, Barbot J: Contact hysteroscopy. *Clin Obstet Gynecol* 1983; 26:219.

Baggish MS, Barbot J: Contact hysteroscopy for easier diagnosis. *Contemp Obstet Gynecol* 1980; 16:3.

Baggish MS, Dorsey JH: Contact hysteroscopic evaluation of the endocervix as an adjunct to colposcopy. *Obstet Gynecol* 1982; 60:107.

Barbot J, Parent B, Dubuisson JB: Contact hysteroscopy: Another method of endoscopic examination of the uterine cavity. *Am J Obstet Gynecol* 1980; 136:721.

Barbot J, Parent B, Doeler B: Hysteroscopie de contact et cancer de l'endometre. *Acta Endosc* 1978; 8:17.

Dorsey JH, Diggs ES, Baggish MS: Cystourethroscopy with the direct view contact endoscope. *Obstet Gynecol* 1981; 57:115.

Dubuisson JB, Henrion R, Barbot J: Embryoscopie de contact. *J Gynecol Obstet Biol Reprod (Paris)* 1979; 8:39.

Hertig AT, Sommers SC: Genesis of endometrial carcinoma: 1. Study of prior biopsies. *Cancer* 1949; 2:946.

Parent B, Barbot J Dubuisson JB, et al: Hysteroscopie de contact. *Encycl Med Chir Paris* 1978; 72-B-10.

Parent B, Toubas C: Une nouvelle technique d'exploration de la cavite uterine: l'Hysteroscopie de contact. *Concours Med* 1973; 95:1635.

Sugimoto O: Hysteroscopic diagnosis of endometrial carcinoma. A report of fifty-three cases examined at the women's clinic of Kyoto University hospital. *Am J Obstet Gynecol* 1975; 121:105.

15

Hysteroscopy and Microcolpohysteroscopy in Gynecologic Oncology

Luca Mencaglia, M.D.

Antonio Perino, M.D.

MICROCOLPOHYSTEROSCOPIC EVALUATION OF BENIGN AND PREMALIGNANT LESIONS OF THE CERVIX

Intraepithelial dysplasias or neoplasias of the uterine cervix make up a group of well-defined morphologic lesions whose accurate and early diagnosis is essential prior to therapeutic intervention.

The technique of choice for mass screening of precancerous lesions of the cervix is cytology by means of cervical scraping and endocervical brush or swab sample. This is an extremely useful diagnostic method since it is simple to perform and is relatively inexpensive to process.

Although cytology is considered the method of choice for screening cervical neoplasia and its precursors, it should be remembered that it is not sufficient for the overall clinical and prognostic evaluation of disease. In fact this technique does result in some false positive, as well as false negative, readings ranging from 5% to 25%. Obviously cytology renders insufficient information to allow histologic grading, localization, or data about the extent of the lesion. Abnormal pap smears must be clinically evaluated by other more accurate methods. In the past, patients with abnormal cytologic results, routinely underwent diagnostic conization. "Conization" should be utilized sparingly for diagnostic purposes because of its invasiveness and consequent potential complications (bleeding, cervical stenosis and incompetence, difficult follow-up). Diagnostic

and therapeutic management of patients with abnormal pap smears have undergone a complete revolution since the popular acceptance of colposcopy by gynecologists throughout the world. Colposcopy enables the observer to view the uterine cervix at high magnification and to combine this with directed biopsy. This excellent technique allows greater accuracy and less invasiveness for identifying precancerous and cancerous lesions of the cervix. Unfortunately, although colposcopy permits the most satisfactory examination of the outer aspect of the cervix, the endocervical canal remains virtually inaccessible to direct vision. It is common knowledge that the location of the squamocolumnar junction (SCJ) varies in relation to the age of the patient and it is clearly located within the endocervical canal in a certain percentage of women. In particular, it is extremely important that the identification of the transformation zone, the SCJ, and the limits of a lesion, is requisite for a satisfactory colposcopic examination. An unsatisfactory colposcopy is discouraging to the patient who presents with an abnormal smear since it really or potentially will subject her to more radical and invasive diagnostic procedures. For example, it has been suggested that all patients must receive a thorough circumferential curettage as well as the punch biopsies. Factually, endocervical curettage (ECC) is not always reliable, since it does not allow the identification of the site from which the biopsy is taken. Furthermore ECC is a painful method of sampling when compared to other techniques. The goal of this chapter is to present the alternative technique of microcolpohysteroscopy (MCH) in diagnosing cervical diseases, particularly those involving the endocervical canal.

General Information on the Technique

The Instrument

The MCH is a relatively new endoscope which was invented and introduced by J. Hamou and extensively evaluated in Italy by the authors of this chapter. The instrument offers a wide range of magnifications ranging from ×1 to ×150 (Table 15–1). Magnifications in the order of ×1 to ×20 give a panoramic view similar to that obtained by colposcopy and traditional hysteroscopy. The higher magnifications offer an "in vivo" microscopic view similar to colpomicroscopy. Views at the lower magnifications (×1 to ×20) do not require special tissue preparation. The higher magnifications (×60 to ×150) require the application of vital staining (Lugol solution and Watermann blue) directly to the mucosal surface. After the aforesaid preparation, it is possible to observe the pattern of the superficial cell layers comprising the epithelia of the human cervix (Plate 101). Gentle pressure on a switching button easily allows one to change from one magnification to another. Since the instrument is small (4.5 mm in external diameter) and easy to handle, it is possible to observe adroitly both the endocervical canal and the endometrial cavity without trauma to the delicate tissues. With higher magnifications, light contact is made between the objective lens of the hysteroscope and the tissue to be viewed, there-fore no distending gas (CO_2) is required. With lower magnifications, panoramic vision is obtained and CO_2 is continuously insufflated through a sheath surrounding the barrel of the telescope. Flow rates of 30 cc/minute achieve the necessary dilatation to displace the lateral walls of the endocervical canal, and 40 to 50 cc/min will usually distend the endometrial cavity. No mechanical dilatation of the cervix or anesthesia is desired or required. The wide range of information that can be obtained with this instrument is shown schematically later in Table 15–2.

Exocervix and Vaginal Fornices

At low magnification MCH images are similar to the pictures observed with a colposcope. Colposcopy, however, provides a more detailed pattern, a wider view, and less distortion than that obtained by way of the oblique vision at 30° with the MCH. On the other hand, with contact vision, high magnification, and vital staining, the images obtained from the exocervix and endocervix are completely different, as follows. (1) The native squamous epithelium is characterized by a surface cell layer characterized by copious cytoplasm and pyknotic nuclei (Plate 102). (2) The transformation zone and the metaplastic epithelium contain less voluminous cells, with moderate cytoplasm and enlarged but quite regular nuclei (mature and immature metaplastic cells). The border area between the native squamous epithelium and the immature metaplastic epithelium is sharply demarcated because of the marked contrast produced

TABLE 15–1.

Magnification and Resolution Range From the Naked Eye to the Light Microscope

Means of Observation	Magnification	Depth of Angle of the Field	Resolution (μm)	Area of Investigation
Eye	1	450 mm	75	Exocervix
Colposcopy	6 to 40*	3 cm	15	Exocervix
Hysteroscopy position 1	1	4 cm	17	Exocervix, endocervix
Hysteroscopy position 2	20	1 cm	8	Exocervix, endocervix, uterine cavity
Microcolpohysteroscopy position 3	60	1.8 mm	2	Exocervix, endocervix, uterine cavity
Microcolpohysteroscopy position 4	150	1.1 mm	2	Exocervix, endocervix, uterine cavity
Light microscope (intermediate magnification)	150	1.3 mm	2	Cytology and histology

*Optimum at ×10.

by the iodine dark and iodine light cells (Plate 103). (3) The SCJ is easily identified since the squamous epithelium is blue, while the columnar cells do not take up the dye and have a clear papillary "finger in glove" aspect (Plates 104 and 105).

Endocervical Canal

Panoramic vision with lower magnification gives good information about the overall morphology of the endocervical canal: after application of 3% acetic acid it is often possible to detect the SCJ. The SCJ is always identified using the higher magnifications, finishing with a direct contact examination of the mucosal surface.

Endometrial Cavity

Detailed information obtained by panoramic MCH, for examination of the uterine cavity, has previously been reported by our team. Contact vision with higher magnification is rarely performed because of technical difficulties.

Clinical Study

We reported the experience of our unit, based on 506 unselected women who underwent MCH. Every patient had a pap smear and a colposcopic examination. Our first goal was to diagnose in each case the physiologic and pathologic parameters of the endocervix. Second, we determined the geography of each endocervical lesion, in order to improve prognosis and increase therapeutic accuracy. Out of the 506 cases, 25 patients with cervical intraepithelial neoplasia (CIN) were studied in detail.

These cases of CIN were studied according to the following criteria: (1) the presence or absence of viral cytopathic effects (Plate 106); (2) degree of cellular abnormalities (Plates 107 and 108); (3) the upper limit of CIN involvement (Plate 109); (4) the lower extent of the CIN area; and (5) the location of the epicenter of the lesion, that is, where the cytological abnormalities were most evident. Our observations were classified according to the criteria suggested by us in collaboration with J. Hamou and J. De Brux (Table 15–2).

Results

The results of MCH observation in our first series of 506 unselected patients are shown in Table 15–3. Cellular abnormalities of the transformation zone classified as D1 or D1+ were observed in 91 of 387 patients who were both cytologically and colposcopically negative for CIN, and in 54 of 60 cases with cytologic or colposcopic inflammatory abnormalities. Very marked cellular alter-

TABLE 15–2.

Classification of Microcolpohysteroscopic Observations*

D0	Transformation zone > 2mm
D1	Transformation zone < 2mm
	Irregular disposition of superficial cells with or without altered nucleo-cytoplasmatic ratio
	Anisonucleosis without severe nuclear alterations
	Dyscariosis with altered nucleo-cytoplasmatic ratio
	Atypical vessels
D1+	Atypical vessels with inflammation
D2	The alterations besides those in D1 with very frequent nuclear alterations: nuclei appear irregular in shape, increased in volume and hyperchromatic with evident mitotic activity.

*After J. Hamou and J. De Brux.

ations (D2) were observed in 12 of 38 cases of CIN grades I to II and in 18 of 20 cases of CIN grade III disease as well as in the only case of invasive carcinoma.

The results of the second series of MCH observations focused on 25 of 56 CIN cases detected in the first series. Results may be summarized as follows.

1. Viral cytopathic effects were suspected in seven (28%) cases.
2. The degree of cellular abnormalities is as summarized in Table 15–3.
3. The upper limit of the lesion was entirely exocervical in 17 (68%) cases and in part exocervical (on the anterior or posterior lip) in 4 (16%) cases (i.e., the lesion did not extend into the endocervical canal for more than 5 mm. In 4 (16%) cases the SCJ was endocervical.
4. The lower limit of lesion was localized less than 5 mm from the SCJ in 22 (88%) cases; in 2 (8%) cases it was located on the exocervix more than 5 mm from the SCJ; in 1 case (4%) the lesion involved the right lateral vaginal fornix.
5. The epicenter of the lesions was identified near to the SCJ in every case.

TABLE 15–3.

Microcolpohysteroscopic Observations in 506 Patients

Cytologic and Colposcopic Diagnosis	Microcolpohysteroscopic Classification			
	D0	D1	D1+	D2
Normal	296	58	33	—
Inflammation	6	26	28	—
CIN I to II without viral cytopathic effects	1	3	14	8
CIN I to II associated with viral cytopathic effects	—	—	8	4
CIN III	—	—	2	18
Invasive cancer	—	—	—	1

Apart from purely benign conditions (e.g., polyps, myomata, benign hyperplasia) and premalignant conditions (e.g., atypical hyperplasia), the most significant disease seen in these patients is endometrial neoplasia. Hysteroscopy has proved to be an extremely reliable method for the diagnosis of this group of diseases. The endoscopic pattern of endometrial cancer is reasonably obvious and is rarely confused with other lesions. In its initial stage the adenocarcinoma shows a germinative picture, with irregular, polylobate, friable projections that are usually necrotic and bleed easily (Plates 114 and 115). Vascularization is irregular and bizarre (Plate 116). In some cases a distinct zone between the neoplasia and the normal endometrium can be seen. It is sometimes possible to see focal lesions, often in the cornu where they could easily be missed with the use of blind sampling techniques. The macroscopic view of the endometrium can correlate with changes in the glandular structure, which are likewise observed by microscopic examination. Seventy percent of our cases were categorized as stage I disease, (i.e., limited to the uterine corpus) (Plates 117 and 118). Spread to the cervical canal (Plate 119) was identified hysteroscopically with high accuracy. In 17 patients with confirmed histologic diagnosis of endometrial neoplasia in the cervix, hysteroscopic diagnosis agreed in 94.2% of cases (Plates 117 through 119).

In conclusion, although the diagnostic accuracy of hysteroscopy was extremely high, it should not be considered an end unto itself but rather as a portion of the investigation to be used in concert with endometrial biopsy. Hysteroscopy can be used for the selection of those patients who are at risk for malignant disease of the endometrium as well as to help direct the biopsy in order to establish an accurate diagnosis. In the same vein, hysteroscopy is a useful tool for excluding further investigations in those patients who show no evidence of disease. The number of cases in which hysteroscopy observation is sufficient, without the help of a subsequent biopsy for reaching a diagnosis, will depend directly on the endoscopist's experience. It is possible,

TABLE 15–5.

Incidence of Menometrorrhagia and Endometrial Histomorphology in 1,295 D&C Patients*

Condition	%
Functional or asynchronous endometrium	66.6
Hypoatrophy	72.5
Adenomatous hyperplasia	77.4
Endometrial polyps	78.1
Glandular hyperplasia	79.3
Adenocarcinoma	97.2
Cystic hyperplasia	100.0

*From Zampi G, et al: *Morfologia delle lesioni preneoplastiche dell'endometrio: In apporto alla ricerca di base all controllo della crescita neoplastica.* Napoli, Idelson, 1981. Used with permission.

even after substantial practice in the use of hysteroscopy, to identify patients suffering from benign or malignant endometrial disease with a 20% rate of false positive but no false negative diagnoses. It is therefore clear that the association of hysteroscopy and biopsy can approach 100% accuracy in the diagnosis of endometrial neoplasia and its precursors. The technical features of the method, shown in Table 15–4, illustrate that a combination of hysteroscopy and directed biopsy offer the best technique, for the early detection of endometrial neoplasia and its precursors.

In dealing with benign and malignant endometrial lesions, account must be taken that in a great number of cases the first symptom is bleeding. Zampi et al. analyzed the incidence of menometrorrhagia linked to the endometrial histomorphology in a series of 1,295 women (Table 15–5). It is interesting to note that although cystic hyperplasia and endometrial neoplasia both produced bleeding in an extremely high number of cases, other lesions were heralded by the same symptom. It can therefore be stated that hysteroscopy is a reasonable technique for the examination of women 45 years or older who are suffering from abnormal bleeding. Its application in association with endometrial biopsy is particularly useful for the early detection of endometrial adenocarcinoma, but it can also render a correct diagnosis for benign disorders which similarly result in abnormal bleeding.

TABLE 15–4.

Technical Features of Hysteroscopy

Fairly invasive technique
Fairly expensive
Very accurate in the diagnosis of all benign and malignant lesions
Possible association with endometrial biopsy, with resulting increase in diagnostic accuracy
Performed without anesthesia or cervical dilatation as an office procedure
Acceptable by the patient
Very few complications

BIBLIOGRAPHY

Antoine T, Grunberger V: Kolpomicroscopic. *Klin Med* 1949; 4:575.
Cittadini E, Allegra A, Perino A: *L'Endoscopia Ginecologica.* Palermo, COFESE Publisher, 1983.

Cronje HS: Diagnostic hysteroscopy after postmenopausal uterine bleeding. *S Afr Med J* 1984; 20:773.

Dargent D, Scasso JC: Hysteroscopy-curettage under local anesthesia in the exploration of abnormal uterine bleeding. *Rev Fr Gynecol Obstet* 1984; 4:293.

Deutschmann C, Lueken RP, Lindemann HJ: Hysteroscopic findings in postmenopausal bleeding, in Siegler AM, Lindemann HJ (eds): *Hysteroscopy: Principles and Practice.* Philadelphia, J B Lippincott Co, 1983.

Dexeus S, Labastida R, Galera L: Oncological indications of hysteroscopy. *Eur J Gynaec Oncol* 1982; 2:61.

Donegan WL, Wharton JT: Carcinoma of the endometrium: A survey of practice. *Am Coll Surg Bull* 1984; 68:5.

Ferenczy A: Management of the patients with an abnormal pap smear, in Ballon SC (ed): *Gynecologic Oncology Controversies in Cancer Treatment.* Boston, G K Hall, 1981, p 141.

Gasparri F, Scarselli G, Mencaglia L: Studio pilota per l'attuazione dello screening per il carcinoma dell'endometrio. *Oncol Ginecol* 1984; 3:5.

Hamou JE: Microhysteroscopy. A new procedure and its original application in gynecology. *J Reprod Med* 1981; 26:375.

Hamou JE: Hysteroscopie et microhysteroscopie avec un instrument nouveau: le microhysteroscope. *Endosc Gynecol* 1980; 2:131.

Larsson G: Conization for preinvasive and early invasive carcinoma of the uterine cervix. *Acta Obstet Gynecol Scand* (suppl)114, 1983.

Mencaglia L, Perino A, Hamou JE: Hysteroscopy in perimenopausal and postmenopausal women with abnormal uterine bleeding. *J Reprod Med* 1987; 32:577.

Mencaglia L, Scarselli G: Etat precanceroux et canceroux de l'endometre, in Hamou JE (ed): *Hysteroscopie et Microcolpohysteroscopie.* Palermo, COFESE Publisher, 1985, p 143.

Mencaglia L, Scarselli G, Tantini C: Hysteroscopic evaluation of endometrial cancer. *J Reprod Med* 1984; 29:791.

Mencaglia L, Tantini C, Del Prete G, et al: La metrorragia nella donna in menopausa: Prospettive di un nuovo approccio diagnostico e terapeutico, in Atti del LWI Congresso della Societá Italiana di Ginecologia ed Ostetricia, Monduzzi, Bologna, 1982, Vol I, p 196.

Perino A, Cittadini E: Metrorragies, in Hamou JE (ed): *Hysteroscopie et Microcolpohysteroscopie.* Palermo, COFESE Publisher, 1985, p 117.

Perino A, Cittadini E: Metrorragies, in Hamou JE (ed): *Hysteroscopie et Microcolpohysteroscopie.* Palermo, COFESE Publisher, 1983, p 117.

Zampi G, Colafranceschi M, Taddei G: *Morfologia delle lesioni delleéndometrio: In apporto alla ricerca di base al controllo della crescita neoplastica.* Napoli, Idelson, 1981.

16

Hysteroscopy and Hysterosalpingography

Jacques Barbot, M.D.

Has hysterography become an obsolete method of diagnosis, and will hysteroscopy replace it? Since the renewed interest in hysteroscopy, this question has been commonly asked. For a long time, hysterography was the only feasible method to visualize the uterine cavity, and a high degree of refinement was attained in the interpretation of the hysterogram. On the other hand, hysteroscopy was considered a curiosity without practical value. As the efficiency of hysteroscopy was increasing, its confrontation with hysterography gradually showed the weak points of the radiologic method. Today the current has reversed in the same excessive way, and the tendency is to consider hysterography as an outmoded technique that has lost its utility.

Long experience with the two techniques and a constant comparison of the results provided by each of them has shown that each technique has inherent defects and strength; often the two are complementary. Certainly hysteroscopy is the most direct method of investigation that integrates all the richness and nuances of the visual sense in enabling one to reach the right diagnosis. Shape, contours, relief, colors, vasculature, consistency, and mobility are sight-oriented parameters. Hysterography is an indirect method, using a contrast medium in an attempt to disclose the contour of the uterine cavity and providing only black-and-white shadows. Nevertheless, this technique of investigation is very delicate, and the contrast medium is often able to find its way into structures that remain out of reach of visual examination.

TECHNIQUE OF HYSTEROSALPINGOGRAPHY

The technique of hysteroscopy is fully described in this book and will not be redescribed. The methodology of hysterosalpingography (HSG) is simple, but it is worthwhile to specify certain points of importance. HSG provides valuable information only when the procedure is performed with technical perfection. We will not describe the technique in detail but will emphasize the main points that are essential for a correct interpretation of the x-ray images.

A water-soluble contrast medium should be used to obtain the most discriminating images of the uterine cavity and the fallopian tubes. The spreading of the medium must be observed under fluoroscopic control in order to time the x-ray images at definite stages of the filling, with each stage providing specific information. With this technique, five judiciously taken films are amply sufficient for a complete investigation. The first image is taken during initial filling; very little dye is instilled in order to obtain a halftone image that reveals the details of the mucosa and small filling defects. The second is taken after complete filling of the uterine cavity. This image is used to determine uterine contour, size, and general configuration. It may demonstrate an abnormality of the uterus such as congenital malformation, endometrial polyp, myoma, or endometrial carcinoma. It also reveals the anatomy and patency of the tubes. Normally the dye should reach the distal end of the tubes and spill freely into the pelvis. The third is an anteroposterior image. It provides information about the position of the uterus and can enable detection of displacements such as retroversion. It is also needed to determine the exact location of a filling defect with respect to the anterior or posterior wall of the uterus. The course of the tubes is also visualized. The fourth image is taken after removal of the cannula during evacuation of the dye. It gives an overall view of the genital tract and allows optimal study of the internal os and endocervix. The fifth image is very important for infertility evaluation. It is taken 15 to 20 minutes after removal of the cannula. It will enable one to confirm whether the tubes are normally patent, with dye dispersing freely into the abdominal cavity, or whether the dye is trapped within diseased tubes (e.g., in the case of hydrosalpinx) or has become loculated in the peritoneal cavity (e.g. in the case of adhesions).

Some technical mistakes are not uncommon when performing HSG and may be responsible for erroneous interpretation. The investigation should be performed during the proliferative phase of the menstrual cycle. The atony of the uterus due to the action of progesterone may be misleading. Uterine bleeding is a contraindication, since blood clots cause artificial filling defects on the imaging study. The introduction of air bubbles during filling by way of the cannula may cause artifacts suggestive of intrauterine disease. In the same way a cannula that is not tightly sealed at the cervix may cause leakage of the contrast medium and artifacts. Failure to apply enough traction on the cervix in order to correct for anteversion or retroversion will not allow adequate exposure of the uterus perpendicularly to the x-rays and results in distortion and foreshortening of the image. Nonremoval of a radiopaque speculum after fixing the cannula to the cervix will obtund meaningful evaluation of the endocervical canal. All of these mistakes can be easily avoided.

APPEARANCE OF THE NORMAL UTERINE CAVITY AS VISUALIZED BY HYSTEROGRAPHY AND BY HYSTEROSCOPY

What is seen of the uterine cavity on the radiograph is in fact the geometric projection of this cavity on a flat surface (the radiographic plate). The uterus should be parallel to the plate to maintain the right proportions in the final image. An accurate mapping of the cavity is obtained with a small enlargement because the film is not in contact with the uterus (Fig 16–1).

On the normal hysterogram the endocervical canal appears as a fusiform cavity tapering toward the internal os. The pattern of the arbor vitae stands out as a net-

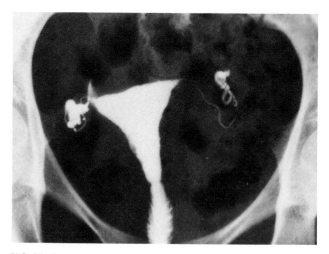

FIG 16–1.
Normal hysterogram. Note the irregular pattern of the endocervical canal due to the "plicae palmitae" and the mucous glands. The two chambers of the endometrial cavity are indicated by the change in direction of the lateral contours.

work of denser lines. The contours are made irregular by the injection of crypts and mucous glands forming oblique diverticula. These irregularities are variable and inconstant, and often make the evaluation of the endocervix difficult. The isthmus is a narrow channel with a stricture at each end. The endometrial cavity appears as a triangle, roughly isoceles, with the short base up. In fact, the lateral sides of the hysterogram are not straight lines but are made up of two segments forming an angle about halfway between the internal os and the tubal ostium, with the upper segment diverging out. Thus the endometrial cavity is divided into two parts. The lower part above the internal os is rather narrow and funnel-shaped. The upper part widens out and includes the fundus in the middle and the two cornua laterally. The tubal ostia are often marked by a stricture followed by a dilated triangle corresponding to the initial portion of the tube. We will not describe the tube further as it cannot be investigated hysteroscopically, and no comparison is possible.

The hysteroscopic panoramic view of the uterine cavity is radically different. The cavity is seen in perspective in a lengthwise direction and the proportions are no longer maintained, the foreground being enlarged compared with the background. The distortion is dramatically increased by the optical instrument through which the inside of the uterus is scrutinized. If this situation is advantageous for the study of small details, a mental correction is always necessary to restore the true size and extent of each structure relative to the others. With panoramic hysteroscopy the endocervical canal appears as a barrel-shaped cavity. Its cross section is circular (Plate 120). It is best examined during the removal of the endoscope, after the endometrial cavity has been evaluated. The leakage of the distending medium is less important than passage through the isthmus where distention must be optimal. The relief of the arbor vitae, made up of longitudinal and oblique folds separated by furrows, is nicely displayed. The internal os appears as a dark, round hole; its size depends on the pressure of the distending medium (Plate 121). After the isthmus is passed, the endometrial cavity is viewed as a suite of two chambers connected by a large opening (Plate 122). The lower chamber, which is cone-shaped with the vertex down, often appears cylindrical because of the distortion of the optical system. The upper chamber is composed of a central portion, the fundus, and two lateral conical alcoves, which are the cornua joined by the tube at the vertex (Plate 123). The communication of the two main chambers corresponds to the angulation we described on the hysterogram lateral outlines. Hysteroscopically it is an oval or circular opening with blunt or sharp edges depending on the degree of divergence of the two horns. The thickness, color, vasculature, and consistency of the mucous membrane covering the uterine cavity vary with the time of the menstrual cycle. Hysteroscopy has demonstrated that the stricture followed by a dilated triangle—often visible at the origin of the tube on the hysterogram and considered at one time as a sphincter—was in fact a mucosal fold (Fig 16–2). Hysteroscopically the tubal ostium may show various appearances. It may be circumscribed by a circular mucosal fold followed by a dilated portion. In that case the first millimeters of the intramural portion of the tube can be evaluated, and small tubal polyps may be disclosed. The mucosal fold can be incomplete (i.e., semi-

circular). Sometimes the ostium is reduced to a plain, narrow hole without any fold or dilatation (Plate 124). In reality the tubal ostium is often punctiform, as can be established by contact hysteroscopy. Only the pressure of the distending medium makes it appear wide open.

We have now described two different representations of the same uterine cavity. The hysterographic perspective has cartographic qualities and we can refer to it each time we want to know the exact configuration of the premises. The hysteroscopic perspective is the eye within the cavity, which provides the details accurately.

TYPICAL APPEARANCE OF THE MOST COMMON ABNORMALITIES AS VISUALIZED BY HYSTEROGRAPHY AND BY HYSTEROSCOPY

The achievement of the correct diagnosis based on the hysterogram necessitates study of direct signs resulting from the presence of the lesion itself, such as a filling defect or a diverticulum, as well as the study of indirect signs due to the repercussion of the lesion on the uterine cavity. Some of those signs have been described as typical of a definite lesion. The hysteroscopic approach is different, since the lesion is seen directly, and the collection of information is much greater and varied.

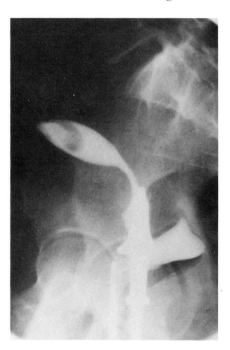

FIG 16–3.
Hysterogram with a filling defect typical of a polyp. This antero-posterior film is necessary to demonstrate the site of implanation of the polyp. The pedicle is located on the posterior wall near the fundus.

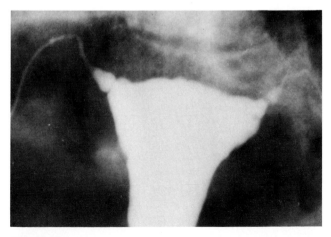

FIG 16–2.
Hysterogram demonstrates the initial portion of the tubes marked by a stricture followed by a dilated triangle. This aspect was thought at one time to be due to a sphincter.

Emphasis will be placed on the hysterographic signs, since the hysteroscopic appearance of most lesions has been thoroughly described in the chapter concerning abnormal uterine bleeding.

Endometrial Polyps

On the hysterogram the direct sign of endometrial polyps is a filling defect having a contour which is regular but not too sharp and which tends to fade as the instillation of the contrast medium increases (Fig 16–3). This defect is also mobile during the filling of the uterine cavity (Fig 16–4). The pedicle is sometimes visible and its implantation is determined on the anteroposterior film. The outline of the uterine cavity is not distorted but quite normal, this being in favor of a soft formation. However, in the case of a very large polyp, a distorted hysterogram may be suggestive of a myoma (Fig 16–5).

The diagnosis of a polyp is practically never missed by the hysteroscopic examination (Plate 125). The appearance of the overlying mucosa allows one to determine whether it is functional or nonfunctional (Plate 126).

Submucous Myomas

In the case of submucous myomas the typical hysterogram demonstrates a round, regular filling defect (Fig 16–6). The base of implantation, which appears on the anteroposterior film, is broad. The location of the defect does not change during the filling of the cavity. The main feature is the distortion of the hysterogram which results from the firmness of the lesion, the con-

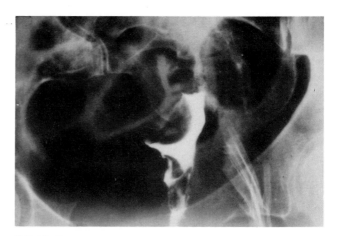

FIG 16–5.
Hysterogram shows a large circular but regular filling defect typical of a submucous myoma.

tours becoming convex. Sometimes the whole cavity seems blown up. In the case of a purely intramural myoma no filling defect is visible, and only the distortion of the hysterogram is suggestive of the lesion.

The hysteroscopic diagnosis of a myoma is easy (Plate 127). The hemispheric protrusion bulging into the uterine cavity is regular, smooth, firm, and covered with atrophic endometrium and dilated vessels. The pedunculated fibroid is less typical and may resemble an endometrial polyp. The purely intramural myoma is difficult to detect, as the distortion of the endometrial cavity is its only sign and is not hysteroscopically obvious.

Endometrial Hyperplasia

Diffuse endometrial hyperplasia is typically characterized by numerous regular filling defects of different

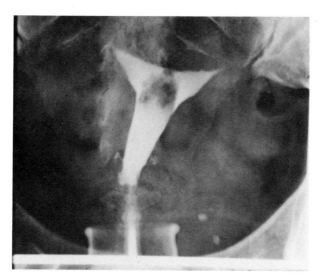

FIG 16–4.
Polyp with filling defect in the uterine cavity.

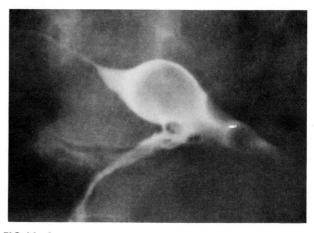

FIG 16–6.
Circular filling defect suggestive of a submucous myoma as the endometrial cavity is distorted.

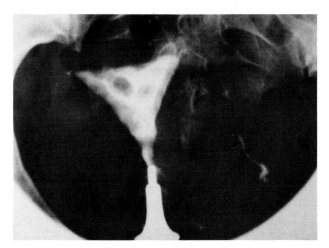

FIG 16–7.
Hysterogram demonstrates a typical diffuse endometrial hyperplasia characterized by numerous regular filling defects.

sizes and separated by denser outlines (Fig 16–7). The whole hysterogram looks dappled and the contours are often hazy or indented, but the cavity is not distorted. The diagnosis of focal hyperplasia is much more difficult and is often missed. The only sign may be an inconstant defect appearing on the initial filling and then disappearing.

Although the diagnosis of hyperplasia may be difficult hysteroscopically, the visual examination usually provides extra information concerning the type of hyperplasia—which can be plain, polypoid, or cystic (Plate 128). It is most important to find any areas of atypical hyperplasia that might be undetectable on the hysterogram (Plate 129).

Endometrial Carcinoma

The extended carcinoma usually exhibits characteristic features on the hysterogram (Fig 16–8). The filling defect is not uniform and has a jagged contour. Many terms have been commonly used in Europe to depict it, such as "boggy" or "moth-eaten." A portion of the hysterogram may appear to be "amputated." The intravasation of the contrast medium is not uncommon, and its consequences concerning dissemination of cancer cells may alarm some physicians. Additionally, the early carcinoma does not always present a typical appearance, and the diagnosis may be missed. Staging of the tumor can also be established on the hysterogram, but it has already been demonstrated that hysteroscopy yields more accurate results.

Several hysteroscopic patterns of invasive endometrial carcinoma have been described, among which the

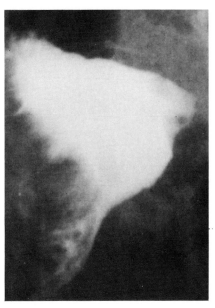

FIG 16–8.
Hysterogram is suggestive of an endometrial carcinoma displaying a very irregular, "ragged" filling defect especially along the right lateral outline.

vegetating type is the most common (Plate 130). The main advantage of visual control is to provide directed sampling of small, uncertain lesions and thus allow earlier diagnosis (Plate 131).

Endometrial Atrophy

In the case of endometrial atrophy the hysterogram shows a small, narrow endometrial cavity with thin, elongated horns (Fig 16–9). The uterine outline is often unsharp and irregular with spicules or diverticula (Fig 16–10). A double contour is sometimes apparent. Filling defects and even disappearance of a part of the uterus are not unusual. These result from intrauterine adhesions of atrophic origin. Trophic disturbances can also contribute to intravasation of the contrast medium. These signs of involution, which are usual in elderly women, may take on alarming appearances, simulating adenocarcinoma. In any case, such a hysterogram generally incites further investigation (Fig 16–11).

The hysteroscopic appearance of the atrophic endometrial cavity does not have an alarming appearance. The endometrium is reduced to a thin, transparent layer that clings tightly to the relief of the underlying myometrium (Plate 132). The recesses between the muscular bundles are not filled in by the thickness of the mucosa, accounting for the irregular contours of the hysterogram. Nowhere is there an outgrowth of mucosa,

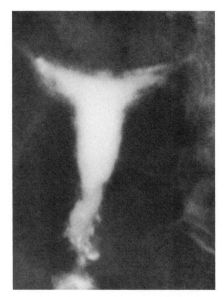

FIG 16–9.
Hysterogram suggestive of endometrial atrophy. The uterine cavity is small with narrow horns and the outline is hazy, displaying here a double contour.

thereby ruling out the possibility of adenocarcinoma. Should the hysteroscopist have any doubt, the curette will usually recover no material.

Adenomyosis

Adenomyosis is an abnormality that occasionally may be demonstrated by the hysterogram (Fig 16–12,A and B). The direct finding of diverticula appear typically as right-angle branchings from the uterine contour and terminate as small, round, pinhead-like dilatations. Only foci of adenomyosis that are in direct continuity with the mucosal surface are thus revealed. Isolated lesions whose presence are not visible tend to generate sufficient surrounding fibrosis so as to modify the general shape and elasticity of the uterine walls. Indirect radiologic findings may therefore suggest adenomyosis, for example, a swollen, enlarged horn or a distorted uterine cavity composed of rigid segments making sharp angles. The "tuba erecta" image is characterized by the initial portion of the oviduct turning upward in an unusual manner (Fig 16–13).

The hysteroscopic signs of adenomyosis are not so diverse. The entrance of the diverticula can be visualized provided the mucosa is not too thick. Systematic scrutiny of the endometrial surface allows the endoscopist to determine the number and the shape of the orifices (Plate 133). Obviously details within the uterine wall such as length and direction of the diverticula cannot be evaluated hysteroscopically. Additionally, the ef-

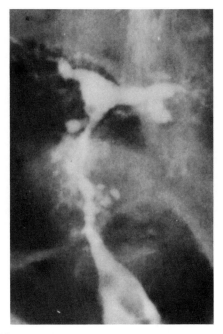

FIG 16–10.
This hysterogram displays a small uterine cavity with numerous diverticula.

fect of the disease on the uterine walls is not perceived (Plate 134).

Intrauterine Adhesions

The hysterographic features of Asherman's syndrome are well documented (Fig 16–14). The synechiae appear as sharply outlined filling defects forming various geometrical designs such as triangles and lozenges. They are constant in shape and demarcation on all the film images. This is an important feature, since a polyp,

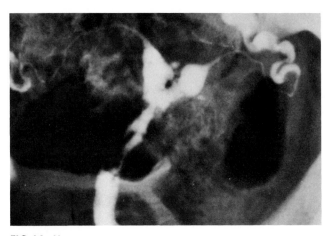

FIG 16–11.
The uterine cavity is small and narrow and displays numerous diverticula.

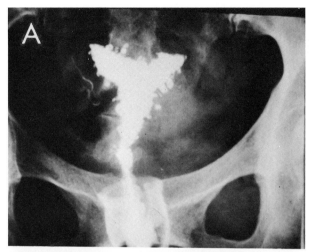

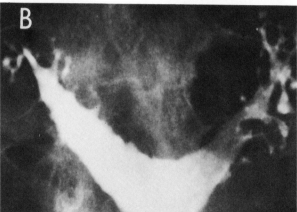

FIG 16–12.
A and **B,** hysterograms show direct signs of adenomyosis. The contrast medium has injected numerous diverticula.

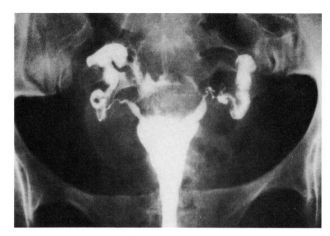

FIG 16–13.
Indirect sign of adenomyosis: the "tube erecta" image.

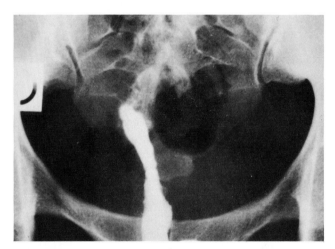

FIG 16–14.
Extensive adhesions obliterate more than 50% of the uterine cavity.

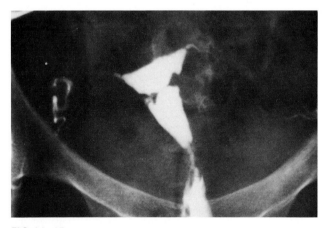

FIG 16–15.
Filling defect typical of a marginal synechia. In this case the adhesion is circular and is visible on both lateral contours of the hysterogram.

for example, will more or less fade as the filling advances. Adhesion location may be endocervical, corporeal, central, or marginal with respect to the uterine walls. In more severe cases, a combination of central and marginal defects will form the hysterogram in such a way that the pattern is virtually beyond description (Fig 16–15). A large part of the uterine cavity may be missing, but the remaining part can usually be accurately delineated. A gradation of disease severity has been proposed based on the estimated surface (as seen on the hysterogram) that has disappeared. A complete blockage at the internal os will not allow the condition of the uterine cavity to be demonstrated.

Hysteroscopy demonstrates not only the location, shape, and size of the adhesions but also their nature. These can be mucosal, fibrous, or myometrial. The endoscopic view also evaluates the status of the remaining endometrium (i.e., functional or nonresponsive to hormones). This extra information is of great value for the

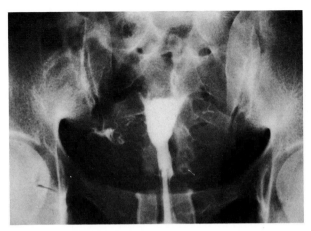

FIG 16–16.
Postoperative hysterogram of patient in Plate 135 three months after treatment.

treatment and subsequent prognosis of the disease. The unique central adhesion is the easiest to visualize. It stands like a column with broadening ends connecting the opposite uterine walls. The marginal adhesion, which is more or less embodied into the lateral uterine wall, is more difficult to perceive. It appears like a crescent or a half-drawn curtain which hides a cornu and creates an asymmetric aspect to the uterine cavity. The mucosal adhesion has the same color as the surrounding endometrium and is easily broken by the pressure of the hysteroscope. The prognosis is excellent. The fibrous or myometrial bands are whitish in color and resistant (Plate 135). Their treatment may be difficult. The complex marginal central scars can divide the uterine cavity into several smaller chambers some of which are concealed to visual examination (Fig 16–16). In such a case, thorough preoperative evaluation of the disease is not possible hysteroscopically. Special mention should be made of the intrauterine adhesions resulting from tuberculosis (Netter's syndrome). This diagnosis may be suggested by the appearance of a network of small alveoli coating the uterine walls. The fundus indeed looks like a honeycomb. The hysterosalpingogram details involvement of the tubes similarly suggestive of pelvic tuberculosis.

Location of an Intrauterine Device

Hysterography has been proposed for the location of an IUD when the filament of the device is no longer visible. A plain radiograph or pelvic ultrasound scan should be obtained first to rule out an unnoticed expulsion. If the device appears on the film, injection of dye and comparison between a front and an anteroposterior film will allow one to know whether the IUD is within or outside the endometrial cavity. More accurate information concerning the exact position of the device is difficult to infer from the hysterogram (Fig 16–17).

Hysteroscopy has now replaced hysterography in the search of a "lost IUD." The visual examination provides substantial additional information concerning the situation of the filament which is not visible on the radiograph, the extent of the displacement, and possible embedment or fragmentation (Plate 136). Visual examination is also recommended in cases of poor tolerance for the IUD, creating abnormal bleeding or pain. Hysteroscopy has even been proposed as a procedure to check the wear of the device at regular intervals in order to decide the correct moment for replacement.

COMPARATIVE ACCURACY OF HYSTEROGRAPHY AND HYSTEROSCOPY

Concerning the accuracy of hysterography, let us recall the study of Sweeney published in 1958. Sweeney analyzed 1,000 hysterograms obtained at the Lying-in Hospital of New York between 1948 and 1957. All the hysterograms had been jointly interpreted by a gynecologist and a radiologist. The preoperative radiologic diagnosis as well as the surgical and pathologic findings were compared. Fifty-five percent of radiologic diagnoses were wrong. At the time this result came as a great surprise to the gynecologic community.

Many investigators have now compared the diagnosis made on the hysterogram to their endoscopic findings. Several of the published studies appear on Table

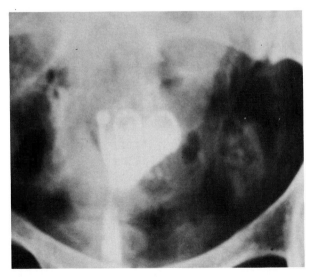

FIG 16–17.
Hysterogram shows a Lippes Loop penetrating the myometrium.

TABLE 16–1.

Accuracy of Hysterography Compared With Hysteroscopy

Year	Authors	No. of Cases	Confirmation of Hysterography (%)
1956	Norment	50	60
1957	Englund et al.	21	52
1970	Guerrero et al.	41	65
1973	Neuwirth and Levine	10	60
1973	Porto	76	58
1974	Porto	134	70

16-1. It may be seen that the hysterogram diagnosis is confirmed in only 50% to 70% of the cases. We made such a comparison in 139 cases in which a preoperative hysterogram was available together with the results of the hysteroscopic examination and the postoperative pathologic findings. All the hysterograms were reviewed by a radiologist and two gynecologists having no knowledge of the hysteroscopic and pathologic results; after discussion, the most likely diagnoses were selected. The endoscopic diagnosis was established by contact hysteroscopy. The lesions submitted for pathologic analysis were either hysterectomy specimens or were recovered by curettage or direct removal under hysteroscopic control. Half of the diagnoses established by hysterography were confirmed by the pathologist vs. 86% for the diagnoses established hysteroscopically. This study was performed 10 years ago with hysteroscopic data obtained during our early experience with contact hysteroscopy. It is likely that such a study carried out nowa-

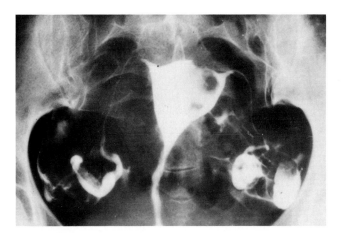

FIG 16–18.
Hysterography was performed for abnormal bleeding. The hysterogram exhibits an irregular filling defect located near the right horn. It is very difficult on this image to establish a proper diagnosis.

days with more advanced instrumentation and increased experience would yield still more conclusive results in favor of hysteroscopy.

It is interesting to note that among the 50% of incorrect hysterographic diagnoses, nearly half (23%) were established with hysterograms displaying noncharacteristic filling defects for which no agreement could be reached by the three reviewers (Fig 16–18). Only 2% of the hysteroscopic diagnoses were perceived as uncertain to the operators. This emphasizes the fact that different abnormalities may produce similar filling defects as two different persons may cast the same shadow. This analogous comparison focuses on the limitations of hysterography. Hysteroscopy is more discriminating where the only limitation is the ability of the viewer to extrapolate the histologic pattern from his or her gross examination (Plate 137).

The most common errors inherent to each technique will now be examined.

HYSTEROGRAPHIC ERRORS

Detection of Small Incipient Endometrial Carcinoma and Evaluation of the Extent of the Tumor

There are several examples of hysterograms considered within normal limits when an endometrial carcinoma was actually beginning to develop. In a group of women who were referred with obvious extensive carcinoma, review of the hysterograms obtained some years before because of abnormal bleeding demonstrated minor irregularities that had been overlooked. The risk of missing early signs is more apt to happen when the carcinoma develops within hyperplastic mucosa. In these cases the hysterogram displays irregular, unsharp contours in a nonuniform background which renders the individualization of an early carcinoma very difficult (Fig 16–19). Women at risk of developing endometrial carcinoma who experience abnormal bleeding will not be guaranteed a negative diagnosis by hysterography, and the investigation must be pursued by performing hysteroscopy with directed biopsy (Plate 138).

The corollary of highly abnormal hysterographic results due to the presence of a coexisting eye-catching lesion such as submucous myoma or a large polyp may also provide a scenario in which an incipient carcinoma could be overlooked. The physician's attention is consumed by the obvious abnormality, which is assumed to cause the symptoms that prompted the hysterographic examination. Additionally, the diagnosis may be com-

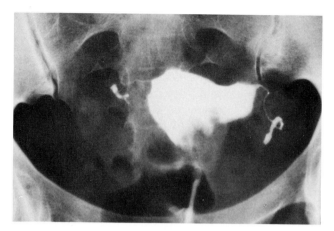

FIG 16–19.
Hysterography performed after an episode of bleeding.

pletely overlooked because the submucous myoma may screen a small carcinoma from the curette.

The evaluation of the extent of endometrial carcinoma, particularly the knowledge of spread to the internal os and endocervical canal, is also inaccurate when based solely on the hysterogram. Based on long-term hysteroscopic experience and comparing its results to the hysterogram, we have often noticed that the superficial spread of the tumor from its main site within the endometrial cavity to the internal os was frequently absent on the hysterogram (Fig 16–20). Thus the staging of the tumor based on hysterography results is grossly inaccurate, particularly as relates to stage II disease involving the cervix.

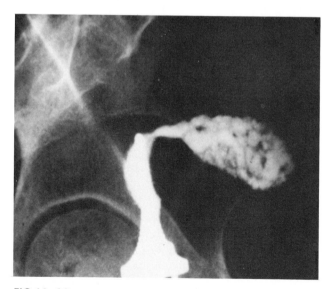

FIG 16–20.
The hysterogram has an alarming appearance (suspicious of neoplasia) although it is difficult to give an accurate diagnosis.

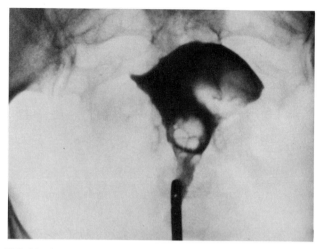

FIG 16–21.
Hysterogram shows a distorted endometrial cavity with two filling defects.

Hysterograms Displaying Noncharacteristic or Misleading Filling Defects

Failure to match a filling defect with a definite lesion because of its lack of specificity is the most common cause of wrong diagnoses (Fig 16–21). It accounts for half of the errors in our series. Obviously it is hazardous to attempt differentiation between polyp, submucous myoma, focal hyperplasia, blood clots, air bubbles, or even carcinoma. It is wise not to surmise but instead to recommend further investigation. The air bubble is usually easy to identify because of its circular shape and its tendency to move up as observed in consecutive films and deform on reaching the cornu. The old blood clot sticks to the uterine wall and usually appears as an irregular filling defect suggestive of various lesions such as placental retention, submucous myoma undergoing secondary changes, or even carcinoma. The fact that hysterography has been performed after an episode of bleeding is never an argument to exclude consideration of this lesion. Only the hysteroscopic examination will clear up the confusion (Plate 139).

One of the common areas of confusion arises between a large area of focal hyperplasia and a real polyp. The polyp is usually more sharply delineated, but this feature is not constant. When several filling defects are present the diagnosis of polypoid hyperplasia is considered as well as polyposis. Unfortunately the nebulous criteria allow no clear differentiation. Focal hyperplasia may produce irregular filling defects, which may also be confused with endometrial carcinoma. Cystic hyperplasia sometimes reveals an alarming hysterogram composed of multiple small filling defects with irregular folds that can puzzle the radiologist or the gynecologist. No definite diagnosis can be inferred from this pattern. The differentiation between polyp and myoma is theoretically easier since the former does not deform the hysterogram as does the latter. A very large polyp may cause distortion, and a small submucous myoma may produce no change in the contour of the endometrial cavity. The confusion cannot be avoided.

The filling defects due to synechiae are undoubtedly the easiest to match with the corresponding disorder since their pattern is typical. However, the characteristic appearance may be misread. Asherman himself reported that he expected to find a submucous myoma after examining the hysterogram. He subsequently performed a hysterotomy and found synechia. Zondek and Rozin reported that filling defects typical of synechiae may be the result of local contraction of a uterus having an otherwise perfectly normal endometrial cavity.

Old placental retention can create unusual filling defects associated with abnormal bleeding (Plate 140). The interval between the antecedent abortion or delivery and the hysteroscopy may be a lengthy one, and no relation between the two is established. The filling defect is irregular and could be confused with endometrial carcinoma. The age of the patient generally rules out this possibility. It should be noted that an old placental polyp is very adherent at the uterine wall, and blind curettage may also prove inadequate for the diagnosis (Plates 141 and 142). Endometrial ossification is a strange disease producing calcified structures within the uterine cavity. Because it may be responsible for infertility, a hysterogram is usually obtained as part of the infertility work-up (Fig 16–22). We have collected a number of these case results and know that the diagnosis is impossible by viewing the hysterogram. The calci-

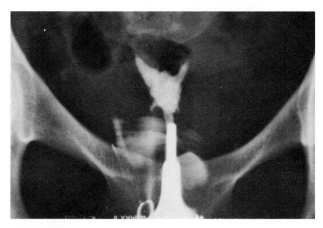

FIG 16–22.
This hysterogram has an irregular outline, but no definite lesion is demonstrated.

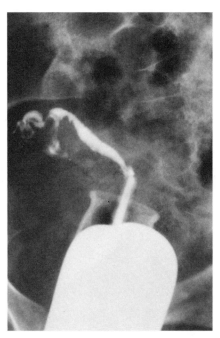

FIG 16–23.
Hysterogram suggestive of a unicornuate uterus. In fact, hysteroscopy revealed the presence of large synechiae obliterating the left uterine horn.

fied structures are too thin to appear on a radiograph, thus the hysterogram appears normal. Every disorder producing the above uncertain or misleading hysterograms are easily identified by hysteroscopy (Plate 143).

Congenital Uterine Malformation and Intrauterine Adhesions

When synechiae completely obliterate the uterine horn, the remaining portion of the endometrial cavity closely simulates a unicornuate uterus (Fig 16–23). A central synechia located in the middle of the cavity extending to the fundus may cause the uterus to appear as bicornuate on the hysterogram (Fig 16–24). We also have seen a case in which two opposite marginal adhesions located symmetrically below each cornu resulted in a hysterogram mimicking a bicornuate uterus. The practice of a systematic hysteroscopy jointly with hysterography in the work-up of any uterine malformation will obviate the confusion.

Assessment of the Endocervical Canal

We have been impressed by the fact that many patients who are referred for a hysterogram and who demonstrate abnormal distortion or filling defects within the endocervical canal hysteroscopically have a perfectly

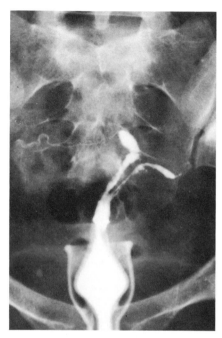

FIG 16–24.
Hysterogram suggestive of a bicornuate uterus. Hysteroscopy demonstrated a long central adhesion reaching the fundus.

normal canal. In fact the evaluation of the endocervical canal by hysterography is difficult for reasons that are both technical and related to the anatomy of this structure (Plate 144). The endocervix is fully visible after removal of the cannula during the evacuation of the dye; however, this moment in time is brief and is difficult to produce properly on the film (Fig 16–25). Its surface is very uneven because the plicae palmitae and glandular recesses create a very irregular outline. Small cysts due to the retention in the mucous glands may also cause

filling defects. A mucous plug may be forced deep into the canal by the pressure of the contrast medium and result in a misleading filling defect. Finally, marked anteflexion or retroflexion of the uterus may cause the opposite walls to obstruct the internal os and prevent the injection of this area. Any abnormality of the endocervical canal seen on the hysterogram must therefore be checked hysteroscopically before any conclusion can be drawn.

HYSTEROSCOPIC ERRORS

Assessment of the General Configuration of the Uterine Cavity

An object seen in perspective through an optical instrument such as a hysteroscope may be the source of visual distortion. This has an adverse effect on accurate mapping of the uterine cavity. For example, assessment of the exact shape of a bicornuate uterus is difficult (Plate 145). Viewed from the internal os, the proximal end of the septum appears very wide since it is close to the objective, and the two horns seem very thin and narrow due to their relative distance. Moreover the two horns cannot be investigated simultaneously, which makes comparison of their respective sizes and direction difficult. All these important deficiencies are immediately remedied by glancing at the hysterogram (Fig

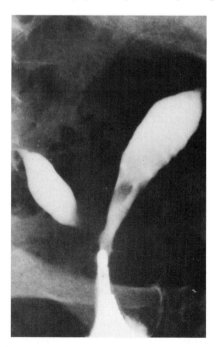

FIG 16–26.
The hysterogram gives an accurate mapping of the malformation shown in Plate 145. It reveals that the horns are not symmetrical. The left horn is more developed than the right horn.

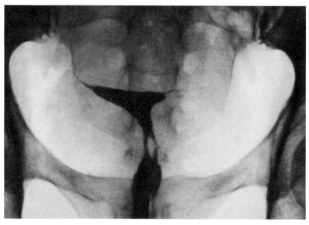

FIG 16–25.
Filling defect occupies the endocervical canal. Hysteroscopy proved that this defect was an artifact.

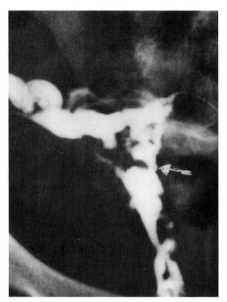

FIG 16–27.
The hysterogram reveals that the upper part of the endometrial cavity is not completely obliterated but is connected with the lower part through a narrow channel *(arrow).*

16–26). The handicap of hysteroscopy is even greater when the disorder is such that it hides part of the uterine cavity. In this case the upper chamber may be totally out of reach of the hysteroscope (Plate 146). This is particularly true in the case of complex synechiae of traumatic or tuberculous origin which split the endometrial cavity into chambers and recesses connected by narrow orifices and canals. Hysterography is then invaluable in revealing the details of this complex architecture (Fig 16-27). The water-soluble medium is able to pass through minute openings and fill all the secluded spaces as long as they are not completely obliterated. Intraoperative film images may be obtained to guide the dissection of scars during operative hysteroscopy.

Assessment of the Lesions Branching Off From the Endometrial Cavity Through the Uterine Walls

As a rule, hysteroscopy enables better assessment of abnormalities that protrude into the endometrial cavity (e.g., submucous myomas or polyps). Such lesions will not be missed, since they will appear in the field of the panoramic endoscope or hit the contact hysteroscope as it moves forward. On the contrary tubular, slitlike, or pouchlike disorders branching from the endometrial cavity through the uterine walls will not attract the viewer's attention, especially when their opening is narrow and not located in the fundus. These abnormalities are

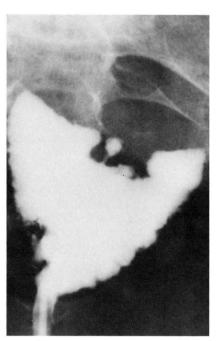

FIG 16–28.
Large focus of adenomyosis is located within an adhesion in the uterine fundus. This association cannot be clearly demonstrated hysteroscopically.

fortunately less common than the protruding ones and are essentially represented by adenomyosis, perforation, or caesarean section scars, all of which are better evaluated by hysterography (Fig 16–28).

PREFERENTIAL INDICATIONS OF HYSTEROGRAPHY AND HYSTEROSCOPY

After reviewing the advantages and disadvantages of each technique it seems possible to determine the circumstances in which each investigation is advisable.

A history of allergy to iodine is a contraindication to hysterography because of the risk of shock. In the case of infertility, when visualization of the tubes is important, the investigation may be attempted after proper sensitivity testing and under close monitoring. Otherwise hysteroscopy is an excellent substitute to hysterography. CO_2 may be selected as the distending medium, since anaphylactic reactions are possible with dextran.

Hysterography is contraindicated during an episode of bleeding because of the artifacts caused by blood clots. Hysteroscopy is the best method of investigation in that case; if bleeding is profuse, contact hysteroscopy or Hyskon panoramic hysteroscopy should be selected.

TABLE 16–2.

Comparative Qualities* of Hysterography and Hysteroscopy

Use	Contact Hysteroscopy	Panoramic Hysteroscopy	Hysterography
Emergency (metrorrhagia)	3	2	1
Infection risks	3	2	1
Allergic risks	3	1	2
Dissemination risks	3	2	1
Evaluation of endocervical canal	3	3	1
Evaluation of intrauterine configuration	1	2	3
Accurate study of mucosa	3	2	1
Detection of early carcinoma	3	2	1
Evaluation of extent of carcinoma	2	3	1
Diagnosis of protruding lesions	2	3	1
Diagnosis of hollow lesions (diverticula, recesses, etc.)	1	2	3
Diagnosis of intramural myoma	1	1	3
Evaluation of the fallopian tubes	1	1	3

*3 = best; 1 = worst.

Although hysterography does not seem to be hazardous insofar as an increase in the rate of recurrences or metastases in cases of endometrial carcinoma, the danger of dissemination of cancer cells through the tubes and the vascular channels is an argument to prefer hysteroscopy. Contact hysteroscopy is the technique least likely to disseminate the disease.

Hysteroscopy is the most accurate method for precise analysis of endometrial mucosal changes. Although the differential diagnosis of benign focal hyperplasia, atypical hyperplasia, and an early stage of adenocarcinoma is not easy even for an experienced hysteroscopist, this visual examination has the outstanding advantage of allowing pinpoint tissue sampling at the correct site. In the same way the extent of the tumor is more accurately delineated with hysteroscopy, particularly in relation to the isthmus. All abnormalities bulging into the uterine cavity will be easily identified by hysteroscopy since their visual appearance is more characteristic than the filling defects produced on the hysterogram. Hysterography will yield more accurate information when it is necessary to know the general configuration of the uterine cavity, mainly in cases of malformation, genital atrophy, and complex synechiae. The evaluation of adenomyosis, caesarean section scars, and sequelae of uterine perforation also requires hysterography.

In conclusion, we have seen that hysterography and hysteroscopy are not mutually exclusive but are often complementary. The comparative qualities of each technique are summarized on Table 16-2. Hysterography is a simple and safe technique that can easily be performed by any radiologist and remains an excellent screening method provided it is completed by hysteroscopy when necessary. Hysteroscopy is an invaluable procedure more accurate than hysterography in many ways. However, it has limits, and the help of the hysterogram may be required.

In the present situation and after excluding the contraindications of each technique, we believe that either hysterography or hysteroscopy can be performed as the primary procedure. However, the only way to avoid missing an incipient lesion is to complete the investigation by a hysteroscopy each time the hysterogram seems normal in spite of abnormal uterine bleeding. In the same way, hysteroscopy is mandatory each time the hysterogram displays nontypical filling defects, in order to avoid a wrong diagnosis. Hysterography must complete hysteroscopy in cases of uterine malformation, adenomyosis, and complex synechiae. The combination of both investigations gives maximal information.

Concerning the infertile patient, it has been suggested that the combination of hysteroscopy and laparoscopy makes HSG unnecessary. In fact, only HSG is able to assess the lumen of the fallopian tube and is required for any infertility work-up prior to laparoscopy.

BIBLIOGRAPHY

Asherman JG: Traumatic intrauterine adhesions. *Br J Obstet Gynecol* 1950; 57:892.

Baggish MS, Barbot J: Contact hysteroscopy for easier diagnosis. *Contemp Obstet Gynecol* 1980; 16:3.

Barbot J: L'hysteroscopie de contact. Paris, these, 1975.

Englund SE, Ingelman-Sundberg A, Westin B: Hysteroscopy in diagnosis and treatment of uterine bleeding. *Gynecologia* 1957; 143:217–222.

Frangenheim H: Vergleichende Untersuchungen Zwischen dem Wert der Hysterosalpingographie und die Coelioskopie bei der Sterilitats diagnostik. *Arch Gynaekol* 1967; 20:167.

Guerrero RQ, Duran AA, Aguilar RE: Histeroscopia (reporte preliminar). *Gynecol Obstet Mex* 1970; 27:683–691.

March CM, Israel R, March AD: Hysteroscopic management of intrauterine adhesions. *Am J Obstet Gynecol* 1978; 130:653.

Musset R: Precis d'hysterographie. Quebec, Les presses d Universite Laval, 1977.

Neuwirth RS, Levine RV: Evaluation of a method of hysteroscopy with the use of 30% dextran. *Am J Obstet Gynecol* 1972; 119:696–703.

Norment WB: The hysteroscope. *Am J Obstet Gynecol* 1972; 119:696–703.

Parent B, Barbot J, Doerler B: Hysteroscopie de contact. Paris, Documentation scientifique laboratoires Roladn-Marie s.a., 1976.

Parent B, Barbot J, Dubuisson JB: Synechies uterines. *Encycl Med Chir Paris Gynecol* 1981; 3:140-A10.

Porto R: Hysteroscopie. *Encycl Med Chir Paris Gynecol* 1974; 72-A10.

Siegler AM: Hysterosalpingography. New York, Hoeber, 1967.

Sugimoto O: Diagnostic and therapeutic hysteroscopy. New York, Igaku-Shoin, 1978.

Sweeney WJ: Accuracy of preoperative hysterosalpingograms. *Obstet Gynecol* 1958; II:640.

Toaff R, Ballas S: Traumatic hypomenorrhea-amenorrhea. *Fertil Steril* 1978; 30:379.

Valle RF, Sciarra JJ, Freeman DW: Hysteroscopic removal of intrauterine devices with missing filaments. *Obstet Gynecol* 1977; 49:55.

Zondek B, Rozin S: Filling defects in the hysterogram simulating I.U. synechiae which disappear after denervation. *Am J Obstet Gynecol* 1964; 88:123.

17

Hysteroscopy for Infertility

Charles M. March, M.D.

From its humble beginnings more than 100 years ago, hysteroscopy has become a sophisticated procedure which is invaluable in the management of certain intrauterine diseases that cause infertility. The instruments to be considered in this chapter on infertility treatment are the panoramic operating hysteroscope, the contact hysteroscope, the microhysteroscope, and the steerable hysteroscope. Each of these has advantages and disadvantages in the management of the infertile woman.

Hysteroscopy has been recommended as a procedure to replace hysterosalpingography (HSG). However, hysteroscopy and HSG should be considered complementary rather than competing techniques (see Chapter 16). First, HSG is a relatively inexpensive procedure that provides important information about the endocervical canal, the region of the internal os, the uterine cavity, and the entire course of the fallopian tubes. For the infertile patient, the latter information is invaluable. Second, HSG outlines the uterine contour more clearly than is possible with hysteroscopy and is far superior to hysteroscopy in the detection of adenomyosis. Finally, HSG may reveal information that would alter the patient's management. The finding of very large hydrosalpinges not amenable to reconstructive surgery may cause the work-up to be discontinued and referral made for in vitro fertilization and embryo transfer. An illness such as bilateral tubal obstruction secondary to pelvic tuberculosis may be suspected initially only by HSG. In this instance other studies would be performed, and if the diagnosis were confirmed, the work-up would be terminated.

A comparison of HSG and hysteroscopy is shown in Table 17–1. This table clearly demonstrates the advantages of hysteroscopy over HSG. However, as a screening procedure and because of lower cost and morbidity as well as the additional information it provides, HSG should not be abandoned. Although some authors have suggested that hysteroscopy will frequently reveal lesions in infertile patients whose HSGs show normal results, the significance and nature of these findings is suspect. If HSG demonstrates a normal endometrial cavity (including views taken early during the uterine filling phase, and provided the axis of the uterus is parallel to the film plate), hysteroscopy need not be performed. However, if HSG reveals an intrauterine defect, hysteroscopy is mandatory.

Although the hysteroscope is an important instrument for the diagnosis of some causes of infertility, its main value lies in that of treatment. Intrauterine diagnosis and surgery for the infertile patient should be confined to the six procedures listed in Table 17–2. Of these, the use of hysteroscopy for both the diagnosis and treatment of intrauterine adhesions was the first procedure proved as being mandatory. Simultaneous hysteroscopy and laparoscopy to treat the septate uterus has made the Tompkins and Jones procedures obsolete; however, this anomaly is more likely to cause pregnancy loss than infertility. Fewer data are available to support the use of hysteroscopy to resect submucous myomas, but ongoing studies have provided evidence of the value of hysteroscopy in selected cases. Polyps probably do not cause infertility or pregnancy loss but often cannot be diagnosed with certainty by HSG, and hysteroscopy permits complete removal with less endometrial trauma than does curettage. An indication that is still investigational is that of cannulation of the fallopian tubes by way of their ostia. Hysteroscopy is necessary only on occasion to remove an embedded foreign body, most commonly an intrauterine contraceptive device (IUD). The routine use of hysteroscopy for all "missing string" IUDs is not advised. Rather, a limited role such as that outlined in Figure 17–1 is recommended.

TABLE 17–1.

Comparison of Hysteroscopy and Hysterosalpingography (HSG)

Hysteroscopy	HSG
• Direct visualization of endometrial cavity	• Cavity outlined by contrast medium
• Definitive diagnosis of "tumor"	• Presumptive diagnosis only
• Lesions mapped accurately	• Localization difficult
• Intrauterine surgery possible	• No uterine surgery
• Uterine study only	• Tubal study also
• Cost moderate	• Cost low

INTRAUTERINE ADHESIONS

The manifestations of intrauterine adhesions (IUA) include menstrual aberrations such as hypomenorrhea or amenorrhea, pregnancy wastage (including both first and second trimester abortions), missed abortion, intrauterine fetal demise, and errors of placental implantation (such as placenta accreta, increta, and percreta), and, finally, infertility. The frequency of IUA is unknown, and it is likely that some patients with IUA are asymptomatic and have normal fertility and reproductive performance.

Prior to the advent of hysteroscopy, the diagnosis of IUA depended on historical criteria, physical findings, laboratory data, and HSG. Suspicion is aroused whenever there is a history of hypomenorrhea or amenorrhea following curettage. The pregnant or recently pregnant uterus is extremely vulnerable to injury. If curettage is performed between the 2nd and 4th weeks following delivery or if curettage is performed because

TABLE 17–2.

Types of Hysteroscopic "Infertility" Surgery

Lysis of intrauterine adhesions
Resection of a septum
Resection of myoma(s)
Resection of polyp(s)
Cannulation of tubal ostia
Removal of foreign bodies

of a missed abortion, the risk of IUA is extremely high. If the patient is amenorrheic but has cyclic changes that suggest normal ovarian function, the likelihood that she has adhesions is high. Studies utilized to document ovulation include a basal body temperature record and serial serum progesterone levels. If the patient is ovulating, the former will be biphasic but may look atypical because the initial values may not be obtained early in the follicular phase, as "cycle day 1" will not be known. The progesterone determinations are obtained at weekly intervals until one value in excess of 3 ng/ml is obtained. The failure to have withdrawal bleeding despite ovulatory cycles is strongly suggestive of the presence of IUA. Further studies to suggest the presence of IUA are: difficulty in sounding the endometrial cavity, the presence of fibrosis in an endometrial biopsy, and failure to bleed after the administration of a progestin or the sequential administration of an estrogen and a progestin. If a hysterosalpingogram reveals single or multiple irregular filling defects, the diagnosis of IUA is relatively secure. However, because all of these criteria are occasionally positive in the absence of IUA, the di-

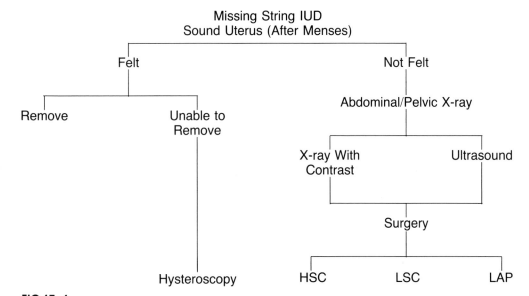

FIG 17–1.
Schema to localize and remove "missing string" IUDs. LAP = laparotomy; HSC = hysteroscopy; LSC = laparoscopy.

TABLE 17–3.

Treatment Objectives for Intrauterine Adhesions

Goal	Means
Restore uterine architecture to normal	Lysis under direct vision
Prevent readherence	Intrauterine splint
Promote endometrial overgrowth	High-dose estrogen
Verify cavity normalcy	Follow-up hysterogram or hysteroscopy

agnosis may be made with certainty only by direct inspection of the uterine cavity.

After the diagnosis of IUA has been made, the treatment goals (Table 17–3) are to restore uterine architecture to normal, to prevent readherence of the uterine walls, to provide stimulation for endometrial growth over the freshly dissected surfaces, and to verify that the uterine cavity is normal prior to permitting the patient to attempt to conceive.

Although there is no information to show that the results of early therapy for intrauterine adhesions are better than those of treatment provided many years after the development of adhesions, most patients who have menstrual disturbances wish to be treated even if pregnancy is not an immediate goal or if the patient wishes long-term contraception. The woman who is not interested in pregnancy should be advised that she cannot use amenorrhea and the presumed presence of intrauterine adhesions as an effective contraceptive. For these reasons, most patients are treated shortly after the diagnosis has been suspected.

Prior to the advent of hysteroscopy, treatment for intrauterine adhesions consisted of an attempt to disrupt the adhesions bluntly using a uterine sound or small curette. If this was not possible, other procedures including endometrial transplants and hysterotomy were performed. When transcervical approaches were used, many authors advocated simultaneous laparoscopy in an attempt to reduce the frequency of uterine perforation. These blind transcervical approaches frequently resulted in the restoration of normal menstrual periods. Although results varied, between 49% and 90% of patients with menstrual disturbances had normal flow restored following therapy.

However, after blind approaches to IUA, pregnancy rates remained quite low. In most large series and in literature reviews, pregnancy rates between 35% and 60% were reported. Of even greater significance, however, is the fact that fewer than 50% of these pregnancies resulted in a term delivery and that between 20% and 35% of those women who were delivered at term

had serious complications of placental implantation. Thus, blind approaches to the treatment of IUA were not successful in achieving a good gestational outcome.

Early hysteroscopic attempts to treat intrauterine adhesions led to an overall pregnancy rate of about 40%, but fewer than 60% of these patients were delivered at term. In addition, in this same series by Sugimoto, the reported frequency of placental complications was 17.8%. This report was rather discouraging because despite the fact that diagnosis was made with certainty and despite the fact that most of the adhesions were being disrupted under direct vision, the outcome was no better than that achieved with earlier techniques, with the possible exception of a lower rate of placental complications. The failure to achieve good pregnancy rates and the high rate of placental problems may be related to the technique utilized. Sugimoto used the outer sleeve of the hysteroscope to disrupt the adhesions bluntly. This technique is likely to be successful for most adhesions located in the center of the uterine cavity. However, those scars that are present along the lateral aspects of the uterus and at the top of the fundus—that is, so-called marginal adhesions—cannot be lysed using this technique. Therefore, Kelly forceps were utilized to disrupt the adhesions after they had been localized with the hysteroscope. Again, a blind technique was being utilized. It is likely that this approach led to either excessive endometrial trauma or to incomplete lysis of adhesions; therefore, the gestational outcome and the complications of pregnancy were worse that might be expected.

Table 17–4 provides data on our first 175 patients who underwent treatment for IUA. These patients ranged in age from 19 to 41 years. Although 168 of them had been pregnant on one or more occasions, only 92 had delivered an infant. In this group of patients the most common antecedent factor was curettage for elec-

TABLE 17–4

Antecedent Factors for the Development of Intrauterine Adhesions

Cause	No. of Patients
Dilatation and curretage	
Elective first-trimester abortion	74
Spontaneous incomplete abortion	70
Postpartum hemorrhage	14
Diagnostic	6
Hydatidiform mole	2
Cesarean section	4
Metroplasty	2
Unknown	3
Total	175

tive pregnancy termination. Most of these procedures were performed by a suction technique which was followed frequently by sharp curettage. Curettage for an incomplete abortion was the second most common etiology, and other causes included curettage for postpartum hemorrhage and a diagnostic dilation and curettage (D&C). With the realization that even a diagnostic D&C can result in adhesions, it would be prudent to refrain from the routine use of D&C at the time of diagnostic laparoscopy for infertility. If performed during the follicular phase of the cycle, this procedure does not provide useful information. If the laparoscopy is done during the luteal phase and if endometrial dating is the goal of endometrial sampling, an adequate histologic sample may be obtained by an endometrial biopsy, and full curettage is not necessary. Unusual antecedent factors for the development of IUA are cesarean section and metroplasty. In three of our patients, no antecedent factor could be detected.

Other causes of IUA are pelvic irradiation, endometrial tuberculosis, and septic abortion. Although the combination of pelvic infection and endometrial curettage has been reported to be the most common cause of adhesions, this has not been our experience. No patient had clinical evidence of infection, and many received "prophylactic" antibiotics. If the postpartum uterus is curetted, adhesions are most likely to develop if the procedure is performed between the 2nd and 4th weeks after delivery. Among postpartum patients, concomitant breast feeding increases the risk of adhesion formation. Women who nurse remain amenorrheic and estrogen deficient for a prolonged period; thus, the stimulus to endometrial regeneration is missing. Recent data suggest that adhesions occur more often after curettage for a missed abortion than after curettage for a spontaneous, incomplete abortion. Adhesions were found after curettage in 13 (30.9%) of 42 women who had a missed abortion, compared with only 5 (6.4%) of 78 who had an "early" abortion.

Among our patients the most common menstrual pattern was that of amenorrhea (Table 17–5). Twenty-eight other patients complained of hypomenorrhea, and

TABLE 17–5.

Menstrual Patterns in 175 Patients With Proved Intrauterine Adhesions

Menstrual Pattern	No. of Patients
Amenorrhea	105
Hypomenorrhea	28
Oligomenorrhea	5
Normal	37

TABLE 17–6.

Classification of Intrauterine Adhesions by Hysteroscopic Findings*

Class	Findings
Severe	More than three fourths of uterine cavity involved; agglutination of walls or thick bands; ostial areas and upper cavity occluded
Moderate	One-fourth to three-fourths of uterine cavity involved; no agglutination of walls, adhesions only, ostial areas and upper fundus only partially occluded
Minimal	Less than one-fourth of uterine cavity involved; thin or filmy adhesions; ostial areas and upper fundus minimally involved or clear

*From March CM, Israel R, March AD: Hysteroscopic management of intrauterine adhesions. *Am J Obstet Gynecol* 1978; 130:653. Used by permission.

five had oligomenorrhea. Those with oligomenorrhea were treated with clomiphene citrate and resumed normal menstrual patterns. Therefore, 42 of the 175 patients (24%) had normal menstrual flow. Thus, the dictum which suggests that the occurrence of bleeding following the administration of progesterone in oil or the sequential administration of an estrogen and progestin rules out the diagnosis of intrauterine adhesions is not valid.

One great value of hysteroscopy is that it allows the operating surgeon to classify the extent of the disease (Table 17–6). By classifying adhesions under direct vision, their extent and degree of vascularity may be known with certainty. The use of a uniform classification based on direct inspection of the cavity is superior to classification systems based on HSG and permits comparison of treatment techniques.

Figures 17–2 through 17–4 demonstrate the appearance of hysterosalpingograms showing minimal, moderate, and severe adhesions, respectively. In this series, 134 patients had an HSG prior to undergoing hysteroscopy. There was fair correlation between the radiographic findings and those seen by hysteroscopy (Table 17–7). Frequently, the HSG tended to exaggerate the extent of the disease. However, in no instance did the HSG demonstrate less severe adhesions than were found by direct uterine inspection. The most dramatic example of this fact was in two women with endometrial sclerosis who had no adhesions at all although the HSG suggested complete obliteration of the endometrial cavity. As would be expected, there was good correlation between the extent of the adhesions and the menstrual pattern (Table 17–8). The great majority of patients who

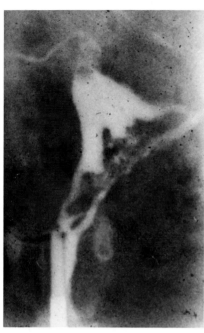

FIG 17–2.
Hysterosalpingogram demonstrates minimal intrauterine adhesions.

had amenorrhea had either severe or extensive adhesions. However, it is important to note that nine patients who had moderate adhesions and five women who had extensive adhesions had either normal menses or oligomenorrhea. Treatment consisted of direct visualization of the adhesions (Plate 147).

Hysteroscopy was performed in the follicular phase for those patients who were menstruating. More than half of the procedures were done under local anesthesia

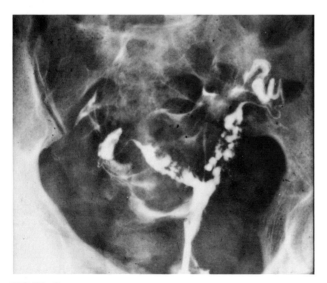

FIG 17–3.
Hysterosalpingogram demonstrates moderate intrauterine adhesions.

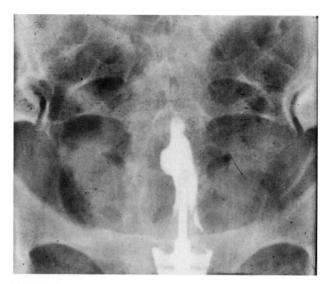

FIG 17–4.
Hysterosalpingogram demonstrates filling of only the endocervical canal and a portion of the lower uterine segment in a patient with extensive intrauterine adhesions.

utilizing a paracervical block with 1% Xylocaine without epinephrine and analgesia consisting of 50 mg of meperidine intravenously. The endometrial canal was dilated to 6 mm and the hysteroscope, which had been prefilled with Hyskon, was inserted to the level of the external os and, if possible, advanced into the cavity under direct vision. The cavity was inspected, and miniature scissors were passed through the operating part of the hysteroscope. All adhesions were lysed under direct vision (Plates 148 and 149). An IUD, almost always a Lippes Loop C or D, was inserted into cavity. Inert devices are preferred to copper-bearing IUDs because they have a larger surface area and cause less intrauterine reaction. If a device could not be placed, a 10-F Foley catheter was inserted and its 3-cc balloon inflated. Catheters are retained for 1 week only, and 100 mg doxycycline twice daily is prescribed. The patient received 2.5 mg conjugated estrogens twice daily for 60 consecutive days. On days 56 through 60 of the estrogen therapy, medroxyprogesterone acetate, 10 mg/day, was added. Following withdrawal bleeding, the IUD was removed. After the drug-induced withdrawal bleeding, the pa-

TABLE 17–7.
Correlation Between Radiographic Findings and Extent of Adhesions at Hysteroscopy in 134 Patients

HSG Findings	No. of Patients	Hysteroscopy Findings		
		Severe	Moderate	Minimal
Severe	80	53	23	4
Moderate	25	0	20	5
Minimal	29	0	0	29

TABLE 17–8.

Correlation Between Presenting Menstrual Pattern and Extent of Adhesions at Hysteroscopy

Menstrual Pattern	No. of Patients	Extent of Intrauterine Adhesions		
		Severe	Moderate	Minimal
Amenorrhea	105	54	37	14
Hypomenorrhea	28	8	17	3
Oligomenorrhea	5	1	1	3
Normal menses	37	4	8	25

TABLE 17–10.

Outcome of Pregnancies Before and After Treatment for Intrauterine Adhesions in Women With No Known Cause for Pregnancy Loss

Before/After Lysis of Adhesions	Gestational Outcome (No Other Cause)		
	n	Term	Abortion
Before	84	14 (16.7%)	70
After	39	34 (87.2%)	5

tient's cavity was reinvestigated. This second investigation was usually by HSG. However, if the initial procedure was very difficult, or if persistent adhesions were suspected, follow-up was by hysteroscopy. Of those patients who underwent a second study of the cavity, 90% had a normal cavity. Some method of verifying that the uterine architecture is normal is mandatory prior to allowing the patient to conceive. It is likely that the poor gestational outcome which followed earlier treatment methods was secondary to residual adhesions.

In 90% of patients it was possible to restore normal uterine architecture at the first procedure. However, some patients with extensive adhesions did require repeat procedures and/or simultaneous laparoscopy, and in one instance hysteroscopic therapy was carried out on five occasions before the uterus could be normalized. We have not used simultaneous laparoscopy routinely as recommended by Levine and Neuwirth and have reserved its use only for the most difficult procedures.

Of greatest importance, however, is the gestational outcome. Of the patients who have wished to conceive and in whom no other infertility factors could be identified, 75% have done so. In Table 17–9 the gestational outcomes following so-called traditional methods of treatment at this medical center following hysteroscopic therapy are compared. Fifty-eight women delivered vaginally, there were ten cesarean sections for obstetrical indications, and 14 pregnancies terminated in abortion, ten of which were first trimester. Nine first trimester abortions were spontaneous. Three of the four second-

trimester abortions occurred in two women who were known to have cervical incompetence. Following treatment of their intrauterine adhesions, patients were returned to the initial referring physician. However, cervical cerclage was not performed, and these pregnancies were terminated by painless abortions in the second trimester. One therapeutic abortion was performed in a patient known to have a balanced translocation. Following amniocentesis at 13 weeks, the karyotype of the fetus was determined to be abnormal, and an infusion of prostaglandins was performed to terminate the pregnancy. A subsequent pregnancy in this patient was normal, and the fetus was delivered at term. None of the patients in this series have had errors of placental implantation, but one required manual removal of the placenta. Before lysis of adhesions, in our first 38 women who conceived, only 14 of 84 wanted pregnancies, and 16.7% resulted in a term gestation. Known causes of loss, such as chromosomal defects and cervical incompetence, were excluded. The corrected term pregnancy rate after treatment of the women was 87.2% (34/39) (Table 17–10). Thus, hysteroscopy permits the diagnosis of intrauterine adhesions to be established with certainty and the extent of the disease to be classified. It also permits complete lysis of adhesions. This safer, more accurate technique results in a gestational outcome which surpasses that achieved by earlier therapeutic regimens and should replace all other treatment methods for the management of intrauterine adhesions.

LEIOMYOMATA AND ENDOMETRIAL POLYPS

For the infertile patient who has a cavity defect demonstrated by HSG (present in about 10% of infertile patients), hysteroscopy allows the diagnosis to be made with certainty. For the woman with endometrial polyps (Plate 150), a lesion which cannot always be differentiated from submucosal myomas by HSG (Figs 17–5 and 17–6), hysteroscopy is invaluable. Moreover, under direct vision, the hysteroscope allows the surgeon to resect the polyps with certainty. Plate 151 shows an endo-

TABLE 17–9.

Gestational Outcome After Treatment for IUA

Method	No. of Pregnancies	First and Second Trimester Losses	Term
Traditional*	369	104 (28%)	147 (40%)
USC†	82	14 (17%)	68 (83%)

*Includes blunt disruption of adhesions. Data from Jewelewicz R, Halaf S, Neuwirth RS, et al: Obstetric complications after treatment of intrauterine synechiae (Asherman's syndrome). *Obstet Gynecol* 1976; 47:701.
†University of Southern California.

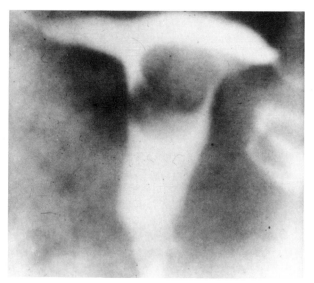

FIG 17–5.
Radiographic view of endometrial polyp. See Figure 17–6.

metrial polyp in a patient who had undergone curettage on six occasions. It was resected easily by hysteroscopy.

The infertile patient with one or more submucosal myomas may also complain of pregnancy wastage. As with polyps, a definitive diagnosis cannot always be made by hysterosalpingogram (Fig 17–7). Under direct vision the surgeon can evaluate the nature of the cavity defect and be certain of its extent and proximity to other important structures such as the internal os or a tubal ostium (Plate 152). Following the initial description by

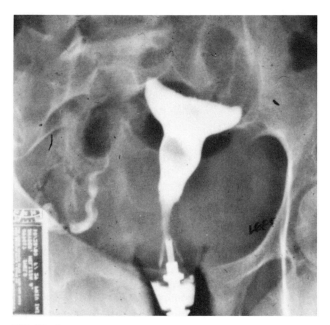

FIG 17–6.
Radiographic view of submucosal myoma. See Figure 17–5.

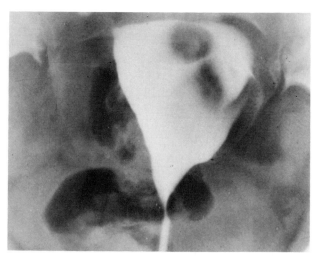

FIG 17–7.
Hysterosalpingogram of patient with submucosal myoma and recurrent abortion.

Neuwirth, other investigators have demonstrated the value of hysteroscopy for the treatment of submucosal myomas. The technique utilized by Neuwirth is outlined in Table 17–11. The resectoscope is 8 mm in diameter, and the cutting loop (Plate 153) is utilized to "shave" the myoma. In our experience, it has not been necessary to perform simultaneous laparoscopy. This is because the myomas are resected using the miniature scissors that pass through the operating channel of the hysteroscope, rather than by using a resectoscope. If cautery is used to resect a large cavity defect, simultaneous laparoscopy is advisable to avoid possible thermal injury to the large or small bowel. The long-term follow-up of patients who have undergone hysteroscopic myomectomy for submucosal myomas is uncertain. In the short term, the recurrence rate has been very low, and the pregnancy rate is excellent. The main value for those patients who have undergone myomectomy and subsequently conceive is that they may be permitted to labor normally and undergo cesarean section only for obstetric indications. In a large series of patients with abnormal bleeding studied at the Los Angeles County–University of Southern California Medical Center, many of whom were infertile, the complaints and findings most

TABLE 17–11.

Hysteroscopic Management of
Submucosal Myomas

Uteri ≤ 10 cm in depth
Simultaneous laparoscopy
Resectoscope to "shave" myoma to
   endometrial base

likely to be associated with submucosal myoma were menorrhagia that had been present for at least 6 months, some degree of uterine enlargement or surface irregularity, hematocrit below 33 vol%, and evidence of ovulatory function, that is, either a biphasic basal body temperature or an endometrial biopsy which demonstrated secretory endometrium. Myomas that are pedunculated (Plate 154) are resected with great ease. Those myomas with a significant intramural component (Plate 155) pose a more difficult challenge. Extensive dissection utilizing the miniature scissors is necessary, and this procedure generally takes a significant amount of time. In these instances and for myomas larger than 5 cm, resection using a resectoscope or laser is superior to the use of scissors.

CONGENITAL ANOMALIES

The role of hysteroscopy for women with one type of congenital uterine anomaly is not certain. Although our experience with the diethylstilbesterol-induced anomaly (Fig 17–8) is small, it is our impression that hysteroscopy offers little with respect to either diagnosis or therapy in these patients. Although some investigators have incised the narrow side walls of patients with a T-shaped uteri in order to increase uterine volume, the side walls readhere because the area of dissection involves muscle, not fibrous tissue.

Reproductive failure is the most common symptom in patients with uterine anomalies. Uterine defects rarely cause infertility. More common symptoms are premature labor and abnormal fetal presentations. Although

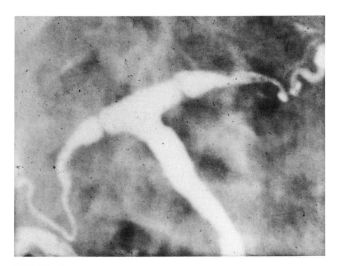

FIG 17–8.
Hysterosalpingogram demonstrating T-shaped uterus in patient exposed to diethylstilbestrol in utero.

60% of pregnancies in women with uterine duplication progress to term, abortion has been reported to occur in as many as 90% of pregnancies in women with septate uteri.

A complete infertility investigation is mandatory before surgical intervention for a uterine anomaly, so that other infertility factors can be ruled out. Depending on the severity of the defect, 5% to 55% of women who have uterine anomaly also have a urinary tract anomaly. Thus, an intravenous pyelogram should be obtained.

Laparotomy with uterine unification by incision or excision of the septum was formerly the procedure of choice for women with this anomaly and a history of recurrent abortion. The procedure advocated by Tompkins spares more uterine tissue than does that of Jones. In the Tompkins procedure, which uses a midline uterine incision, the nonfunctional endometrium overlying the fibromuscular system is removed, and the cornual portion of the uterus is avoided.

More recently, hysteroscopy has been used not only to assess the size and extent of the septum (Plate 156) but also to treat the anomaly. In fact, the ease and success of this procedure have caused it to replace other methods of therapy. Prior to planning hysteroscopic therapy for these women, laparoscopy is required to verify that the anomaly is that of a septate uterus which is unified externally. A finding of uterine septum may also be associated with a bicornuate uterus, and hysteroscopic dissection would obviously be inappropriate for this patient.

If a uterine septum is the only defect, hysteroscopy may be performed and incision accomplished easily. The miniature scissors is utilized to divide the septum in the center. The septum consists of a fibroelastic band that retracts quite easily with only scant bleeding. For septa that are 3 cm wide or less at the top of the fundus, the incision is carried cephalad from the most inferior point of the septum and directed laterally as the most superior aspect of the uterus is approached. For patients with larger septa, a different approach was used. The incision is begun at the lowermost portion of the septum and carried cephalad along one side until that margin is incised up to 0.5 cm from the junction with normal myometrium (Plate 157). Next, the other lateral margin is incised up to the same level, and subsequently each new lateral aspect is incised alternately until the original, very wide, V-shaped septum is converted to a short, broad notch between the tubal ostia. Finally, the notch is incised beginning at one cornual recess and progressing to the other. This approach is taken because minimal bleeding usually ensues as the junction between septum and muscle is incised. By leaving this part of the dissection for the end of the procedure, blood

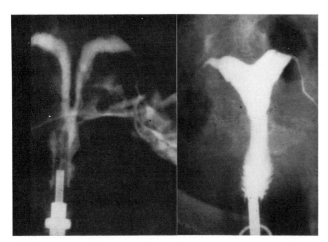

FIG 17–9.
Hysterosalpingogram before *(left)* and after *(right)* hysteroscopic metroplasty.

loss is minimized and an impeccable view is maintained. The dissection is complete when the hysteroscope can move freely from one cornual recess to another without intervening obstruction, when both tubal ostia can be visualized simultaneously, even when the hysteroscope is in the middle or upper fundus, and/or when the laparoscopist observes that the entire uterus "glows" uniformly, even when the distal end of the hysteroscope is located in one cornual recess. An intrauterine splint is not necessary.

Conjugated estrogens, 1.25 mg/day, is prescribed for 25 days, together with medroxyprogesterone acetate at 10 mg/day the last 5 days of the estrogen treatment. Following the first spontaneous bleeding, a HSG is performed to verify that the cavity is normal. Figures 17–9 through 17–12 demonstrate preoperative and postoperative hysterosalpingograms in patients with septate uteri treated by hysteroscopic incision. Multiple studies have demonstrated the value of this approach. Although some have advocated that a resectoscope be used to divide the septum, the reported rate of uterine unification is about

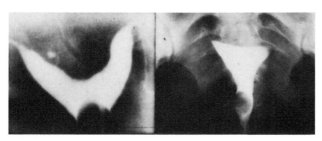

FIG 17–10.
Hysterosalpingogram before *(left)* and after *(right)* hysteroscopic metroplasty.

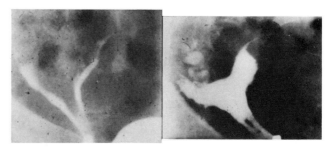

FIG 17–11.
Hysterosalpingogram before *(left)* and after *(right)* hysteroscopic metroplasty.

70%, well below that achieved by scissors incision. Table 17–12 depicts the obstetric outcome after hysteroscopic metroplasty in 63 patients who had conceived previously. A comparison of hysteroscopic therapy and treatment by laparoscopy demonstrates the advantages of the endoscopic approach (Table 17–13). The value of hysteroscopic metroplasty for the patient with repeated pregnancy wastage has been proved and is well estab-

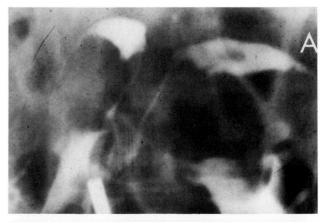

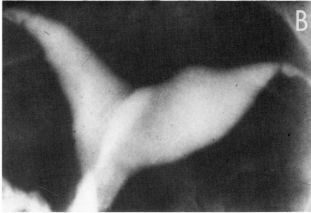

FIG 17–12.
Hysterosalpingogram before **(A)** and after **(B)** hysteroscopic metroplasty.

TABLE 17–12.

Gestational Outcome in 63 Patients Before and After Hysteroscopic Metroplasty (All Had Conceived at Least Once Before Surgery)

Outcome	Preoperative (n = 240)	Postoperative (n = 63)
Term, survived	7	51
Premature, survived	5	4
Premature, NND or SB*	16	0
Abortion	212	8
Successful	12 (5.0%)	55 (87.3%)

*NND = neonatal death; SB = stillbirth.

lished. The role of metroplasty for a patient with primary infertility remains controversial. However, because of the ease with which hysteroscopy can be performed, because of the procedure's low morbidity, and because of its potential benefits, that is, normal delivery, it is likely that the indications for resection of a uterine septum will be liberalized.

Some investigators have advocated the use of hysteroscopy for the cannulation of fallopian tubes. This procedure is not as simple as it appears. Although it is easy to cannulate tubal ostia, the intramural portion of the fallopian tube frequently takes a very circuitous route, and it is likely that uterine perforation will occur even with attempts to pass the finest catheters into the tubal isthmus and ampulla. The tubal damage thus induced may add a second cause for the infertile patient's failure to conceive. However, other investigators have demonstrated that simultaneous laparoscopy and hysteroscopy with selective cannulation of the tubal ostium and passage of a guide wire through interstitial portion of the tube may establish tubal patency, thus obviating the need for laparotomy. This technique needs more study before its ultimate value will be known.

The rigid 7-mm panoramic operating hysteroscope with a 30° foreoblique lens is the instrument utilized most often for investigation and treatment of the infertile patient. Operating instruments are either flexible or semirigid and are suitable for all types of surgery. A

TABLE 17–13.

Comparison of Abdominal Metroplasty and Hysteroscopic Incision of Uterine Septum

Reason	Abdominal Metroplasty	Hysteroscopic Incision
Hospitalization	Yes	No
Surgery	Major	Minor
Avoid pregnancy	3–6 mo	1 mo
Delivery route	Cesarean section	Vaginal

modification of these instruments is the so-called "optical" scissors, grasping forceps or biopsy forceps that are rigid and are fixed to the sheath of the endoscope. These instruments are heavy and therefore more resistant to breakage, but the lack of movement reduces their versatility. Another modification is a deflecting mechanism located at the front edge of the sheath which allows the operator to direct a catheter more easily into a tubal ostium.

Because it offers a clear view of the cavity, because it is not miscible with blood, and because of reduced patient discomfort when administered in intermittent pulsatile doses of 5 ml, Hyskon, a 32% solution of dextran with an average molecular weight of 70,000, in 10% glucose and water is the medium of choice for hysteroscopy. Even after the extensive intrauterine surgery has been carried out, the hysteroscopist's view remains clear. This advantage is not present when saline, glucose and water, or carbon dioxide are used, although all of these media achieve excellent uterine distension and visualization.

The contact hysteroscope, which is discussed by Dr. Baggish, is an excellent screening tool that may be used in the office to establish the diagnosis of many cavity defects with certainty and to detect and remove retained foreign bodies. This 6-mm telescope that is used may often be passed without cervical dilation or anesthesia. Although few surgical procedures can be performed at this time using the contact hysteroscope, it is useful as a screening procedure. If contact hysteroscopy detects a lesion, the surgeon can limit panoramic hysteroscopy to only those cases in which intrauterine surgery is necessary. Another value of the contact hysteroscope in the infertile patient is to be able to differentiate luteal phase spotting secondary to an endocrine disorder from that which occurs secondary to an endometrial polyp.

The microhysteroscope and its role in the infertile patient is not clear. The only medium for the instrument is CO_2. It is possible that this instrument will allow us to learn more about the preimplantation phases of the endometrium, especially in patients with unexplained infertility. It has also been advocated by some as an adjunct for embryo transfer in patients undergoing in vitro fertilization. However, this indication is only in a planning stage at this time.

The steerable hysteroscope, developed 15 years ago, has a tip that can be aligned perfectly with a tubal ostium. This instrument was originally developed for hysteroscopic sterilization; however, problems with cost, weight, and maintenance made it infeasible, and the instrument was withdrawn while still in an investigative stage.

BIBLIOGRAPHY

Adoni A, Palti Z, Milwidsky, et al: The incidence of intrauterine adhesions following spontaneous abortion. *Int J Fertil* 1982; 27:117.

Brueschke EE, Wilbanks GD: A steerable fiberoptic hysteroscope. *Obstet Gynecol* 1974; 44:273.

Chervenak FA, Neuwirth RS: Hysteroscopic resection of the uterine septum. *Am J Obstet Gynecol* 1981; 141:351.

Cumming DC, Taylor PJ: Combined laparoscopy and hysteroscopy in the investigation of the ovulatory infertile female. *Fertil Steril* 1980; 33:475.

Daly DC, Walters CA, Soto-Albors CE, et al: Hysteroscopic metroplasty: Surgical technique and obstetric outcome. *Fertil Steril* 1983; 39:623.

DeCherney AH, Russell JB, Graebe RA, et al: Resectoscopic management of müllerian fusion defects. *Fertil Steril* 1986; 45:726.

Guerrero RQ, Duran AA, Ramos RA: Tubal catheterization: Applications of a new technique. *Am J Obstet Gynecol* 1972; 14:674.

Israel R, March CM: Hysteroscopic incision of the septate uterus. *Am J Obstet Gynecol* 1984; 149:66.

Jewelewicz R, Halaf S, Neuwirth RS, et al: Obstetric complications after treatment of intrauterine synechiae (Asherman's syndrome). *Obstet Gynecol* 1976; 47:701.

Klein SM, Garcia C-R: Asherman's syndromes: A critique and current view. *Fertil Steril* 1973; 24:722.

Klein TA, Richmond JA, Mishell DR Jr: Pelvic tuberculosis. *Obstet Gynecol* 1976; 48:99.

Levine RU, Neuwirth RS: Simultaneous laparoscopy and hysteroscopy for intrauterine adhesions. *Obstet gynecol* 1973; 42:441.

March CM, Israel R: Hysteroscopic management of recurrent abortion caused by septate uterus. *Am J Obstet Gynecol* 1987; 156:834.

March CM, Israel P: Gestational outcome following hysteroscopic lysis of adhesions. *Fertil Steril* 1981; 36:455.

March CM, Israel R: A comparison of steerable and rigid hysteroscopy for uterine visualization and cannulation of tubal ostia. *Contraception* 1976; 14:269.

March CM, Israel R: Intrauterine adhesions secondary to elective abortion: Hysteroscopic diagnosis and management. *Obstet Gynecol* 1976; 48:422.

March CM, Israel R, March AD: Hysteroscopic management of intrauterine adhesions. *Am J Obstet Gynecol* 1978; 130:653.

Novy MJ, Thurmond AS, Uchida CT, et al: Diagnosis and treatment of cornual obstruction by transcervical coaxial retrograde cannulation. Abstract 033. Presented at the 43rd Annual Meeting of the American Fertility Society, September 28, 1987.

Neuwirth RS: A new technique for an additional experience with hysteroscopic resection of submucous fibroids. *Am J Obstet Gynecol* 1978; 131:91.

Neuwirth RS, Amin HK: Excision of submucous fibroids with hysteroscopic control. *Am J Obstet Gynecol* 1976; 126:95.

Rock JA, Jones HW Jr: The clinical management of the double uterus. *Fertil Steril* 1977; 28:798.

Schenker JG, Margalioth EJ: Intrauterine adhesions: An updated appraisal. *Fertil Steril* 1982; 37:593.

Semmens JP: Congenital anomalies of female genital tract. *Obstet Gynecol* 1962; 19:328.

Stein AL, March CM: The outcome of pregnancy in women with müllerian duct anomalies (submitted for publication).

Sugimoto O: Diagnostic and therapeutic hysteroscopy for traumatic intrauterine adhesions. *Am J Obstet Gynecol* 1978; 131:539.

Sweeney WJ III: The interstitial portion of the uterine tube—its gross anatomy, course and length. *Obstet Gynecol* 1962, 19:3.

Taylor PJ, Cumming DC: Hysteroscopy in 100 patients. *Fertil Steril* 1979; 31:301.

Valle RF, Sciarra JJ: Hysteroscopic treatment of the septate uterus. *Obstet Gynecol* 1986; 67:253.

Wood J, Pena G: Treatment of traumatic uterine synechias. *Int J Fertil Steril* 1982; 37:593.

18

Hysteroscopy for Abnormal Bleeding

Jacques Barbot, M.D.

Abnormal uterine bleeding is the oldest and the most frequent indication for the performance of hysteroscopy. Let us recall that the first successful hysteroscopy was performed by Pantaleoni in 1869 on a postmenopausal woman suffering from uterine bleeding. He discovered an endometrial polyp and cured his patient. Let us also keep in mind that for more than a century, blood has been the main hindrance to clear viewing of the uterine cavity, and this has delayed the development of hysteroscopy. Consequently, curettage and, later, hysterography have remained until recently the two main procedures for the investigation of metrorrhagia. Nowadays blood is no longer a visual problem, and hysteroscopy has become the most accurate method available to evaluate the endometrial cavity. Should only one of the increasing indications for hysteroscopy be retained, abnormal bleeding, because of its frequency and potential seriousness, would constitute that singular indication.

PLACE OF ABNORMAL UTERINE BLEEDING AMONG THE INDICATIONS FOR HYSTEROSCOPY

Abnormal bleeding is one of the most common gynecologic disorders which prompt a patient to consult a physician. This should not be a surprise since most intrauterine abnormalities sooner or later generate this alarming symptom. The emergence of new indications and the resulting diversification in the use of hysteroscopy have tended to reduce the indications related to metrorrhagia in young women. In postmenopausal women in whom disease related to reproduction is minimal, abnormal bleeding constitutes the major indication for intervention. Of course the number of hysteroscopies performed for abnormal bleeding will vary, depending on each physician's particular orientation in the field of gynecology.

Metrorrhagia was the primary indication for hysteroscopy in 48% of the 500 cases published by Porto in 1970. It accounted for 49.6% of 320 patients reported by Sciarra and Valle in 1977. This symptom was the indication for hysteroscopy in 37.5% of 680 examinations performed by Hamou et al. In a series of 810 contact hysteroscopies we performed in patients with problems not related to pregnancy, abnormal bleeding was the main complaint in 64.8% of the cases. In a recent series of 1,500 hysteroscopies, it accounted for 52.1% of the patients. Essentially one hysteroscopy out of two is performed because of abnormal bleeding.

TECHNIQUE OF HYSTEROSCOPY: PARTICULAR POINTS RELATED TO UTERINE BLEEDING

Is the technique of hysteroscopy different when the investigation is performed because of abnormal bleeding? When the endoscopic examination is performed in the absence of blood, the technique is, of course, very straightforward and quite routine. To perform the examination during an episode of bleeding—either because of an emergency or because medical treatment cannot stop the bleeding—requires greater skill. The difficulties will be variable, depending on (1) the magnitude of the bleeding, (2) the available instrumentation, (3) the technique used, and (4) the experience of the hysteroscopist.

With CO_2 as the distending medium, the presence of blood can cause the formation of gas bubbles, which make vision hazy or may even obtund the whole field of view. Some artifices are useful to know to cope with this particular situation. It is advisable to use a hysteroscope sheath provided with a gas channel opening at the tip of the telescope. The gas flow will clear the optic surface, blowing away bubbles and blood. This device

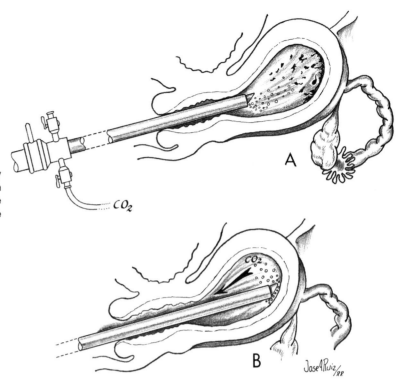

FIG 18–1.
A, the force of CO_2 gas flow tends to blow away the blood, having a "windshield wiper" effect on the lens of the telescope. **B,** simply touching the telescope to the uterine mucosa may also clear the lens sufficiently to allow clear viewing.

was described by Semm as having a "windshield wiper" effect (Fig 18–1,A). When this action is incapable of providing clear viewing one should touch the end of the telescope to the mucosa of the uterine fundus. This simple maneuver often restores satisfactory vision (Fig 18–1,B). In cases of failure it will be necessary to remove the instrument and clean the tip of the telescope with gauze soaked in sterile saline or water. Another problem associated with profuse bleeding that causes poor vision is obstruction of the gas channel by blood clots. This causes the uterine cavity to collapse and a red curtain appears to cover the front of the telescope. The obstruction may be confirmed by removing the endoscope and submerging it in liquid: no bubbles are produced. The gas channel is unclogged by connecting a syringe to the inflow stopcock and injecting liquid under pressure through it. In other circumstances the field will remain clear but the gas pressure will force a pool of blood to spread out over the posterior wall of the uterine cavity and submerge the cornua. Abnormalities located in those areas will remain undetected until the blood is removed. The easiest remedy is to introduce a catheter connected to a syringe through the operating channel and aspirate the blood under visual control (Fig 18–2). In case of bubble formation, the hysteroscopist must remain patient. Sometimes, after a short wait, the field will suddenly clear up and the bubbles will disap-

pear. This event can be hastened by varying the gas pressure (either increasing or decreasing it). Since the clear view of the uterine cavity may last only a short time, the endoscopist must be ready to make a rapid diagnosis. When vision is severely restricted to the point of precluding a complete and reliable investigation, another distention technique should be used.

The use of dextran as the distending medium is not common in Europe. Hyskon is worth trying in cases of

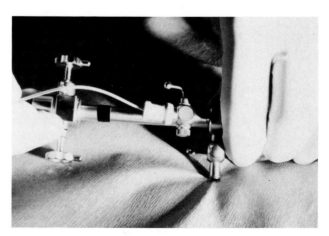

FIG 18–2.
An aspiration cannula is introduced by way of the operating sheath to aspirate blood away from the operative field.

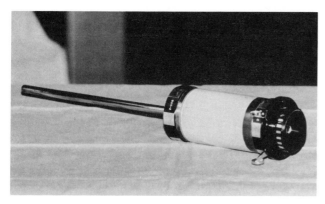

FIG 18–3.
The contact hysteroscope maintains mucosal contact, and bleeding is no longer a problem.

severe bleeding either as the first technique or following the failure of CO_2. Hyskon flow is used first to clear the uterine cavity of blood; then, vision is maintained because of lack of miscibility of this solution with blood.

Another alternative is to use a contact hysteroscope (Fig 18–3). When the instrument maintains mucosal contact, bleeding is no longer a problem regardless of the quantity of blood within the uterine cavity. The interpretation of the image is, however, different from that of panoramic hysteroscopy. Contact hysteroscopy may be selected in the first place whenever difficulties are anticipated with panoramic hysteroscopy because of bleeding. Since the presence of blood does not modify the standard technique, a quick diagnosis is ensured. The only limitation to this instrument is the proficiency of the operator to interpret contact vision correctly.

HYSTEROSCOPIC FINDINGS IN PATIENTS WITH ABNORMAL BLEEDING

The findings in a series of 768 hysteroscopies performed for abnormal bleeding appear in Table 18–1. During the women's reproductive years, submucous myomas, endometrial hyperplasia, and endometrial polyps were the most common lesions detected. These accounted for more than half of all the findings (54% in this series). Pregnancy-related bleeding was the next most common diagnosis. In postmenopausal women, hyperplasia, polyps, and myomas were frequently found, as were endometrial atrophy and carcinoma. Abnormalities which produce uterine bleeding are numerous and provide a microcosm of the whole catalog of intrauterine disease conditions.

TABLE 18–1.

Hysteroscopic Findings in 768 Patients With Abnormal Uterine Bleeding

	Age Classification	
Findings	Reproductive Age	Postmenopausal
Myomas	93	27
Endometrial hyperplasia	91	27
Endometrial polyps	82	70
Endocervical polyps	20	13
Normal cavity	68	38
Placental polyps	58	0
Decidua (ectopic pregnancy)	6	0
Endometrial atrophy	7	25
Adenomyosis	8	2
Endocervical carcinoma	4	4
Endometrial carcinoma	3	38
Other	47	37
Total cases	487	281

CONTRIBUTION OF HYSTEROSCOPY ACCORDING TO DISORDERS INVOLVED IN ABNORMAL UTERINE BLEEDING (EXCLUDING PREGNANCY-RELATED BLEEDING)

Endometrial polyps, submucous myomas, and endometrial hyperplasia account for the majority of benign intrauterine disease conditions. They have several features in common. The primary presenting symptom is usually abnormal bleeding. The gynecologic examination, including speculum examination and bimanual palpation of the uterus, does not usually lead to their diagnosis. It is now well documented that the standard diagnostic procedures designed to detect and differentiate these lesions are unreliable. The interpretation of abnormal shadows appearing on the hysterogram is uncertain or wrong in 30% to 50% of cases. Dilatation and curettage cannot remove the fibroids and often misses the polyps. An accurate diagnosis is absolutely necessary to direct the correct treatment, which is in fact different for the three lesions. Endometrial hyperplasia requires curettage and perhaps hormonal therapy. A polyp requires precise division of its pedicle at the base, followed by its removal with forceps. A pedunculated myoma can be managed as a polyp, but the sessile variety requires either delicate hysteroscopic excision or conventional surgical removal. In the absence of accurate diagnosis, frustration is the rule and the patient history is characterized by recurrent bleeding, abnormal filling defects persisting on the hysterogram, and repetitive curetting, culminating in an unnecessary hysterectomy.

Endometrial Polyp

Diagnosis

A functional polyp is lined with mucosa responsive to ovarian hormones and changing with the menstrual cycle. The structure is generally small in size, as it unevenly participates in menstrual shedding (Plate 158). Typically, the polyp is relatively broad-based and soft. Its color and vasculature resemble that of the surrounding endometrium (Plates 159 and 160). It may be mistaken for an area of focal hyperplasia (Plate 161). Contact hysteroscopy is of great value in doubtful cases, as it demonstrates the presence of a central vascular axis and the tissue cohesion characteristic of a real polyp (Plate 162).

The nonfunctional polyp is insensitive to progesterone but still responds to estrogens, which support its growth. It can grow to a large size and, as its pedicle lengthens, becomes flattened between the opposing uterine walls. It may become triangular in shape. This variety of polyp is red-yellow in color, and its distal end is sometimes ecchymotic (Plate 163, A and B). CO_2 gas pressure applies it along the posterior uterine wall. Since it is very mobile, it tends to slip away from the contact hysteroscope. Therefore, it can be overlooked during a hasty examination with this instrument (Plates 164 and 165).

The polyp of the older woman is covered by a layer of white, atrophic endometrium (Plate 166). It is usually broad-based, and its surface appears uneven because of small bluish translucent cysts.

Contribution of Hysteroscopy

The hysteroscopic examination permits accurate gross diagnosis. The proficient hysteroscopist can accurately anticipate the microscopic pattern, but the last word is always reserved for the pathologist. The ability to recover the entire polyp under visual control will also result in more reliable histologic examination. Blind curettage removes polyps in fragments together with strips of endometrium, making detection difficult for the pathologist. Hysteroscopy obviates the danger of overlooking adenocarcinoma developing within an initially benign polyp, or spreading from a nearby endometrial area. Likewise, a thorough visual study of the uterine cavity can reveal other lesions coexisting with endometrial polyps, for example, endometrial hyperplasia or submucous myoma. Ultimately, after elective removal of a polyp, it is advisable in women over the age of 40 to complete the procedure by a thorough sampling to make certain that no incipient lesion has been left behind. Reinsertion of the hysteroscope ensures the operator that the uterus has been thoroughly emptied.

Submucous Myomas

Diagnosis

The diagnosis of a submucous myoma is usually easy. It most typically appears as a round protrusion bulging toward the uterine lumen (Plate 167). The overlying endometrium is often atrophic and lighter in color than the surrounding mucosa. A network of dilated vessels can be seen on its surface (Plate 168). Its hard consistency is demonstrated by the resistance it offers to the pressure of the hysteroscope tip. It constitutes an obstacle that cannot be pushed away but only passed around.

As the myoma becomes pedunculated its appearance is less characteristic, and its differentiation from an endometrial polyp may be difficult. When it extends toward the cervix, the myoma becomes flat and the tip appears more reddish. The intramural myoma produces a slight protrusion in the overlying endometrium, which otherwise does not differ from the surrounding mucosa. It can be easily overlooked. The asymmetric appearance of the uterine cavity when viewed from the internal os may be the only sign of this lesion.

Contribution of Hysteroscopy

Hysteroscopy is of great value for the diagnosis of submucous myoma, especially the small tumors which are consequently missed by the pelvic examination but which may cause heavy bleeding because of their intracavitary location (Plate 169). When hysterography is precluded because of persistent bleeding, hysteroscopy can provide an immediate diagnosis and save an unnecessary curettage. The presence of a submucous myoma can occasionally be suspected by the "feel" of the curette, but in most cases the diagnosis will be missed, and the abnormal bleeding will persist because the myoma has been eroded by the scraping. Sometimes a myoma is discovered by manual palpation of the uterus, but one must not be too hasty to implicate it as the cause of the bleeding. Frequently hysteroscopy, if performed, will avoid an inaccurate diagnosis by demonstrating a coexisting abnormality within the uterine cavity, for example, endometrial hyperplasia, polyp, or carcinoma.

Hysteroscopy is very useful in determining the proper treatment and can aid in avoiding unnecessary laparotomy or hysterectomy when conservative management of the uterus is possible. Pedunculated submucous myomas can easily be removed accurately and atraumatically by operative hysteroscopy (Plate 170). The hysteroscopic removal of sessile myomas is difficult. The embedded part of the tumor is often left in the myometrium, and the value of this procedure has still to be proved by long-term follow-up of patients who have undergone this surgery. When surgical myomectomy has been selected, prior hysteroscopy shows the exact location of the submucous myoma. It enables the surgeon to incise the myometrium at the right place in the least traumatic way. When the myoma is purely intramural, hysteroscopy rules out the presence of a coexisting intracavitary myoma and avoids entering the endometrial cavity merely for diagnosis (Plate 171).

Benign Endometrial Hyperplasia

Diagnosis

Benign endometrial hyperplasia may be defined as an increase in the number and density of the components of the normal endometrium, glands and stromal cells; but this increase remains harmonious, and a normal ratio between those two elements is maintained. This differentiates benign hyperplasia from atypical or adenomatous hyperplasia in which the endometrial glands tend to replace the normal supporting stroma. Given this general definition, several types of benign hyperplasia may be described. Simple hyperplasia appears as a simple increase in the thickness of the normal endometrium (Plate 172). In polypoid hyperplasia the surface of the endometrium becomes wavy and can simulate polyps (Plates 173 and 174). In benign cystic hyperplasia the glands are enlarged and dilated, accounting for the characteristic "Swiss cheese" pattern seen on histologic sectioning. Moreover, diffuse hyperplasia has to be distinguished from focal hyperplasia in which an isolated patch of hyperplastic mucosa is found within the normal endometrium (Plate 175). The hysteroscopic diagnosis of endometrial hyperplasia may be difficult. The first difficulty arises from the very definition of hyperplasia with reference to normal endometrium. The normal endometrium undergoes continual changes throughout the menstrual cycle, and the difficulty is to recognize at which phase of normal endometrial growth hysteroscopic examination can enable a diagnosis of hyperplasia. At the end of the late proliferative phase when the mucosa reaches its peak of thickness but has not undergone changes secondary to progesterone secretion, the appearance of the endometrium is close to that of hyperplasia. A knowledge of the appearance of the normal endometrium throughout the menstrual cycle is therefore necessary to make a proper diagnosis. Although hysteroscopy cannot compete with the microscopic examination, it is possible with experience to recognize the different physiologic stages of the endometrium. This determination is based on four criteria, which include thickness, color, vasculature, and consistency of the mucous membrane.

Another difficulty relates to the technique of hysteroscopy. A normal endometrium examined on the same day of the cycle appears dramatically different depending on whether it is viewed by contact, with a liquid medium, or with a gaseous medium. Contact hysteroscopy is undoubtedly the closest to reality because no artificial distention of the uterine cavity is produced. At the end of the proliferative phase, the mucosa appears thick and undulated. The presence of numerous folds on the endometrial surface is not in this case related to polypoid hyperplasia but simply to the fact that the uterine cavity is by nature potential and this character is preserved by contact hysteroscopy. The mucosa appears pale pink in color and shows scarce and tiny vessels. Its cohesiveness is weak, and fragmentation occurs under the pressure of the hysteroscope.

During the secretory phase, the mucosa is still thick and wavy but the color becomes darker, more grayish, and translucent, the vessels are more numerous, appearing wider in caliber and sinuous in shape, and the coherence increases so that no fragmentation occurs. All these changes constitute evidence of progesterone activity, which creates stromal edema and increases vascularity. With panoramic hysteroscopy using CO_2 as distending medium, the same mucosa will appear uniformly flat and its degree of thickness is no longer perceptible. The expansion of the uterine cavity created by the pressure of the gas on the mucous membrane causes the natural folds to disappear. Now when panoramic vision is achieved by using a liquid medium, the mucosal folds reappear and seem larger. In spite of uterine cavity distension, the mucosa retains the natural tendency to spread out like seaweed with its outgrowths quivering in the liquid current. A good hysteroscopist must take these changes into account to avoid either a false positive or a false negative diagnosis of endometrial hyperplasia. When viewed through a contact hysteroscope, simple endometrial hyperplasia closely resembles preovulatory endometrium in regards to color, vascularity, and consistency. The abnormally high thickness results in more numerous folds, which pile up in parallel layers. The diagnosis of simple endometrial hyperplasia is even more difficult with panoramic CO_2 hysteroscopy, since the mucous membrane remains flat in spite of the increased thickness. Porto has advocated producing a furrow within the endometrium utilizing the tip of the endoscope to properly assess thickness. The diagnosis of polypoid hyperplasia is easier to make because its characteristics are viewed more objectively. By contact hysteroscopy the uterine cavity displays a characteristic contour made of numerous lobes packed together because of the absence of uterine distension. These projections do not disappear with the distension of the uterine cavity, and a positive diagnosis by panoramic hysteroscopy is feasible. However, the severity of the condition is dependent on the degree of distension, since the more the uterine cavity is distended, the less prominent the projections appear. Cystic hyperplasia is clearly visible by contact hysteroscopy.

Contribution of Hysteroscopy

Hysteroscopy is the only method which enables the examiner to perceive the living mucous membrane as a whole "in vivo." The mental reconstruction inferred from the outlines and defects of a hysterogram is incomplete. Random tissue sampling provides only limited information. The curette blindly destroys the endometrial organization and collects small fragments for the pathologist. Direct vision of the uterine cavity prior to any trauma provides an accurate classification and mapping of hyperplasia, whether plain or polypoid, diffuse or focal. Focal hyperplasia can be diagnosed when hysteroscopy is routinely performed (Plate 176). It is often missed on the hysterogram, appearing as a noncharacteristic occult defect seen during initial filling but disappearing as more dye is injected. Likewise, it is not often detected at curettage. It is nevertheless a common finding at hysteroscopy, but its significance is not as yet clear. When an area of focal hyperplasia is discovered during routine hysteroscopy for abnormal bleeding, its relationship to the bleeding should be considered with caution and other causes searched for (Plate 177). It is essential not to miss an area of atypical hyperplasia or an early cancer hidden in the hyperplastic mucosa. The presence of atypical vessels should lead to directed biopsy. Since endometrial hyperplasia is often associated with hyperestrogenic states, its coexistence with other estrogen-stimulated lesions should be considered. One of the advantages of hysteroscopy is to allow the endoscopist to review the endometrium thoroughly before initiating sampling or therapy. Focal hyperplasia may occasionally resemble a polyp. If doubt exists, differentiation can easily be made by contact hysteroscopy. A true polyp has a pedicle with a stromal core and typical axial vessels. It is firmly attached to the uterine wall and resists the pressure of the hysteroscope. An outgrowth of focal hyperplasia has no organized structure, no consistency, and will be easily torn off by the hysteroscope.

Hysteroscopy is invaluable to follow up the efficacy of treatment for endometrial hyperplasia. For severe diffuse hyperplasia, repeat hysteroscopic control of the curettage ensures that a significant quantity of mucosa has been removed. This procedure is supported by the fact that approximately 25% of the endometrial surface is not cleared by conventional blind curettage. If hormonal therapy has been elected, the response to progesterone can be accurately assessed by hysteroscopic examination following a few months of treatment.

Atypical Hyperplasia and Endometrial Carcinoma

Diagnosis

Atypical endometrial hyperplasia is considered a premalignant lesion that is likely to progress to endometrial carcinoma if left untreated. An attempt should be made to diagnose endometrial carcinoma hysteroscopically not only when the tumor is invasive and displays an obvious malignant appearance, but also at an early stage of carcinoma in situ. The distinction between atypical adenomatous hyperplasia, carcinoma in situ, and early invasive carcinoma may be difficult even for the most experienced pathologist, and it is out of the question to differentiate these lesions hysteroscopically. The diagnostic approach should be similar to that of colposcopy, which is to identify the most suspicious area for biopsy. Unfortunately, no chemical agents (e.g., acetic acid and Lugol's solution) are available to reveal atypical hyperplasia and early carcinoma of the endometrium during the hysteroscopic examination. Attempts to develop a clinical stain for use in selecting biopsy sites in the endometrium have to date failed. A thorough knowledge of the hysteroscopic appearance of the normal endometrium and of the various types of benign hyperplasia is required before detection of a more serious abnormality is possible. Close attention should be given to areas differing in color, relief, and consistency from the normal surrounding endometrium. The presence of atypical vessels is highly suspicious of significant neoplasia. The use of contact hysteroscopy and magnification increases the accuracy of diagnosis and provides the greatest amount of detailed information.

For technical and anatomical reasons, endometrial carcinoma does not lend itself well to mass screening; consequently, it is frequently extensive at the first hysteroscopic examination performed for abnormal bleeding. The hysteroscopic appearance is rather characteristic and does not present a diagnostic problem (Plate 178). However, this characteristic pattern of endometrial carcinoma as seen by hysteroscopy is also influenced by the technique and instrumentation used for the examination. Contact hysteroscopy eliminates light reflections, emphasizes details and color, reveals the vascular pattern, and provides information about the thickness of the lesion. Panoramic hysteroscopy facilitates the correct location of the tumor, and accurately defines shapes and geographical extent. CO_2 distension provides a luminous atmosphere but flattens the reliefs and makes surfaces smoother. Liquid medium allows the tissues to spread out, but the field of vision appears smaller and the color paler.

With a liquid medium, Sugimoto has described four types of cancer. The *polypoid type* recalls an endometrial polyp, but the surface is uneven and the vessels are dilated and tortuous (Plate 179). The *nodular type* has a wider base of implantation and displays a rough surface with an atypical vascular pattern (Plate 180). The *papillary type* may have a polypoid or nodular appearance but its surface is bristled with multiple projections that spread out and quiver in the liquid medium. This endoscopic appearance is equivalent to the papillary histologic pattern. Ultimately, the surface of each of these types can become ulcerated, thus introducing a fourth type: the *ulcerated* one. With CO_2 hysteroscopy we have observed 87 cases of carcinoma which can be divided into three types of appearance. The *vegetating type* is the most common and consists of whitish outgrowths. This appearance regroups the nodular and papillary types of Sugimoto as, with a gas medium, the papillary projections cannot spread out and are not visible. The *polypoid type* has the narrow base of implantation characteristic of the endometrial polypi, but it differs from the latter by a more cylindrical shape and a rough, uneven surface covered with irregular dilated vessels. The *cerebroid type* is usually extensive and displays irregular whitish protuberances separated by deep grooves, recalling brain tissue (Plate 181). Any of those types can be modified by ulceration, necrosis, or hemorrhage, adding grayish or reddish shades to the normal aspect. Contact examination provides appearances of its own. The analysis of 56 cases has permitted us to individualize several types, which are described in the section on "Contact Hysteroscopy."

Contribution of Hysteroscopy

Hysteroscopic visualization of endometrial carcinoma was reported long ago by Charles David (1907) using a contact hysteroscope. Gauss (1928), using a panoramic water hysteroscope, presented detailed description of the neoplasm and also illustrated it by numerous drawings. However, hysterography and fractional curettage remained the only procedures by which to establish the diagnosis and the extent of the disease. It was not until 1971 that Joelsson et al. in Sweden suggested the use of hysteroscopy as a routine method to evaluate endometrial carcinoma.

Abnormal bleeding is the only symptom in about 80% of women with endometrial carcinoma (Plate 182). Thus, this type of cancer is encountered during hysteroscopies performed for abnormal bleeding in both premenopausal and postmenopausal women. The rate of discovery increases with a woman's age. Sugimoto reported 53 cases of endometrial carcinoma in a series of 1,824 patients examined hysteroscopically for abnormal bleeding. We diagnosed this lesion in 56 of 1,400 contact hysteroscopies performed for metrorrhagia.

Hysteroscopy is currently the most reliable technique that provides the most reliable information about the diagnosis and intrauterine extent of endometrial carcinoma (Plate 183). Endometrial smears provide false negative results, especially in highly differentiated or small tumors. The hysterogram can suggest endometrial carcinoma but often proves to be misleading. Blind curettage is not always accurate. Small carcinomas located deep within the cornu or behind a submucous myoma may be missed by the curette. In most cases, the hysteroscopic examination allows clear visualization of the tumor. The histologic type and the prognosis can often be predicted. The superficial extent from the major focus of the tumor often appears more significant than expected based on the hysterogram. The depth of myometrial invasion remains unknown. Tissue sampling is mandatory, since the visual examination does not replace the pathologic diagnosis.

Staging the tumor is an important part of the hysteroscopic examination, as treatment and prognosis will be entirely different depending on whether the tumor is confined to the corpus (stage I) or whether the cervix is involved (stage II) (Plate 184). Liukko et al. examined hysterectomy specimens and found cervical involvement in 16% of the tumors classified as stage I by fractional curettage. Stelmachow performed hysteroscopy after staging by hysterography and curettage and found that 9 of 22 cases classified as stage I were in reality stage II, and 2 of 9 cases classified as stage II were in reality stage I. These data demonstrate the superiority of hysteroscopy in determining the true extent of the cervical involvement. It is absolutely essential when performing hysteroscopy to examine the endocervical canal prior to cervical dilatation in order to avoid tissue distortion that may lead to mistaken diagnosis.

Whether hysteroscopy can contribute to local extension or metastatic spread of the tumor is a concern to many gynecologists. The question is also pertinent to hysterography and curettage. Peritoneal spillage of the contrast medium visible on some hysterograms suggestive of endometrial carcinoma suggests the passage of cancer cells into the pelvis. Likewise, the intravasation of the same contrast medium appearing on other films highlights the hazard of vascular dissemination. This danger is also present during curettage. Peritoneal spillage of the distending medium during panoramic hysteroscopy can also be demonstrated by concomitant laparoscopy. Likewise, the vascular passage of CO_2

distending medium can be documented by arterial Paco₂ changes when the pressure of insufflation becomes too high. With contact hysteroscopy no distending medium is used, and the risk of cellular spread is minimal. Actually a real question exists as to whether the dissemination of cancer cells will lead to subsequent implantation of the cells and metastasis. Johnsson compared two groups of patients examined for endometrial carcinoma either by curettage and hysterography or by curettage alone and found no significant difference in the rate of metastasis. Regardless of the diagnostic method used, one can conclude that the danger is more potential than real.

Other Pathologic Conditions Causing Abnormal Bleeding

We have seen that endometrial polyps, submucous myomas, endometrial hyperplasia, and endometrial carcinoma are common causes of abnormal bleeding. For women in the reproductive age, pregnancy-related problems constitute a significant cause of bleeding. This will be treated in another chapter of this book. Hysteroscopy may be of help in several other benign conditions in which bleeding is a symptom, for example, endometrial atrophy, adenomyosis, anovulatory bleeding, and contraception-related bleeding.

Endometrial Atrophy

Abnormal bleeding secondary to endometrial atrophy is not uncommon in the elderly patient (Plate 185). However, the likelihood of endometrial cancer in this group requires that this disorder be ruled out. Cytologic and biopsy findings negative for disease are insufficient to exclude its presence. A correct interpretation of the hysterogram in elderly women is difficult because of the uterine involution. A curettage is considered to be mandatory and usually yields no endometrial tissue. These drawbacks can be avoided by simply performing a hysteroscopy. The examination is usually possible on an outpatient basis. The use of a small-caliber hysteroscope and local anesthesia permits the patient to be immediately reassured. The hysteroscopic diagnosis of endometrial atrophy is straightforward. The uterine cavity is small and distends with difficulty; some intrauterine adhesions are not uncommonly seen. The mucous membrane is reduced to a transparent film, revealing the relief of the underlying muscular bundles of the myometrium, producing interlacing columns and recesses and occasionally genuine diverticula. The presence of petechiae attests to the tendency for bleeding. Cystic atrophy in which the dilated glands are covered with atrophic epithelium appear hysteroscopically as numerous translucent blue-gray spheres. Most important, no lesion is viewed within the uterine cavity that necessitates a biopsy procedure, and medical treatment may be safely prescribed. Endometrial atrophy is rare during a woman's reproductive life, but can be induced by therapy. Bleeding secondary to long-term progestagen or Danocrine therapy seldom requires hysteroscopy.

Adenomyosis

Adenomyosis is usually associated with menorrhagia and less often with metrorrhagia. Its discovery in a hysterectomy specimen is not uncommon, but the preoperative diagnosis may be difficult. On the hysterogram the only direct sign of adenomyosis is the presence of diverticula appearing only if the lesions are connected with the endometrial cavity. At hysteroscopy the diagnosis is not easy and necessitates a close scanning of the endometrial surface. Hysteroscopy can only visualize the entrance of diverticula connecting with the cavity and appearing as dark depressions that are variable in size (Plate 186). The number and appearance of those orifices are also subject to variation and range from one large diverticulum to multiple small dots scattered over the endometrial surface (Plate 187). The openings can be concealed by a thick or hyperplastic endometrium. The best time for their detection is immediately after menstruation. Foci of adenomyosis can also be detected hysteroscopically when they are not in continuity with the mucosal surface on condition that they lie not too far from it. They are then viewed transparently and appear as bluish or brownish areas.

Abnormal Bleeding During Contraception or Hormonal Therapy

An increase in the menstrual flow is usual after insertion of an IUD. However, excessive and prolonged menstruation may produce real complications (Plate 188). Bleeding between menstrual periods can also occur. This abnormal bleeding can be premonitory of an organic lesion that otherwise would have been asymptomatic. This bleeding, therefore, should prompt an investigation of the uterine cavity. Rather than blind removal of the IUD, performance of hysteroscopy with the IUD in place is recommended (Plate 189). In the absence of an organic lesion, this procedure enables the gynecologist to detect a cause of bleeding which would otherwise be missed, for example, displacement or partial embedment of the IUD (Plate 190). In this latter case, the retrieval under visual control will avoid the drawbacks of a blind attempt, namely, the rupture of the filament or the device (Plate 191). In other cases the IUD is viewed in good position and no intracavitary abnormality is detected.

For women taking oral contraceptives, the occurrence of breakthrough bleeding is not uncommon. If the abnormal bleeding persists after a shift to other dosages an organic cause should be ruled out before the patient elects another contraceptive method. Hysteroscopy is the fastest and safest method to exclude this possiblity.

Dysfunctional Bleeding

In the absence of contraceptive or hormonal therapy, dysfunctional bleeding can be diagnosed if no intrauterine lesion is present. The diagnostic work-up will depend on the age of the patient.

We have tried throughout this chapter to demonstrate that in every area of gynecology in which abnormal bleeding is involved, hysteroscopy is the key investigative procedure. Unexpected uterine bleeding is often a minor incident in the life of a woman and will usually have no adverse consequences; however, it can also signal a serious disorder that requires prompt diagnosis. The pitfalls are either to be too reassuring, to do nothing, or to prescribe symptomatic treatment hoping that things will settle down. It is tragic to miss a serious disease or equally so to undertake major, radical procedures which are out of proportion to a benign and transitory disorder.

BIBLIOGRAPHY

Baggish MS: Evaluation and staging of endometrial and endocervical adenocarcinoma by contact hysteroscopy. *Gynecol Oncol* 1980; 9:182.

Barbot J, Parent B, Doerler B: Hysteroscopie de contact et cancer de l'endometre. *Acta Endoscop* 1978; 8:17.

Barbot J, Parent B, Dubuisson JB: Contact hysteroscopy: Another method of endoscopic examination of the uterine cavity. *Am J Obstet Gynecol* 1980; 136:721.

Barbot J, Parent B, Dubuisson JB, et al: Guedj H. Hysteroscopie. *Encycl Med Chir Paris Gynecol* 1984; 12:72-A10.

David C: L'endoscopie uterine (hysteroscopie), these. Paris, Jacques, 1908.

Gauss CJ: Hysteroskopie. *Arch Gynaek* 1928; 133:18.

Hamou J, Salat-Baroux J, Henrion R: Hysteroscopie et microhysteroscopie. *Encycl Med Chir Paris Gynecol* 1985; II:72-B10

Joelsson I, Levine RU, Moberger G: Hysteroscopy as an adjunct in determining the extent of carcinoma of the endometrium. *Am J Obstet Gynecol* 1971; III:696.

Johnsson JE: Hysterography and diagnostic curettage in carcinoma of the uterine body: An evaluation of diagnostic value and therapeutic implications in stages I and II. *Acta Radiol* 1973; 326(suppl):I.

Liukko P, Gronroos M, Punnonen R, et al: Methods for evaluating the intrauterine location of carcinoma. *Acta Obstet Gynecol Scand* 1979; 58:275.

Porto R: Hysteroscopie. *Encycl Med Chir Paris Gynecol* 1974; 72:A–10.

Pantaleoni DC: On endoscopic examination of the cavity of the womb. *Med Press Circular* 1869; 8:26.

Parent B, Guedj H, Barbot J, et al: *Panoramic Hysteroscopy.* Baltimore, Williams & Wilkins, 1987.

Roberts S, Long L, Jonasson O: The isolation of cancer cells from the blood stream during uterine curettage. *Surg Gynecol Obstet* 1960; 111:3.

Sciarra JJ, Valle RF: Hysteroscopy: A clinical experience with 320 patients. *Am J Obstet Gynecol* 1977; 127:340.

Siegler AM, Kemman E: Location and removal of misplaced or embedded intrauterine devices by hysteroscopy. *J Reprod Med* 1976; 16:139.

Stelmachow J: The role of hysteroscopy in gynecologic oncology. *Gynecol Oncol* 1982; 14:392.

Sugimoto O: Hysteroscopic diagnosis of endometrial carcinoma. *Am J Obstet Gynecol* 1975; 121:105.

Valle RF: Hysteroscopic evaluation of patients with abnormal uterine bleeding. *Surg Gynecol Obstet* 1981; 153:521.

19

Hysteroscopy for Miscellaneous Diagnoses

Rafael F. Valle, M.D.

Adding a visual dimension to the examination, hysteroscopy provides the ability to explore visually previously inaccessible areas within the uterine cavity and, therefore, adds precision and accuracy in delineating abnormalities even when these are focal or located at the uterotubal cones.

The diagnostic applications of hysteroscopy have paved the way for and served as a background to its therapeutic uses. Because original endoscopes lacked operative capabilities, the original uses of hysteroscopy were diagnostic. As modern hysteroscopy evolved in the early 1970s, the list of diagnostic applications gradually enlarged after more than a century of sporadic but fruitful experience. When the small, simple, safe, and efficient diagnostic endoscopes for office use were popularized in the early 1980s, their diagnostic applications increased.

The most common diagnostic applications of hysteroscopy are for abnormal uterine bleeding in premenopausal and postmenopausal women, infertile patients with abnormal hysterograms, patients with lost or misplaced IUDs, and evaluation of patients with pregnancy wastage (Table 19–1).

Clinical applications of hysteroscopy under evaluation are the study of: cyclic changes of the endocervical mucus in the cervical crypts and possible scarring of this area, evaluation and staging of adenocarcinoma of the endometrium to rule out cervical invasion and map the exact location of the disease, endometrial changes compatible with chronic inflammation, and abnormal growth and maturation of the endometrial lining (dystrophies).

The prevalence of abnormalities found at diagnostic hysteroscopy in several studies has varied from 28.9% to as high as 70%, depending on the selection of patients.

Many of these abnormalities were not diagnosed previously by biopsies or curettage.

In a series of 436 patients undergoing hysteroscopy for a variety of indications, the most common findings were abnormal uterine bleeding in pre- and postmenopausal women, misplaced intrauterine foreign bodies, infertility with abnormal hysterosalpingograms, and repeated pregnancy losses (Table 19–2).

The hysteroscopic findings in these 436 patients are detailed in Table 19–3. In 73.1%, a visually recognizable and/or pathologically suspicious intrauterine abnormality was found. In most but not all patients, the abnormalities explained their symptoms. Three patients were diagnosed as having a focal adenocarcinoma of the endometrium, and biopsy under direct vision confirmed the suspected diagnosis.

The ability to visualize the location, extension, and type of abnormality found in hysteroscopy increases precision of treatment because the lesion can be biopsied directly and/or on some occasions removed transcervically (Fig 19–1).

EVALUATION OF PERSISTENT OR RECURRENT ABNORMAL UTERINE BLEEDING

The most frequent indication for hysteroscopy remains the evaluation of patients with recurrent or persistent abnormal uterine bleeding. Although dilatation and curettage has been used frequently in these situations, the difficulty in completely curetting the endometrial cavity has been one of its drawbacks, particularly when focal lesions, submucous leiomyomas, or endometrial polyps are present. These drawbacks have been amply demonstrated by comparing dilatation and curett-

TABLE 19–1.

Diagnostic Applications of Hysteroscopy

Exploration of the endocervical canal
Suspected endometrial polyps
Suspected submucous leiomyomas
Misplaced foreign bodies
Uterine anomalies
Intrauterine adhesions
Evaluation of endometrial lining
Evaluation of uterotubal junctions
Focal pathologic lesions (adenocarcinoma of
  endometrium and precursors); location and
  extent

TABLE 19–2.

Indications for Hysteroscopy in 436 Patients

	Patients	
Presumptive Diagnosis	No.	%
Abnormal uterine bleeding	131	30.0
Intrauterine foreign body	126	28.9
Postmenopausal bleeding	41	9.4
Primary infertility	35	8.0
Secondary infertility	31	7.1
Suspected uterine anomaly on hysterosalpingogram	30	6.9
Leiomyomatous uterus with bleeding	21	4.8
Habitual abortion	13	3.0
Tubal catheterization prior to tubal reanastomosis	3	0.7
Suspected uterine perforation	3	0.7
Possible incomplete removal of products of conception	2	0.5

TABLE 19–3.

Hysteroscopic Findings in 436 Patients

	Patients	
Findings	No.	%
Normal intrauterine visualization	117	26.8
Intrauterine foreign body	111	25.5
Endometrial polyps	88	20.2
Submucous leiomyoma	40	9.2
Intrauterine adhesions	25	5.7
Uterine septum	16	3.7
Atrophic endometrium	9	2.1
Cesarean section scar defect	7	1.6
Adenomatous hyperplasia	5	1.1
Patulous cervix	5	1.1
Unicornuate uterus	3	0.7
Tubal catheterization prior to reanastomosis	3	0.7
Adenocarcinoma of endometrium	3	0.7
Uterine perforation	3	0.7
Incomplete removal of products of conception	1	0.2

age and hysteroscopy in its diagnostic and therapeutic efficacy. Word demonstrated that one in ten lesions may be missed by the curette. Studies evaluating prehysterectomy curettage have also demonstrated the difficulty in total removal of the endometrial lining. In 50% of uterine curettages performed prior to hysterectomy, more than 60% of the endometrium was left behind (Table 19–4).

With increased use of office biopsies of the endometrium, usually with suction apparatuses such as the Vabra, accuracy and simplicity have been greatly enhanced. Nonetheless, in the presence of focal lesions of the endometrium, these techniques may fail in 5% to 10% of patients. When polyps or submucous leiomyomas are present, the diagnosis is missed even more frequently. When the large portion of the endometrium is affected by a lesion, curettage of the endometrium is diagnostically useful. This is true when examining the endometrium to determine postovulatory changes during the secretory phase. Visual exploration of the entire endometrium helps to obviate the drawbacks. In patients with normal findings, curettage may be avoided altogether (Table 19–5).

The rate of abnormalities found by hysteroscopy in patients evaluated for abnormal uterine bleeding varies from 40% to 85%. In 553 patients who underwent hysteroscopy to evaluate abnormal uterine bleeding, 352 (63.5%) had an abnormality. Of these, in 419 premenopausal patients, 277 (66.1%) had intrauterine abnormalities that could explain their symptoms (Table 19–6).

Table 19–7 details the hysteroscopic findings in 134 postmenopausal patients; 75 of these patients (55.9%) had a visually detectable lesion.

Although patient symptoms may suggest submucous leiomyomas, presently used diagnostic methods have not been satisfactory. Uterine sounding, endometrial biopsy, dilatation and curettage, and hysterosalpingography do not provide consistently accurate diagnosis, particularly if the lesion does not significantly distort the uterine cavity. Hysteroscopy permits direct vision of the topography and symmetry of the uterine cavity, providing easy, accurate diagnosis of intrauterine lesions, as well as permitting direct treatment.

Endometrial polyps frequently cause abnormal uterine bleeding but seldom cause infertility unless they are located at a crucial point in the uterus such as the uterotubal cones, or interfere with sperm migration. A large polyp also may act as a foreign body, impeding implantation. Polyps found in the course of infertility evaluation should be treated, particularly if they are symptomatic. Polyps may be easily overlooked even with hysterograms. Nevertheless, with a fractional injection of radiopaque dye, particularly a water-soluble one under

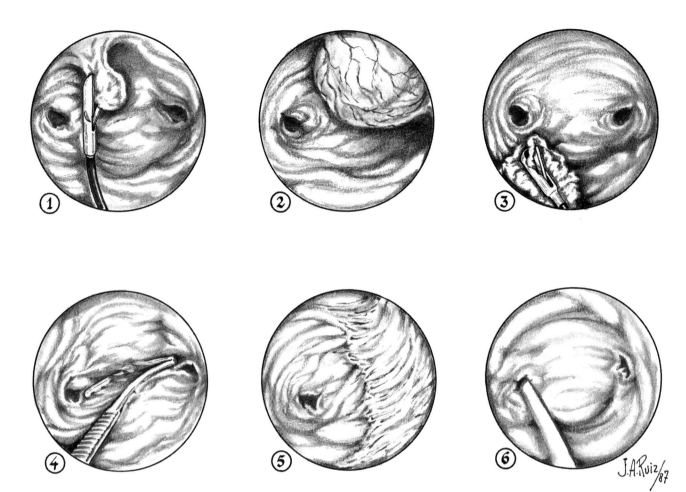

FIG 19–1.

1, pedunculated endometrial polyp. The narrow pedicle is being transected. *2,* sessile submucous leiomyoma. *3,* hysteroscopic biopsy of focal endometrial lesion. *4,* misplaced IUD partially embedded. *5,* partial occlusion of the uterine cavity by a thick adhesion; only right tubal opening is seen. *6,* tubal cannulation.

fluoroscopic view, polyps may be suspected. Hysteroscopy may not only determine the presence of the polyp but aid in its complete removal (Plate 192).

Because submucous leiomyomas and endometrial polyps distort the symmetry of the uterine cavity, they are easily detected under panoramic hysteroscopy (Plate 193). To differentiate between those two entities, the endoscopist must consider not only shape but also color, consistency, and peripheral vascularization; biopsy may be required. An endometrial polyp is soft and can be

TABLE 19–4.

Adequacy of Endometrial Curettage

Study	No. of Patients	Curettage	
		Adequate	Incomplete
Englund et al. (1957) (D&C/hysteroscopy)	124	44 (35%)	80 (65%)
Gribb (1960) (D&C/hysteroscopy)	58	9 (15.4%)	49 (84.6%)
Stock and Kanbour (1975) (D&C/hysterectomy)	50	<½ of cavity in 30 (60%)	<⅔ of cavity in 42 (84%)
Word et al. (1958) (D&C/hysterectomy)	512	10% of lesions missed by curettage	—

TABLE 19–5.
Adequacy of Endometrial Curettage (Polyps)

Study	No. of Patients	% Diagnosed	% Missed
Bibbo et al. (1982) (Vakutage-D&C or hysterectomy)	840	83	17
Burnett (1964) (D&C/hysterectomy)	1,298 specimens; 121 (9.3%) had polyps	53	47
Grimes (1982) (Vabra: review)	111	80–83	17–20
Valle (1981) (hysteroscopy/ curettage)	553 (179 had polyps)	100/10	0/90

easily indented with a probe and biopsied; it can be easily displaced by manipulation or even with a liquid distending medium; the color is uniform and pale. The myoma, on the contrary, is firm in consistency, cannot be biopsied easily, cannot be indented with a probe or

TABLE 19–6.
Hysteroscopic Findings in 419 Patients of Reproductive Age With Abnormal Uterine Bleeding

Findings	No.	%
Normal intrauterine visualization	142	33.9
Endometrial polyps	165	39.4
Submucous leiomyoma	68	16.2
Adenomatous hyperplasia	16	3.8
Intrauterine adhesions	9	2.1
Intrauterine foreign body (unsuspected)	7	1.7
Uterine septum	7	1.7
Cesarean section scar defect	5	1.2

TABLE 19–7.
Hysteroscopic Findings in 134 Patients With Postmenopausal Bleeding

Findings	No.	%
Normal intrauterine visualization	59	44.0
Endometrial polyps	37	27.6
Atrophic endometrium	17	12.7
Submucous leiomyoma	12	8.9
Adenomatous hyperplasia	6	4.5
Adenocarcinoma of endometrium	3	2.3

easily displaced with manipulation; the color is less uniform, and there may be petechiae and necrotic areas. The peripheral vascularization is more evident, and in general, the myoma markedly distorts the uterine cavity.

Although the accuracy of hysteroscopic diagnosis is easy and effective in some conditions, such as endometrial polyps, submucous leiomyomas, uterine anomalies, and intrauterine adhesions, nonetheless, in exploration of endometrial changes, a histopathologic confirmation is mandatory. Therefore, an appropriately targeted biopsy must be performed.

CONFIRMATION OR RECTIFICATION OF ABNORMAL HYSTEROSALPINGOGRAMS

Hysterosalpingography is a simple method of examination of the uterine cavity and fallopian tubes and, as a screening method, remains the method of choice in infertile patients. Nonetheless, because this technique may produce false positive results owing to transient distortion of the uterine cavity, blood clots, mucus, debris, or air bubbles, the interpretation may often be jeopardized. Errors in technique, the selection of dye and the interpretation itself may also add to its inaccuracy. Direct visualization of the endometrial cavity may help to avoid these problems.

The precise diagnosis can be made by obtaining direct biopsies when visualization alone may not provide the exact diagnosis. Abnormal hysterographic findings have been confirmed by subsequent hysteroscopy in from 43% to 68% of cases in different studies comparing these two techniques. Nonetheless, when a hysterogram demonstrates a normal uterine cavity, in general, hysteroscopy will also be normal. This has helped us to draw guidelines in its use. Infertile patients indeed may benefit from hysteroscopy when they have an abnormal hysterosalpingogram. In those patients with normal hysterosalpingograms but unexplained infertility or abnormal uterine bleeding, hysteroscopy is of more limited value.

In Table 19–8, the hysteroscopic findings in 63 infertile patients with abnormal hysterosalpingograms are listed. Twenty patients (31.6%) have a normal intrauterine cavity despite abnormalities seen on a hysterosalpingogram. Although the value of hysteroscopy in patients with pregnancy wastage is unclear, it is evident that the information derived may help in understanding some of the anatomic variations present at the level of the internal cervical os, endocervical canal, and uterine cavity, particularly those related to uterine and cervical anomalies (Figs 19–1 and 19–2; Plates 192 and 193). Hysteroscopy helps in the evaluation and hysteroscopic division of uterine septa (Figs 19–3 and 19–4).

Hysteroscopy, nonetheless, does not exclude the hysterosalpingogram; rather, it complements this method and increases its accuracy. Although hysterosalpingography does not offer direct visualization of the uterine cavity, it offers more areas of examination than hysteroscopy; it also permits evaluation of the fallopian tubes and identification of possible intratubal defects or diverticula, and evaluation of tubal patency (Table 19–9).

TABLE 19–8.

Hysteroscopic Findings in 63 Patients With Abnormal Hysterosalpingograms

	Patients	
Findings	No.	%
Normal intrauterine visualization	20	31.6
Intrauterine adhesions	12	19.0
Endometrial polyps	11	17.5
Submucous leiomyoma	9	14.3
Uterine septum	9	14.3
Unicorunuate uterus	2	3.2

LOCATION OF MISPLACED OR "LOST" IUDs

Although IUD use is decreasing in the United States, problems of misplacement do occur and are difficult to solve by blind transcervical manipulations. Although the advent of ultrasound has helped in locating an IUD misplaced within the uterus, the problem of embedment and/or fragmentation has not been easy to solve even with x-ray examinations. The use of hysteroscopy has facilitated location of misplaced devices, particularly

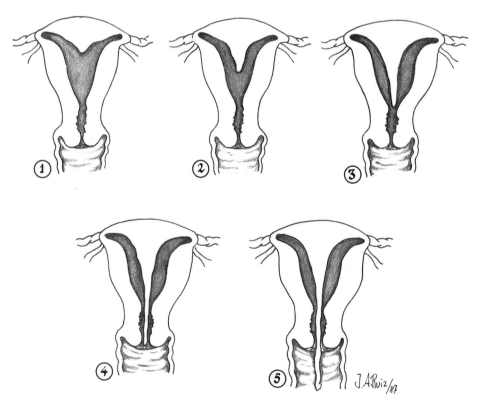

FIG 19–2.
Uterine septa dividing the uterine cavity at different levels. *1,* uterus subseptus. *2,* partial broad uterine septum. *3,* complete uterine septum. *4,* complete uterine septum with septate cervix.

5, complete uterine septum with septate cervix and septate vagina.

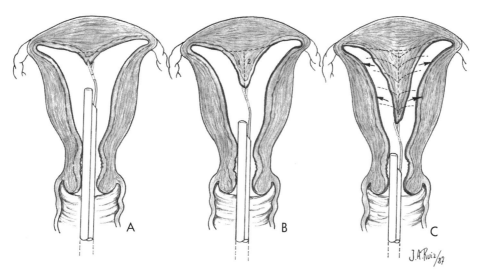

FIG 19–3.
Hysteroscopic division of uterine septum: **A,** division of small thin septum; **B,** division of partial, broad septum (division progresses sequentially from side to side to achieve symmetry); **C,** division of a complete septum.

when partially embedded or fragmented. Outpatient examination of the uterine cavity immediately rules out the intrauterine presence of the device and, when it is absent, a single radiograph of the abdomen would rule out translocation (Plate 194). Many other foreign objects have been retrieved from the uterine cavity by hysteroscopy, such as plastic tips of broken curettes, nonabsorbable suture threads, laminaria tents, and bone fragments from previous incomplete abortions (Plates 195 and 196).

In more than 300 patients evaluated by hysteroscopy for "lost" IUDs, only 6% required a radiograph of the abdomen to rule out translocation. When the IUD was located in the uterine cavity, in all patients it was safely removed under hysteroscopic guidance utilizing local anesthesia (Table 19–10; Plate 197).

After the endocervical canal has been explored, the hysteroscopist can follow lesions from the ectocervix and measure their invasion of this area to allow for more conservative and precise treatment. Furthermore, lesions high in the endocervical canal can be detected appropriately and confirmed by targeted biopsies (Plate 198).

With a panoramic view of the uterine cavity and uterotubal junctions, scars can be seen, and diagnostic or therapeutic systems can be delivered to the fallopian tubes (Plates 199 and 200).

With technological improvements in instrumentation and skill and the tenacity of endoscopists, diagnostic clinical applications of hysteroscopy are increasing.

TABLE 19–9.

Comparison of Hysteroscopy and Hysterosalpingography

Hysteroscopy	Hysterosalpingography
Direct visualization of uterine cavity	Indirect visualization (contrast medium shadow)
Diagnosis and specification of intrauterine lesions	Recognition and presumptive diagnosis
Possibility of targeted biopsies and surgical therapy	No possibility of targeted biopsies and surgical therapy
Localization of abnormalities (polyps, myomas, malformations, carcinoma, etc.)	Localization of abnormalities is difficult
Direct access to tubal lumen (biochemical or biophysical studies, selective chromopertubation)	No direct access to tubal lumen (indirect study, possible spasm . . .)
No evaluation of fallopian tubes possible	Evaluation of tubal lumen, patency, epithelial folds, and abnormalities
Requires special instrumentation, experience; more expensive	Simple instrumentation, easy to perform, less expensive

TABLE 19–10.

Hysteroscopy in Patients With "Lost IUDs"

Findings	Patients	
	No.	%
IUD in uterine cavity	107	87.7
Empty uterine cavity requiring x-ray	15	12.2
Unnoticed expulsions	9	7.3
Translocation	6	4.9

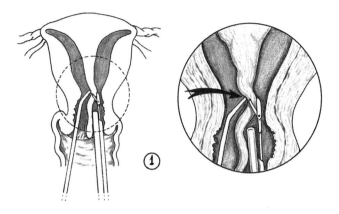

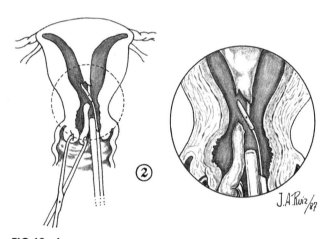

FIG 19–4.
Hysteroscopic division of complete uterine septum with septate cervix: *1,* a window is preformed at level of internal cervical os (inset shows detailed representation); *2,* the cervix not housing the hysteroscope is occluded, and the corporeal uterine septum is divided (inset shows detailed representation).

As diagnostic applications pave the way for therapeutic uses, these two aspects of hysteroscopy are difficult to separate; they ran parallel to one another.

One of the most significant advances in diagnostic hysteroscopy has been the introduction of small endoscopes, less than 4 mm in total diameter, for office use. The smaller size reduces discomfort, eliminating cervical dilatation and trauma to the endocervical canal, and provides a practically painless, simple, and safe office technique. One of the drawbacks related to the size of the instrument is that no manipulations or surgical in-terventions may be performed. Patients with positive findings will require a second procedure for biopsy or treatment with an operating hysteroscope. Nonetheless, because the examination with small endoscopes serves as a screening method, the selected patients who require additional intervention will benefit from this approach.

Modern hysteroscopy has developed rapidly in the last 15 years as a practical and useful technique for the gynecologist. With all its simplicity and safety, however, the technique cannot replace sound clinical, medical judgment and therefore should be used within the framework of specific clinical indications.

BIBLIOGRAPHY

Bibbo M, Kluskens L, Azizi F, et al: Accuracy of three sampling techniques for the diagnosis of endometrial cancer and hyperplasias. *J Reprod Med* 1982; 27:622–626.

Burnett JE: Hysteroscopy-controlled curettage for endometrial polyps. *Obstet Gynecol* 1964; 24:621–625.

Englund SE, Ingelman-Sundberg A, Westin B: Hysteroscopy in diagnosis and treatment of uterine bleeding. *Gynaecologia* 1957; 143:217–222.

Gribb JJ: Hysteroscopy: An aid in gynecologic diagnosis. *Obstet Gynecol* 1960; 15:593–601.

Grimes DA: Diagnostic dilatation and curettage: A reappraisal. *Am J Obstet Gynecol* 1982; 142:1–6.

Hamou J: Microhysteroscopy: A new procedure and its original applications in gynecology. *J Reprod Med* 1981; 26:375–382.

Pantaleoni DC: An endoscopic examination of the cavity of the womb. *Med Press Circular* 1869; 8:26–27.

Stock RJ, Kanbour A: prehysterectomy curettage. *Obstet Gynecol* 1975; 45:537–541.

Valle RF: Indications for hysteroscopy, in *Hysteroscopy: Principles and Practice.* Siegler AM, Lindemann HJ (eds): Philadelphia, JB Lippincott Co, 1984; pp 21–24.

Valle RF: Hysteroscopic evaluation of patients with abnormal uterine bleeding. *Surg Gynecol Obstet* 1981; 153:521–526.

Valle RF: Hysteroscopy: Diagnostic and therapeutic applications. *J Reprod Med* 1978; 20:115–118.

Valle RF, Sciarra JJ: Current status of hysteroscopy in gynecological practice. *Fertil Steril* 1979; 32:619–632.

Valle RF, Sciarra JJ, Freeman DW: Hysteroscopic removal of intrauterine devices with missing filaments. *Obstet Gynecol* 1977; 49:55–60.

Word B, Gravlee LC, Wideman GL: The fallacy of simple uterine curettage. *Obstet Gynecol* 1958; 12:642–648.

20

Operative Hysteroscopy I

Michael S. Baggish, M.D.

Jacques Barbot, M.D.

Rafael F. Valle, M.D.

The ability to intervene surgically with the hysteroscope has substantial advantages for the patient, the physician, and the third party payer. Psychologically, an operation performed without incisions, followed by rapid recovery and diminished pain is perceived by the patient with far less apprehension and greater tranquility than more complex procedures. The physician can perform operations in a more expeditious, exact manner within shorter periods of time. The risk of postoperative complications, for example, wound infection, is greatly diminished, and the chance of some postoperative problems, such as wound dehiscence, is reduced to zero. Hysteroscopic operations, in contrast to open laparotomy, translate to shortened hospitalization, reduced operating time, and reduced costs. Additionally, some operative techniques have been made obsolete by the advent of operative hysteroscopy. Virtually no one performs metroplasty by cutting open the abdomen and incising the uterus; rather, the septum is simply cut by way of the endoscopic approach. A further accrued benefit is that the hysteroscopic approach to treating a uterine septum means that the woman who subsequently conceives can be delivered of her infant by the vaginal route, in contrast to the abdominal metroplasty, which always requires delivery by cesarean section.

PROCEDURE

The choice of the distending medium rests primarily with the individual surgeon. Liquid media have the advantage of being cleared from time to time by aspiration or by flushing. CO_2 is not useful when bleeding is encountered. Similarly, there is substantial individual variation and preference in choice of instruments, for example, rigid, semirigid, or laser. Few experienced hysteroscopic surgeons select flexible instruments because these are simply too fragile and flimsy to perform the job adequately. Clearly, compulsive preoperative preparations may reflect whether the hysteroscopic procedure is easy or difficult, successful or unsuccessful, skilled or amateurish.

Preparation

Every patient deserves and requires a complete preoperative evaluation, including a history and physical assessment. Appropriate laboratory studies and consultations should be arranged. If indicated, hysterograms should be obtained. The authors prefer to perform office hysteroscopy if this is agreeable to the patient to further supplement the diagnostic survey. When the work-up is completed every woman should be given the opportunity for thorough, informed consent including a description of possible side effects and complications of operative hysteroscopy.

When simultaneous laparoscopy is required or desired, the patient should be informed about the abdominal incisions needed for laparoscopy and should be prepared for possible complications associated with this aspect of the procedure. Likewise when the operation is posted with the operating room, a list of instruments and accessories for hysteroscopy should be requested. Suitable time should be allocated for combined procedures. When there is a risk of bleeding (e.g., myomectomy; take-down of extensive adhesions), the patient should have a blood sample drawn for type and hold. Obviously any woman with rheumatic heart disease, prolapsed mitral valve, or any other valid indication should be covered by appropriate antibiotic prophylaxis for genitourinary surgery.

Frequently the timing of the operation determines the success or failure of the hysteroscopic surgery. We prefer to treat our patients with Danocrine or Megace preoperatively to render the endometrium atrophic prior to major hysteroscopic surgery unless these drugs are contraindicated. An alternative to preparation with a drug is to plan the surgery for the early proliferative phase of the cycle. Surgery during the secretory phase is more difficult because vision is suboptimal and also because bleeding is more likely to eventuate.

Depending on the skill of the surgeon, the operation may be performed under direct vision or indirectly by attaching a microchip television camera to the eyepiece of the endoscope and operating by viewing the video monitor (Fig 20–1). The latter offers the advantage of allowing the assistants and nursing staff to fully observe the operation. We have found this technique particularly useful since more effective and efficient assistance can be rendered and a full record of the operation can be obtained. The major disadvantage of video hysteroscopy relates to the two-dimensional view afforded to the surgeon. This technique, however, is a convenience to the laparoscopist when combined operations are done.

For prolonged procedures it is advantageous to request the circulating nurse to record and read out the quantity of liquid medium used. This is of great practical importance when Hyskon is selected as the distending medium. Additionally it is advantageous to inform the anesthesiologist about side effects of the selected medium prior to surgery.

Perhaps the worst difficulty insofar as the technical aspects of operative hysteroscopy are concerned is the inability to maintain uterine distension. This problem is principally encountered when the cervix is overdilated. Although not perfect, this situation may be remedied by the strategic placement of a purse-string suture just below the bladder reflection. Excessive leakage may be prevented by due care when dilating the cervix. Distension may also be lost if there is a faulty seal covering the operating channel (Plate 201).

Positioning of the patient is of prime importance, as is accurate determination of the position of the uterus. Proper positioning of the operator relative to the patient's uterus completes this important phase of the preparation for surgery. The authors subscribe to the luxury of having an operating stool equipped with wheels to allow easy shifting of the surgeon's position. Ideally a hydraulic up and down control will allow even greater facility when the operator desires to change his or her position.

Initially, before inserting the operating hysteroscopic system, a scout diagnostic endoscopic examination should be done. We prefer to do this portion of the hysteroscopy with a 5-mm sheath utilizing CO_2 as the

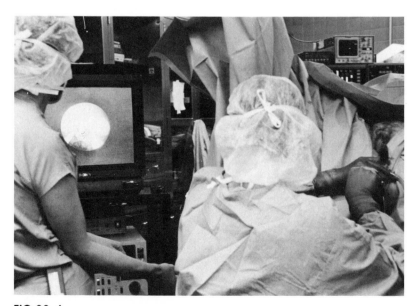

FIG 20–1.
A microchip video camera is attached to the eyepiece of the hysteroscope. Surgery is performed watching the video monitor screen.

distending medium (flow rate, 30 to 40 cc per minute). This rapid-scanning endoscopy gives the surgeon a final view of the uterine cavity prior to initiating the operative portion of the procedure and affords the advantage of last minute adjustments in the surgical plan.

Experienced endoscopists check all operating instruments to be sure they work before beginning surgery.

Choice of Anesthesia

Operative hysteroscopy for minor problems may be performed under local anesthesia because these procedures usually last 30 minutes or less. This type of anesthesia may be administered by paracervical block or, preferably, by injection of the local anesthetic directly into the substance of the cervix (Fig 20–2). Several agents are available, but the simplest drug which provides adequate anesthesia for short procedures is 1% Xylocaine without additives. For longer operations Marcaine may prove to be advantageous. Fewer than 5% of our cases have been done under regional blockade. This has not been a popular anesthetic technique for either physician or patient. General anesthesia has proved to be the safest and most popular method of anesthesia for operative endoscopy. Even high-risk patients may enjoy the safety of cardiac general anesthesia. General anesthesia is beneficial when the patient is expected to be in the uncomfortable lithotomy position for an hour or more.

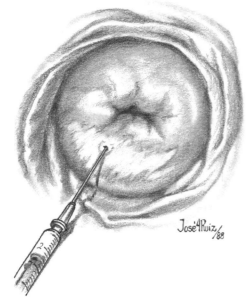

Fig 20–2.
Local anesthesia is injected directly into the cervix by means of a 25-gauge needle.

MAJOR USES
Directed Hysteroscopic Biopsy

There is very little logic in modern obstetrics and gynecology for the performance of a blind dilatation and curettage. The procedure of choice to investigate potential or probable intrauterine disease is hysteroscopy combined with either biopsy sampling or directed curettage. Roberts et al. demonstrated that vigorous curetting of endometrial carcinoma led to the appearance of malignant cells in inferior vena cava blood samples; therefore, selective sampling would appear to be safer for the patient at risk. Additionally, focal lesions, such as polyps, carcinoma in situ, and hyperplasia, may be easily missed by blind curettage. Clearly, the most accurate biopsy is the one that is taken while viewing the lesion with the hysteroscope in a manner analogous to the cervical biopsy performed under colposcopic guidance (Fig 20–3; Plate 202,A). These biopsies are carried out with either a flexible, semirigid biopsy forceps, or rigid biopsy instrument (Plate 202,B). The major disadvantage of the instrumentation relates to the small volume of tissue obtained. The jaws of a semirigid biopsy forceps, for example, hold a total volume of 0.1 cc. Even under ideal circumstances an endometrial section may be difficult for the pathologist to interpret, and when faced with a minuscule sample, the chance for error in diagnosis will be amplified. The rigid biopsy forceps obtains approximately twice the volume of tissue as the smaller flexible instruments, and if more than one piece of tissue is secured, the chance for accurate diagnosis increases (Fig 20–3,C). An alternative acceptable technique utilizes the hysteroscope to identify the lesion in order to establish a presumptive diagnosis as well as to localize the site of the disease process. The endoscope is then withdrawn, a curette is directed to the known location of the lesion, and a plentiful sample of tissue is removed and sent to the pathologist for diagnosis (Fig 20–3,D and E). Still another method retains the hysteroscope in place but relies on the endoscopist to carefully insert a small curette into the cervix and uterine cavity close to the hysteroscope and then obtain a directed sample (Fig 20–3,F). A similar technique may be accomplished with a dual channel operating sheath but substituting a 2-mm sampling cannula with suction under direct vision. The latter technique is analogous to that utilized for chorionic biopsy (Fig 20–3,G).

Removal of Intrauterine Foreign Bodies

The best method to remove "lost" intrauterine devices (IUDs) lying in the endometrial cavity is under di-

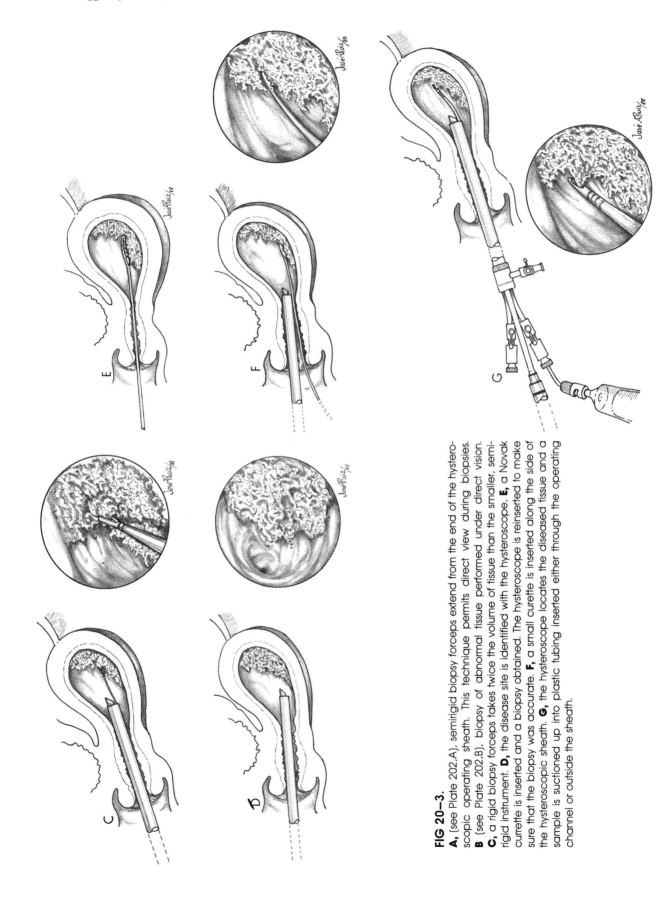

FIG 20–3.

A, (see Plate 202.A), semirigid biopsy forceps extend from the end of the hysteroscopic operating sheath. This technique permits direct view during biopsies. **B** (see Plate 202.B), biopsy of abnormal tissue performed under direct vision. **C,** a rigid biopsy forceps takes twice the volume of tissue than the smaller, semirigid instrument. **D,** the disease site is identified with the hysteroscope, **E,** a Novak currette is inserted and a biopsy obtained. The hysteroscope is reinserted to make sure that the biopsy was accurate. **F,** a small curette is inserted along the side of the hysteroscopic sheath. **G,** the hysteroscope locates the diseased tissue and a sample is suctioned up into plastic tubing inserted either through the operating channel or outside the sheath.

rect hysteroscopic view (Plate 203). Not only can one see where the device is located, but this precise observation also eliminates the trauma of blind probing with resultant bleeding and increased potential for infection. Several methods have been employed to extract the IUD. Utilizing a flexible or semirigid grasping instrument and maintaining the hysteroscope just above the internal cervical os provides a panoramic view of the cavity. The IUD string is sited, seized, and the hysteroscope is withdrawn, dragging the IUD with it through the cervix (Fig 20–4; Plates 204 and 205).

Another method for IUD removal utilizes the grasping forceps to grab the stem of the device (Plate 206) followed by removal through the uterus to the exterior. For the extraction of embedded or fragmented devices the instrument of choice is the powerful rigid grasping forceps. A piece of the IUD is securely grasped, and while the surgeon maintains steady pressure, the sheath and endoscope are pulled down through the uterus and cervix. The experienced surgeon will carefully locate a sturdy part of the fractured IUD; once the forceps is locked onto the device he will not release it or attempt to seek a new point to grasp. Invariably release of the device will be accompanied by bleeding and it may not be possible to locate it again or lock onto it. For imbedded devices a simultaneous laparoscopy is helpful in determining whether the device has penetrated through the uterine serosa (Fig 20–5; Plate 207). The latter may require a transabdominal removal. Similarly, if a device is fragmented and must be brought out piecemeal, the logical plan for removal is plotted (e.g., first, removal of the upper portion, followed by the lower portions).

Nonembedded devices may be easily extracted under local anesthesia; however, embedded or fragmented devices require substantial manipulations as well as ad-

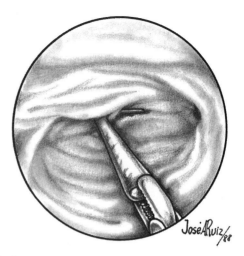

FIG 20–5.
When the device is embedded, a simultaneous laparoscopy should be performed.

junctive laparoscopy and will be best accomplished under general inhalation anesthesia (Plate 208). Valle and Sciarra reported hysteroscopic intrauterine device extraction in 15 women. Successful removal was carried out in 11; 4 women had empty cavities. Siegler and Kemmann reported 10 women who underwent hysteroscopic examination for occult intrauterine devices. Hysteroscopy failed to detect the misplaced devices in 2 women (1 with an embedded device wholly within the myometrium; 1 whose device was obscured by the amniotic sac). An additional case revealed only a small portion of the device visible by hysteroscopy (i.e., the device perforated the lower uterine segment). In the latter instance the device was preferentially removed by laparoscopy.

Removal of Endometrial Polyps

It is well known that uterine polyps are often missed by blind curettage. Valle (1981) reported that polyps were missed in 150 of 179 patients at curettage. Hysteroscopy is a valuable technique enabling one to differentiate between polyps and other space-occupying lesions within the uterine cavity. Additionally, hysteroscopy is the only method by which one can accurately locate the polyp pedicle, with the possible exception of instances where the polyp prolapses through the cervix and is visible to the naked eye or to the magnification of the colposcope (Plate 209). Once the polyp pedicle has been precisely located, operative hysteroscopy may be performed and the pedicle can be cut with semirigid or rigid scissors (Plates 210 and 211). Attention should be drawn to the fact that the polyp(s) is often attached near the fundus, and the approach to the pedicle can be

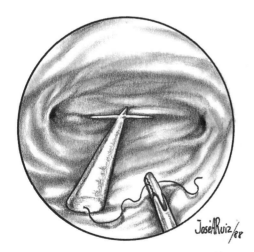

FIG 20–4.
IUD string is grasped under direct vision.

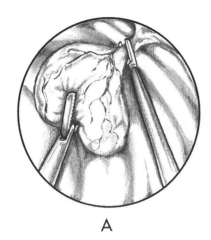

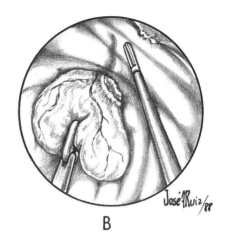

FIG 20–6.
A, utilizing a dual operating channel sheath; the surgeon grasps the polyp with a forceps while cutting the pedicle with a scissors (or Nd-YAG laser fiber). **B,** after the pedicle has been severed, the polyp is removed.

difficult. When the polyp is lying over the posterior wall of the uterus the pedicle is not visible, and the operator may have to push the tip of the endoscope between the polyp and the posterior wall and lift it up. The same problem may be resolved with scissors (i.e., the operator slips the scissors between the polyp and the posterior wall in order to swing the polyp upward).

A double channel operating sheath may be advantageous to use for the extraction of larger polyps and those whose pedicles are difficult to see. Baggish utilizes either the aspiration cannula, which attaches to the polyp by suction, or a grasping forceps to move the polyp until the pedicle is in view. Through the other channel, a Nd-YAG laser fiber or semirigid scissors is inserted (Fig 20–6). The pedicle of the polyp can then be severed under direct vision. Large pedicles contain thick-walled vessels and may bleed heavily. The Nd-YAG laser has an advantage in that the pedicle can be coagulated thoroughly before cutting to separate the polyp from the uterine cavity (Plate 212). When the polyp has been freed, a grasping forceps latches onto a piece of the polyp and the entire hysteroscope with its sheath is removed, carrying the polyp with it. Not uncommonly more than one polyp is seen. In such circumstances the surgeon is well advised to cut all the polyp pedicles before the removal process. Sometimes when the hysteroscope and sheath are reinserted, vision is less than optimal. The latter circumstance rarely interferes with gathering floating polyps but may render accurate transection of the pedicle impossible.

MISCELLANEOUS OPERATIONS

Another less common application of operative hysteroscopy is the removal of endometrial ossifications. These calcified structures can occupy a large portion of the uterine cavity (Plate 213). They usually do not appear on the hysterogram and are seen only by hysteroscopy. According to Barbot they are not as rare as was once thought. Among 20 cases, infertility was the main problem associated with these lesions. Curettage has not been a satisfactory method for removal of these spicules (Plate 214,A). Under hysteroscopic visual control the fragments should be grasped with a forceps and gently withdrawn (Plate 214,B). The procedure is repeated as often as necessary until the uterine cavity is completely clear. If one fragment is left behind, the disease will reappear.

Lysis of Intrauterine Adhesions

Among the applications of operative hysteroscopy, the treatment of Asherman's syndrome was the earliest to be performed routinely and is the most documented.

The protocol is well established and includes four steps: (1) restoration of normal anatomy, (2) prevention of readhesions by inserting an IUD for 2 months, (3) endometrial resurfacing of the resected scars with estrogen therapy, and (4) control of the results after removal of the IUD.

Prior to treatment, it is important to classify the severity of the disease (Plate 215). This classification is useful for prognosis and is the singular method to compare results and determine the best treatment technique. Two classifications have been proposed: one based on hysterography and taking into account the surface of the hysterogram occupied by filling defects (Toaff and Ballas), and one based on hysteroscopy and taking into account not only the surface involved but also the type of the adhesions and the involvement of the fundus and ostia (Plate 216). In fact hysterography

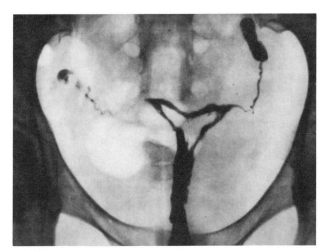

FIG 20–7.
Hysterogram suggests uterine synechiae by the presence of a persistent filling defect.

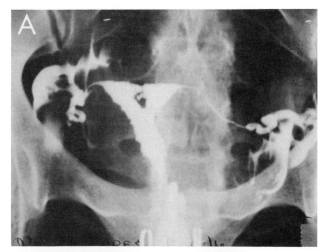

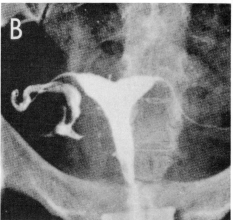

FIG 20–8.
Preoperative **(A)** and postoperative **(B)** hysterograms of the patient shown in Plate 219.

and hysteroscopy are complementary, and both should be used for diagnosis and classification when the adhesions are severe. The hysterogram is more accurate in determining the surface of the cavity involved, and hysteroscopy is more accurate in determining the type of adhesions (Fig 20–7).

Concerning the operative technique, two methods are advocated: the rupture of the adhesions by simply applying pressure on them with the tip of the hysteroscope, or the cutting of the adhesions by means of scissors, electrocautery, or laser beam. The first technique is easy, quick, and simple. It can be done with a diagnostic hysteroscope, either panoramic or contact, and requires little or no dilatation. However, it is less accurate than the cutting method and should be reserved for fresh adhesions that disrupt very easily or older adhesions located within the endocervical canal or in the center of the uterine cavity. The second method is more complicated and takes more time. It requires an operating hysteroscope and dilatation of the cervix. It should be used for old and complex adhesions involving the fundus and the lateral aspects of the uterine cavity.

The treatment of central adhesions of the column-shaped type (i.e., connecting the anterior and posterior walls of the uterus) is easy and, regardless of the technique used, usually successful (Plates 217 and 218). The simplest method is to establish contact between the adhesion and the tip of the hysteroscope, then push the scope forward to break the adhesion (Plates 219 and 220). The operator can see the fibrous bridges stretch, split, and, when the adhesion is completely separated, the two stumps retract on the uterine walls (Plate 221). The contact hysteroscope is a convenient instrument for this procedure because the shaft is strongly built and the vision is always clear. The prognosis for more extensive

central adhesions remains good when the tubal ostia are still visible (Fig 20–8,A and B). However, the treatment is more delicate and is best performed with scissors, resectoscope, or laser.

Marginal adhesions are always difficult to manage. They are easily demonstrated by the hysterogram but may be difficult to detect by hysteroscopy (Fig 20–9). They are usually crescent-shaped and are detected because the uterine cavity viewed from the internal os is not symmetrical and one cornu is not visible. Sharp dissection with scissors is recommended. More complex patterns of adhesions include both central and marginal types that divide the uterine cavity into several chambers communicating by small orifices (Plate 222,A) The hysterogram is very useful for a complete evaluation of the disease. The contrast radiograph clearly demonstrates the extent of the chambers above the orifices that are visible by hysteroscopy. The only feasible technique is to employ an operating hysteroscope and gradually cut the fibrous bands with scissors until a normal uterine

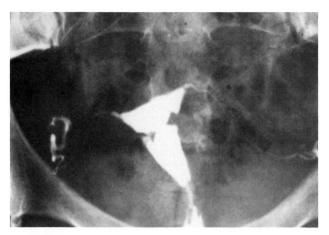

FIG 20–9.
Hysterogram shows marginal adhesions

cavity has been restored (Plate 222,B). In very severe cases the uterine cavity is reduced to a small, narrow tunnel. Normal endometrium has disappeared, and only white fibrous tissue is visible. The hysterogram accurately confirms that the upper fundus and the ostial areas are occluded (grade 4), and the treatment will be very difficult.

Restoration of normal menstruation can be anticipated, whether hysteroscopy is used or not, with an 80% to 90% chance of success. The results are less optimistic for patients who wish to conceive, although accurate analysis is difficult to obtain because most cases are not graded. Data from 40 reports representing more than 1,000 patients who were treated without hysteroscopy reveals a conception rate of bout 50%, and among those conceiving only half carried a term delivery. Hysteroscopic treatment, on the other hand, can achieve a conception rate of 75% and, above all, less pregnancy wastage and fewer delivery complications.

UTERINE SEPTUM

Septate and bicornuate uteri represent developmental defects in müllerian duct fusion and may be seen in up to 5% of women. Clinically, the septate uterus leads to diminished uterine capacity, reduced vascularity within the septum itself, and first and second trimester pregnancy wastage (Plate 223). Various figures have been quoted about the relative risk of abortion or premature delivery in this condition and range from 15% to 95%.

Criteria that should be fulfilled prior to surgical intervention in septum removal include (1) demonstration of reproductive loss, which is defined in most series as

one or more abortions or premature deliveries; (2) complete endocrine infertility evaluation to exclude other causes of pregnancy wastage; (3) complete infectious disease work-up including anaerobic and aerobic organisms, chlamydia, and mycoplasma cultures; (4) intravenous pyelography; (5) preoperative hysterosalpingography.

Prior to the development of modern operative hysteroscopy the accepted surgical techniques required laparotomy with incision into the substance of the uterus and depending on the individual technique either removal (Strassman or Jones) or section (Tompkins) of the septum.

Several hysteroscopic techniques have been described in the direct view take-down of uterine septa. Each technique has its own advocates and detractors. The best results regardless of individual variation will vary with the skill and experience of the surgeon.

March and Israel prefer the flexible scissors introduced through the operating channel of the hysteroscopic sheath. They favor this device over the rigid scissors because the flexible tool does not protrude beyond the endoscopic sheath as do the rigid scissors; because the flexible instrument may be used in a panoramic mode, which provides a wider field of view; and because the operator may maneuver the flexible scissor blades into the cornual recesses and rotate the scissors in eccentrically placed septa (Plate 224).

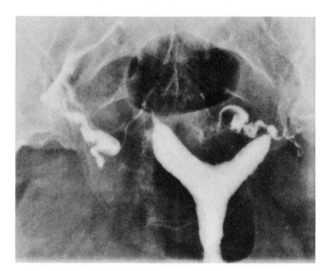

FIG 20–10.
A (above), hysterogram shows pattern compatible with septate uterus. Laparoscopy confirmed that the uterus was *not* bicornuate. **B** (see Plate 225), hysteroscopy confirms presence of the uterine septum. **C** (see Plate 226), semirigid scissors is poised at the central portion of the septum. **D** (see Plate 227), septum is bloodlessly transected. **E** (see Plate 228), the septum has been excised. The myometrium is reddish and has a tendency to bleed. The muscle bundles are apparent. The transected septum on each side is white and does not bleed.

The semirigid scissors have the advantage over flexible scissors of great stiffness and stability. They therefore cut more effectively and still offer the advantage of adjusting the optics either farther back to afford a panoramic view, or close-up for fine, detailed cutting (Fig 20–10; Plates 225 through 228). Thicker septa may be hemisected: that is, one begins at the lower extremity on either the right or left side and progresses upward toward the fundus with one arm of the scissor blades free (on the outer margin of the septum) and the other within the substance of the septum. Because septa have a poor vascular supply, are mainly fibrous tissue, and have a marshmallow-like consistency within the interior, this shearing technique may be done in several increments to completely incise a thick septum (Fig 20–11,A–E). The tendency when cutting either a thin or thick septum is to drift posteriorly as the upper portion of the septum is cut. The operator will be wise to stop cutting from time to time in order to reorient the endoscope to the midline of the uterine axis and then continue the incising operation (Fig 20–12, A and B). If the surgeon drifts too far posteriorly bleeding will be encountered as the myometrium is entered. Chervenak and Neuwirth reported a technique of inserting a fine scissors adjacent to the hysteroscope (i.e., not within the operating sheath) to give greater flexibility of motion.

DeCherney and coworkers utilize a 24 F urologic cystoscope and resectoscope to perform electric cutting of the septum.

Baggish has utilized a fine quartz fiber and the Nd-YAG laser to incise septa. This technique is very handy in the case of thick septa and, like the techniques described earlier, requires simultaneous laparoscopy (Fig 20–13). The laser operation may be performed utilizing an endoscopic video camera attached to the eyepiece of the hysteroscope, with the operator viewing and operating from a high-resolution television monitor (Fig 20–14). The advantage of the laser technique is the speed

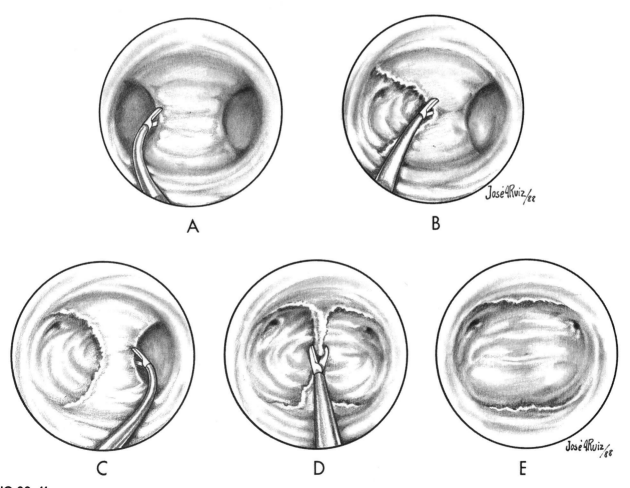

FIG 20–11.
A, when the septum is broad one blade of the scissors cuts into the substance of the septum while the other blade remains in the free cavity. **B,** when the fundus is reached on one side, the other side is transected in a similar manner. **C,** next the center (now thinned) of the septum is transected. **D,** The upper portion septum is cut. **E,** The operation is finished.

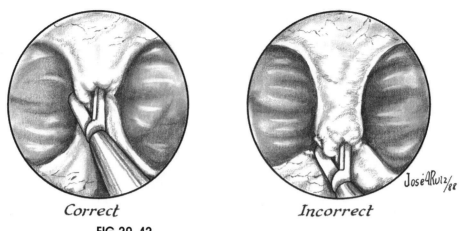

FIG 20–12.
The correct place to cut the septum is in the center.

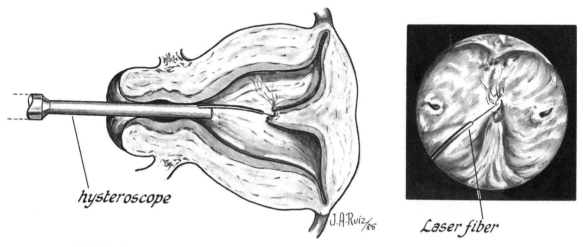

FIG 20–13.
A 600-μm Nd-YAG quartz fiber is inserted into the operating channel of laser hysteroscope.

and bloodless nature of the operation. The quartz fiber is introduced through the operating channel of the hysteroscope sheath. Since the fiber is only 500 to 600 μm in diameter, it makes a narrow cut through the septum (Fig 20–15). Each cornu is identified, and the tubal ostia are visualized. The fiber is engaged in either right or left uterine cornu well medial to the oviduct ostium (i.e., at the farthest lateral extremity of the septum). After the power is set at 25 W and light contact is made with the endometrial surface, the fiber is dragged across the septum, incising as it swings from left to right or vice versa. As with the scissors technique, the operator must constantly orient himself or herself so as not to allow the cutting fiber to drift too far posteriorly (Fig 20–16). In a variation of this technique, a sapphire tip attached to the laser fiber is utilized. The sapphire lens serves to focus the Nd-YAG laser beam to a narrow diameter, increasing the power density sufficiently to allow for more

efficient cutting (Plate 229). The fiber with or without the sapphire lens is swept back and forth from side to side until the desired depth for the septal resection is reached. Obviously, close observation from above with the laparoscope is required to reduce the risk of uterine perforation and to alert the surgeon to stop laser action immediately if perforation occurs.

Postoperatively, most experienced hysteroscopists do not place an IUD or other foreign body within the cavity. Individual preference will mandate the administration of estrogen—with a dosage equivalent to 1.25 to 2.5 mg of Premarin daily. Clearly the administration of prophylactic or therapeutic antibiotics is empirical. Most patients leave the hospital or surgicenter after recovery from anesthesia. We follow patients weekly for 2 weeks, then every other week with office hysteroscopy, followed by a hysterogram at 8 weeks postoperatively (Fig 20–17).

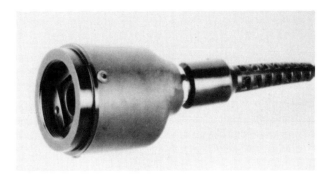

FIG 20–14.
Microchip endoscopy camera attaches to the eyepiece of the hysteroscope.

ENDOMETRIAL ABLATION

Intractable uterine bleeding unresponsive to conservative hormonal therapy or dilatation and curettage has in the past been managed by hysterectomy. During the 1980s, a reasonable alternative to hysterectomy has appeared in the form of transcervical hysteroscopic endometrial ablation. The technique may be carried out by two major techniques: (1) Nd-YAG laser, or (2) the resectoscope technique. Briefly, the laser technique depends on delivery of coherent light by means of a quartz fiber inserted through the operating channel of the hysteroscope (Fig 20–18). Recently, Baggish developed a special dual channel hysteroscope for intrauterine laser surgery. The laser technique depends on the characteristic front scatter of the 1,064-mm output of the Nd-YAG laser. This action penetrates the endometrium and exerts an extensive coagulative effect in the superficial myometrium (Fig 20–19). Additionally, as the laser beam reflects back from the disrupted tissue particles, it

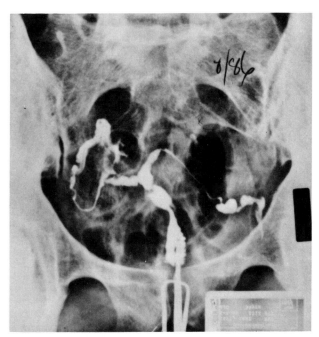

FIG 20–15.
Preoperative hysterogram shows a broad septate uterus.

produces destruction of the surface endometrium (Fig 20–20). The key action of this methodology, however, is based on coagulation of the large radial artery within the myometrium and interruption of the vascular supply to basal and functional layers of the endometrium. The end result is coaptation of the uterine walls and obliteration of the cavity (Fig 20–21; Plate 230).

DeCherney and Polan have described an alternate method of cauterizing the endometrial surface using the wire loop and the handle mechanism of the cystoscopic resectoscope. This procedure was performed on 11 pa-

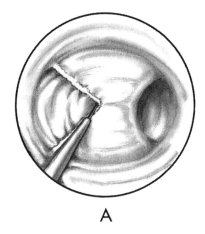

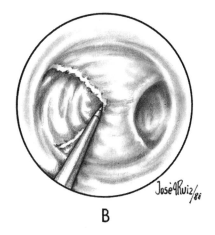

A   B

FIG 20–16.
The laser fiber touches the septum at either the right or left extremity and is swept across the tissue. The energy of the Nd-YAG laser bloodlessly incises the septum. **A,** bare laser fiber. **B,** fiber with attached sapphire tip.

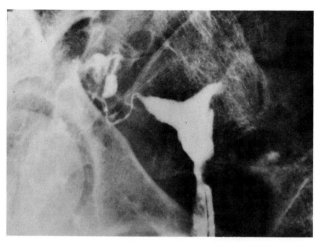

FIG 20–17.
Postoperative hysterogram of patient in figure 20-15.

tients in less than 30 minutes each, with two thirds of a high-risk group of women attaining long-term amenorrhea. In a later report, the New Haven group reported on 21 patients who underwent endometrial cautery excision in which Hyskon was used as the distending medium. Eighteen patients followed for greater than 6 months had no further vaginal bleeding. Interestingly, five patients had significant immediate bleeding, necessitating insertion of a Foley catheter into the uterus for up to 24 hours postoperatively. Three patients in the earlier series required an intrauterine Foley catheter for approximately 6 hours postoperatively to stop bleeding.

Baggish and Baltoyannis have recently reported a series of very high risk women in whom hysterectomy would have been a life-threatening operation and in whom Nd-YAG laser surgery was utilized to stop heavy,

uncontrolled bleeding which led to anemia. Half of these patients were diagnosed as having a major clotting defect. The laser operations differed from other reported series in that the dual channel hysteroscope was utilized simultaneously to aspirate and ablate; the operations were done indirectly, utilizing a video monitor; and Hyskon replaced dextrose in saline as the distending medium (Plate 231). The average time to complete the endometrial ablation was 60 minutes, but none of these women developed significant immediate bleeding and none required placement of a tamponade catheter within the uterus as did the resectoscope patients. The advantages and disadvantages of the two techniques are detailed in Table 20–1. The major deficiency with both operations is lack of long-term follow-up (i.e., more than 10 years) and the fact that only a small pool of women have undergone the surgery, and these have been operated on by an even smaller group of gynecologists.

SUBMUCOUS MYOMATA UTERI

The presence of a submucous myoma in a woman in the reproductive years who desires continued childbearing creates an enigma for the gynecologist (Fig 20–22; Plates 232 and 233). In the past, the conservative approach to therapy has been laparotomy, hysterotomy, and removal of the myoma (Plate 234). Recently, hysteroscopic operative removal has been advocated as a more efficacious and safe procedure. Submucous myomata may present a greater risk to the patient than either the intramural or subserous varieties. Submucous myomata characteristically are associated with chronic

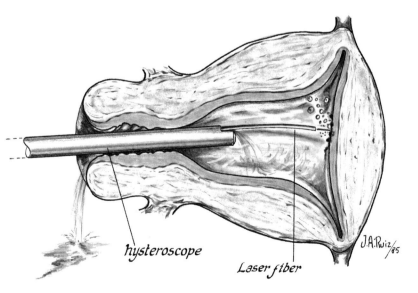

FIG 20–18.
A fine quartz fiber is delivered through the operating channel of the hysteroscope to make light contact with endometrial surface. The Nd-YAG laser energy is carried by way of the fiber.

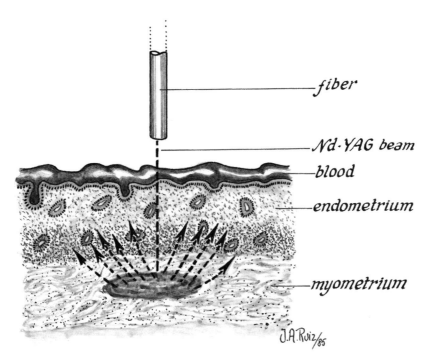

FIG 20–19.
The laser energy penetrates the surface of the endometrium and exerts a maximal coagulative action in the superficial myome- trium. By backscatter the beam reflects backwards to further co- agulate the surface tissues.

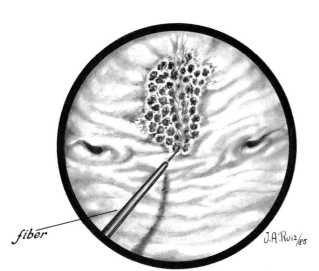

Laser beam coagulating endometrial surface

FIG 20–20.
Schematically, the laser fiber makes light touch in a "pointillism" technique, creating multiple connecting points of damage to the endometrial surface.

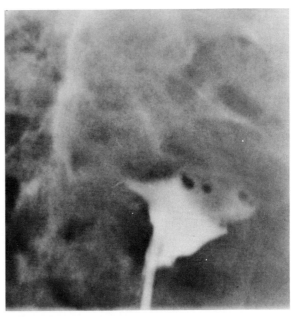

FIG 20–21.
A (see Plate 230), histologic section of uterine wall taken 8 weeks after laser ablation. Carbon particles surrounded by foreign body giant cells and collagen are all that remain of the endo- metrium **B** (above), hysterogram at 8 weeks postablation shows most of the cavity to be obliterated the sound passed to 3 cm then met obstruction of the coated walls of the uterus.

TABLE 20–1.

Comparison of Nd-YAG Laser and Resectoscope for Endometrial Ablation

Category	Nd-YAG Laser	Cystoscopic Resectoscope
Resultant amenorrhea	High	High
Time to complete	Longer (30–60 min)	Shorter (30 min)
Immediate bleeding	Low	High
Delayed bleeding	Low	Unknown
Skill required	High	High
Conduction through tissue	None	Conducts
Simultaneous laparoscopy	None	None
Field of view	Expansive	Reduced
Outpatient	Yes	Yes
Long-term follow-up	6 yr	5 yr

endometritis, have a greater risk for malignant change (leiomyosarcoma), and are prone to bleed (Plate 235). Neuwirth and Amin were pioneers in developing techniques for hysteroscopic treatment of submucous myomata. Initially the lesions were removed by rather rough methods, for example, ovum forceps were used to twist pedunculated myomata off their pedicles, and scissors were inserted outside of the hysteroscopic sheath to cut the myoma pedicle. More recently the techniques have been refined to utilize scissors inserted through the operating sheath of the hysteroscope or the cystoscopic resectoscope to shave sessile myomata to the level of or just below the endometrial surface. Problems associated with these techniques include postoperative bleeding, intraoperative bleeding, and difficulty extracting the excised myoma from the uterine cavity.

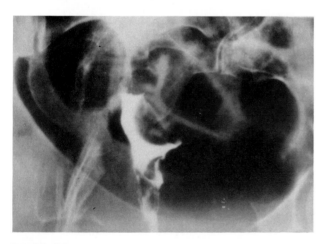

FIG 20–22.
A (above), hysterogram shows a large, round filling defect of the uterine cavity. The lesion is compatible with a submucous myoma. **B** (see Plate 232), submucous myoma as seen by panoramic hysteroscopy. The myoma is located on the anterior wall. **C** (see Plate 233), contact hysteroscopy of the submucous myoma shown in **B. D** (see Plate 234), cross specimen of the myoma seen in **A** to **C**.

Morcellation divides the lesion into smaller pieces which are easier to remove. Neuwirth has crushed excised myomata with ovum forceps in order to deliver them through the cervix. Postsurgical bleeding has been dealt with effectively by the insertion of an intrauterine balloon for 6 to 24 hours postoperatively.

The Nd-YAG laser delivered by a quartz fiber through the operative channel of the operating hysteroscope may be utilized by means of several techniques. First, either the pedicle of a pedunculated myoma or the sessile myoma may be cut off at the base by means of the laser alone. The specimen is grasped with a semirigid forceps and removed by pulling the entire sheath through the cervix. An alternative technique morcellates the myoma, whose component pieces are removed by ovum forceps or grasping forceps. Finally, the laser may be utilized to coagulate the base of the myoma, after which the semirigid scissors is inserted through the hysteroscopic sheath to cut off the myoma. Actually, with the dual channel operating sheath, the laser fiber and scissors may be simultaneously inserted into the uterus. The laser fiber may then be removed so that the coagulated edge of the myoma may be grasped with semirigid forceps and held on tension as the scissors cuts through the tissue. The myoma may then be subdivided to facilitate removal (Fig 20–23,A–C). For vascular lesions a long, flexible, 22-gauge needle may be inserted through the operative sheath and 1:30 Pitressin injected directly into the lesion before the cutting is initiated (Fig 20–24). When greater flexibility is required, a fine scissors may be inserted alongside the hysteroscope for myoma resection.

Most hysteroscopic surgeons have preferred to perform myomectomy utilizing Hyskon as the distending medium because of its lack of miscibility with blood and its optical clarity. Likewise, most surgeons have preferred the additional safety insurance of performing a simultaneous laparoscopy.

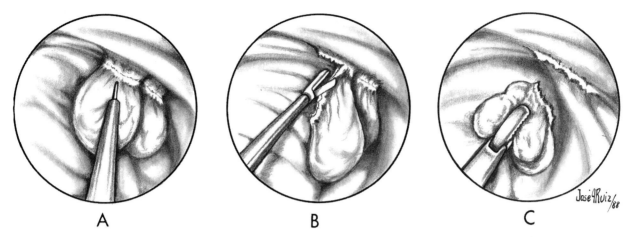

A B C

FIG 20–23.
A, Two submucous myomas are in juxtaposition to each other. The Nd-YAG laser fiber is employed to coagulate the base. **B,** the semirigid scissors then cuts the myoma base. **C,** the pieces of myoma are retrieved for removal by semirigid or rigid forceps.

Pedunculated myomas should be manipulated into a position to allow clear identification of the pedicle (Plate 236). Pitressin (vasopressin) 1:30 injection or Nd-YAG laser coagulation is worthwhile prior to cutting the pedicle. This step will usually eliminate pesky bleeding and relieve the surgeon of the necessity for inserting a balloon into the uterus. Postoperatively the patient should be placed on antibiotics, since these lesions are usually inflamed. Low-dose Premarin is administered to stimulate endometrial growth and epithelialization of the operative site. It is worthwhile to perform an office hysteroscopy with CO_2 to examine the cavity 6 to 8 weeks postoperatively. In some patients the excised myomata will regrow and some patients will require further surgery. Of 26 patients operated on by Neuwirth, 9 required further surgery and 7 underwent hysterectomy. If conception is the goal of the patient this should be attempted within 6 to 8 weeks postoperatively, as tumor regrowth is not predictable.

For pedunculated myomata presenting in the lower uterine segment, cervical dilation and excision with the CO_2 laser delivered through the colposcope may be a reasonable alternative to hysteroscopic removal (Plate 237,A). A diagnostic hysteroscopy is first done, and the site of the myoma is verified. Pitressin 1:30 is injected circumferentially into the cervix. The CO_2 laser delivered by way of a micromanipulator cuts the posterior lip of the cervix and the canal through and through (Plate 237,B). The myoma is grasped with a 10-inch laser hook, and the traction is placed downward on the myoma (Plate 237,C). The pedicle is exposed, injected with Pitressin 1:30, then transected with the laser beam (Plate 237,D). The cervix is repaired with interrupted 3-0 Vicryl sutures (Plate 237,E).

The advantages of hysteroscopic resection of submucous myomata are several. First, the operation may be performed on an outpatient or overnight admission basis, resulting in considerable cost savings. Second, the patient suffers less pain and substantially less operative morbidity. Third, if the patient becomes pregnant, deliv-

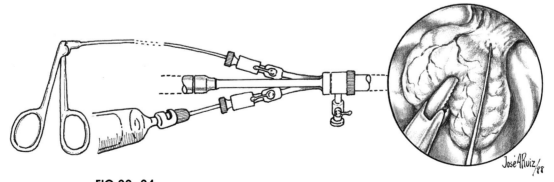

FIG 20–24.
The broad pedicle of a myoma is injected with a dilute solution of vasopressin.

ery by the vaginal route may be anticipated. Although one third of these patients will require more surgery; a window of time can be gained for pregnancy or menopause to supervene. As part of the informed consent, every patient undergoing hysteroscopic myomectomy should be prepared for possible laparotomy.

Barbot has to date treated 60 cases of submucous myoma hysteroscopically (Plate 238). The myoma was completely removed in 36 cases (60%), partially extricated in 13 cases (21%), and unable to be excised in 11 cases (18%). All of the failures were related to large, sessile lesions. Five of the 11 myomata were more than 40 mm in diameter. The only observed complication was uterine perforation, which was followed by abdominal myomectomy. Among the partial removals, four patients had recurrent bleeding and underwent repeat myomectomy or hysterectomy. All the failed cases also underwent repeat myomectomy or hysterectomy. The overall failure rate was therefore 25%.

ULTRASONOGRAPHIC MONITORING

A recently published alternative to simultaneous laparoscopic monitoring of operative hysteroscopy is real-time ultrasonography. One technique describes three contrasts obtained by (1) filling the urinary bladder with fluid, (2) infusing by gravity the cul-de-sac, and (3) distending the uterine cavity with fluid and inserting an operative device. Essentially, real-time ultrasonography provides an indirect visual image of the uterine wall, the lesions, and the hysteroscope.

BIBLIOGRAPHY

Baggish MS, Baltoyannis P: New techniques for laser ablation of the endometrium in high risk patients. *Am J Obstet Gynecol* (in press).

Chervenak FA, Neuwirth RS: Hysteroscopic resection of the uterine septum. *Am J Obstet Gynecol* 1981; 141:351.

DeCherney A, Polan ML: Hysteroscopic management of intrauterine lesions and intractable uterine bleeding. *Obstet Gynecol* 1983; 61:392.

DeCherney AH: Hysteroscopic management of mullerian fusion defects, in Siegler AM, Lindemann HJ (eds): *Hysteroscopy: Principles and Practice.* Philadelphia, JB Lippincott, 1984, p 204.

DeCherney AH, Russell JB, Graebe RA, et al: Resectoscopic management of mullerian fusion defects. *Fertil Steril* 1986; 45:726.

DeCherney AH, Diamond MP, Lavy G, et al: Endometrial ablation for intractable uterine bleeding: Hysteroscopic resection. *Obstet Gynecol* 1987; 70:668.

Ismajovich B, Lidor A, Confino E, et al: Treatment of minimal and moderate intrauterine adhesions. *J Reprod Med* 1985; 30:769.

Israel R, March CM: Hysteroscopic incision of the septate uterus. *Am J Obstet Gynecol* 1984; 149:66.

Joelsson I, Levine RU, Moberger G: Hysteroscopy as an adjunct in determining the extent of carcinoma of the endometrium. *Am J Obstet Gynecol* 1971; 111:696.

Levine RU, Neuwirth RS: Simultaneous laparoscopy and hysteroscopy for intrauterine adhesions. *Obstet Gynecol* 1973; 42:441.

Lin BL, Iwata Y, Miyamoto N, et al: Three-contrasts method: An ultrasound technique for monitoring transcervical operations. *Am J Obstet Gynecol* 1987; 156:469.

March CM, Israel R: Intrauterine adhesions secondary to elective abortion. *Obstet Gynecol* 1976; 48:422.

March CM, Israel R: Hysteroscopic management of recurrent abortion caused by septate uterus. *Am J Obstet Gynecol* 1987; 156:834.

Neuwirth RS, Hussein AR, Schiffman BM, et al: Hysteroscopic resection of intrauterine scars—using a new technique. *Obstet Gynecol* 1982; 60:111.

Neuwirth RS: Hysteroscopic management of symptomatic submucous fibroids. *Obstet Gynecol* 1983; 62:509.

Neuwirth RS, Amin JH: Excision of submucous fibroids with hysteroscopic control. *Am J Obstet Gynecol* 1976; 126:95.

Shalev E, Zuckerman H: Operative hysteroscopy under real-time ultrasonography. *Am J Obstet Gynecol* 1986; 155:1360.

Siegler AM, Kemmann E: Hysteroscopic removal of occult intrauterine contraceptive device. *Obstet Gynecol* 1975; 46:604.

Taylor PJ, Cumming DC, Hill PJ: Significance of intrauterine adhesions detected hysteroscopically in eumenorrheic infertile women and role of antecedent curettage in their formation. *Am J Obstet Gynecol* 1981; 139:239.

Toaff R, Ballas S: Traumatic hypomenorrhea—amenorrhea. *Fertil Steril* 1978; 30:379.

Valle RF, Sciarra JJ: Hysteroscopy: A useful diagnostic adjunct in gynecology. *Am J Obstet Gynecol* 1975; 122:230.

Valle RF: Hysteroscopic evaluation of patients with abnormal uterine bleeding. *Surg Gynecol Obstet* 1981; 153:521.

21

Operative Hysteroscopy II

Robert S. Neuwirth, M.D.

Surgical procedures performed under hysteroscopic control were initially limited to tubal sterilization by cauterization of the ostia, as reported by Lindemann, Quinones, and Neuwirth in 1970. Since these first reports, surgery under hysteroscopic control has expanded. The prerequisites for a good surgical procedure are a diagnosis, clear appraisal of the surgical anatomy, control of the bleeding, adequate exposure, and precise technique with the operative instruments to avoid unintended actions. This chapter will address these issues as they apply to hysteroscopic surgery.

APPLICATIONS

At this time there are clear indications for hysteroscopic surgery in the treatment of Asherman's syndrome, correction of the septate anomaly of the uterus, removal of an embedded or trapped intrauterine device (IUD), and the thorough removal of endometrial polyps. Applications under development are tubal sterilization with Silastic formed-in-place tubal plugs, removal of submucous fibroids, and the treatment of menorrhagia by endometrial ablation in lieu of hysterectomy. In each of these applications an incorrect diagnosis can lead to serious error. For example, a patient with secondary amenorrhea and a false positive hysterogram showing filling defects can be a candidate for hysteroscopic repair of scar under laparoscopic control. Only technically well performed hysteroscopy will enable detection of this error and return the patient for better diagnostic work-up. Retrieval of a lost IUD should be preceded by localizing pelvic radiographs from two angles, with a probe in the uterus to identify the location of the IUD relative to the endometrial cavity. This will avoid fruitless searches for the foreign body as well as prepare the surgeon for what may be encountered in locating and removing the device. Finally, the treatment of abnormal uterine bleeding with a hysteroscope must be preceded always by a patient history, physical examination, Papanicolaou smear, endometrial biopsy, and—when fibroids are thought present—a pelvic sonogram.

SURGICAL ANATOMY

As with any surgical procedure the surgical anatomy in hysteroscopy is critical (Fig 21–1, A and B). Using the hysteroscope to appraise the surgical field can be misleading, as the working distance from objective lens to tissue is short, making the field magnified and limiting the surgeon to small views which must be mentally reconstructed in order to appreciate the surgical anatomy. This problem is most complex in viewing Asherman's syndrome as well as submucous fibroids, where normal landmarks can be distorted significantly. It is also critical to be aware that the myometrial thickness may be 1 cm or less, and the cornual areas may even be less thick. For this reason as well as reducing the potential damage of an accidental perforation, simultaneous laparoscopy is a good idea during the course of major hysteroscopic intervention (Fig 21–2, A and B). This safety measure is obvious before proceeding with a septate uterus in order to rule out a bicornuate anomaly as well, which would contraindicate hysteroscopic repair. During the course of repair of Asherman's syndrome, inadvertent uterine perforation is quite easy, and the laparoscope is very useful. In the removal of submucous fibroids, the knowledge of the serosal side of the uterus is helpful, particularly as a resection of the submucous fibroid or submucous component of an intramural fibroid is proceeding.

In planning for hysteroscopic submucosal myomectomy, careful examination is important to determine the

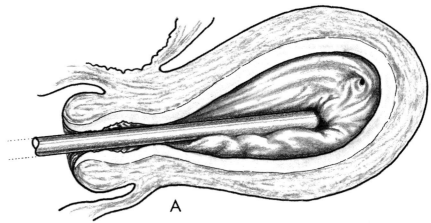

FIG 21–1.
A, the barrel of the hysteroscope may be used to estimate the thickness of the endometrium. **B,** after pressure is placed on the endometrium and the endoscope is raised, a groove can be identified.

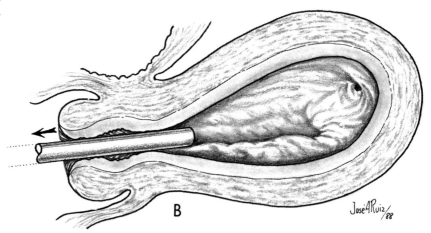

number of fibroids, the size and location of the attachment to the uterine wall, and the location of the fallopian tube orifices. The distance of the tumor from the internal cervical os or top of the fundus is important. As a procedure progresses the operative field becomes disturbed with blood, tissue fragments, and local tissue edema; also, the anatomy changes as the surgery progresses. Therefore, accurate knowledge of surgical anatomy at the start of the procedure is important to success and the avoidance of complications.

SURGICAL MANIPULATIONS WITH THE HYSTEROSCOPE

There are four basic approaches to intrauterine intervention where the hysteroscope can be used. The first and easiest technique is to employ the hysteroscope as a viewing instrument, remove it, and use a curette, an ovum forceps, hook, or scissors to manipulate in a semi-blind manner. This is most applicable to the removal of a polyp or an IUD or for cutting a small adhesive band low in the uterine cavity. Once the maneuver is completed, the hysteroscope is replaced for control of viewing.

A second approach is to employ instruments with clamps, biopsy forceps, and scissors fixed to the distal end of the sheath. These are easy to insert and operate but have the drawback of a close, fixed distance to the objective lens, so that surgery is conducted with great magnification and less of a field of view. These instruments can be used with a variety of distension media, including viscous liquids if bleeding is a problem.

The third approach is to pass instruments through the sheath of the hysteroscope, which permits movement to and from but limits lateral movement. This overcomes the optical problems of a fixed distance to the surgical field. However, the lens is smaller, there are fewer fiberoptic light bundles, and the cannula usually will not have sufficient caliber to allow passage of a vis-

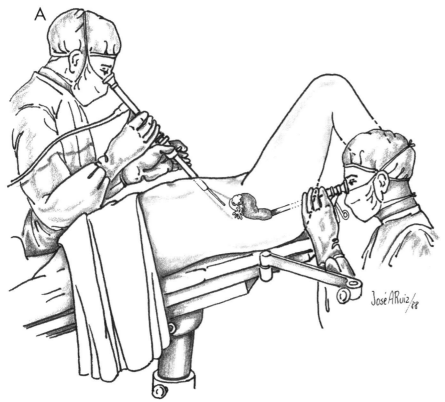

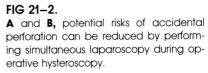

FIG 21–2.
A and **B,** potential risks of accidental perforation can be reduced by performing simultaneous laparoscopy during operative hysteroscopy.

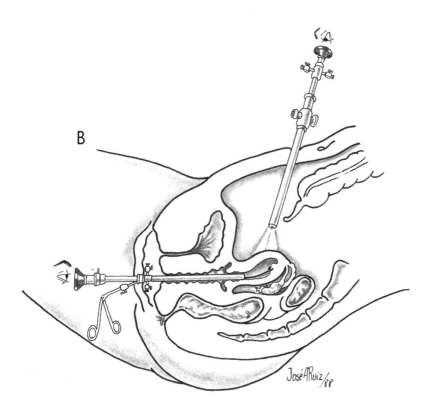

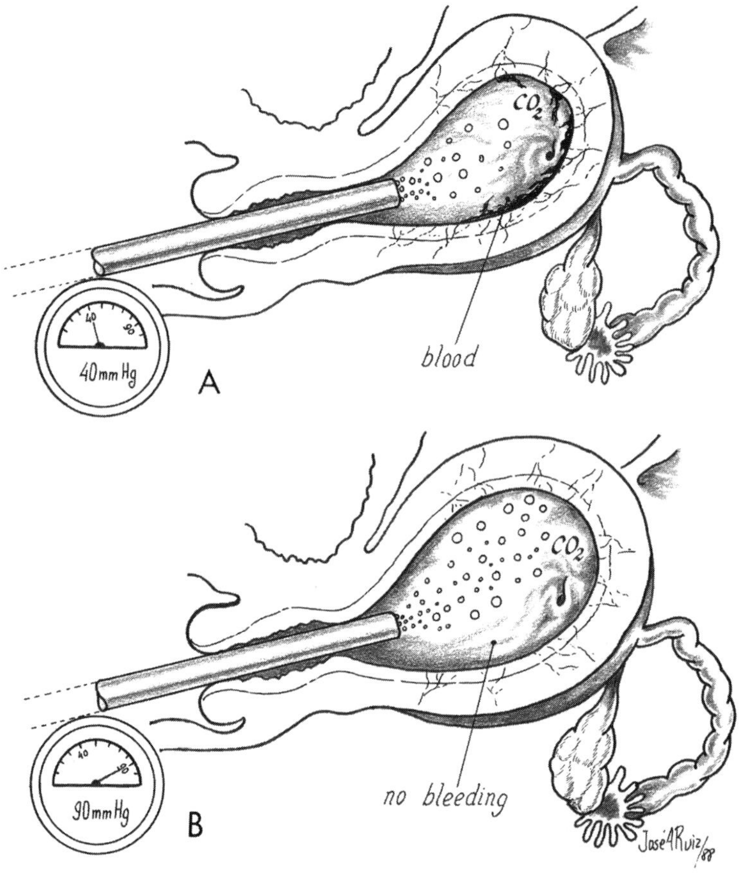

FIG 21–3.
A, when intrauterine pressure is low, bleeding is more apt to interfere with vision during operative procedures. **B,** increasing the flow rate, and hence the intrauterine pressure produced by the distending medium, will quickly arrest endometrial bleeding because the feeding vessels are compressed.

cous medium, such as Hyskon, during the surgical work with mechanical instruments if bleeding becomes a problem. The exception to this is the use of the laser such as the neodymium (Nd)-YAG, which is conducted through a slender fiberoptic bundle and can be operated in low-viscosity or high-viscosity liquids. The other exception is the resectoscope, which has a larger diameter and will accept low- and high-viscosity liquids.

The last alternative is the passage of instruments outside of the hysteroscope sheath—between it and the endocervical canal. This method requires the greatest manual skill but offers free hand motion in the uterine cavity. It requires a high-viscosity liquid to maintain uterine distention. The technique requires withdrawal of the hysteroscope to the external os, insertion of the operating instrument into the cervix, and reinsertion of the hysteroscope. The hysteroscope and operating instrument are advanced together under visual control and aligned to commence the surgery.

None of these techniques is exclusive of the other providing the equipment is available and the surgeon is skilled in each of these options.

CONTROL OF BLEEDING AND ADEQUATE EXPOSURE

In order to see adequately in the uterus, the intrauterine pressure must be above 50 mm Hg. As the pressure rises, it also reduces bleeding from veins and small arterial vessels (Fig 21–3,A and B). This is the primary means of hemostasis during the entire uterine surgery. The flow of the distension medium is important as a lens-washing system in order to clear the field of blood and debris. Liquids with higher viscosity are more effective for lens washing than CO_2; bubbles tend to be a problem in gas. Techniques that employ CO_2 during hysteroscopic surgery have relied on vasospastic agents such as vasopressin to control bleeding and to maintain an operative field. For the most part, however, liquids are a more effective means of accomplishing these objectives.

The problems with liquids are the absorption into the vascular system through the capillary and lymphatic channels open during this surgery. Therefore, whether using Hyskon or lower viscosity fluids, one must be careful to note early signs of hypervolemia and pulmonary edema. Hyponatremia can also occur with nonelectrolyte liquids. If the laser is to be used, the liquid may be of low or high viscosity and need not be a nonelectrolyte. If electrosurgery is to be used, a nonelectrolyte such as 5% dextrose in water, 1.5% glycine, or Hyskon must be employed. The heating inherent in laser or electrosurgery may produce carmelization at the tip of the operating instrument, requiring that it be cleaned off as necessary. However, the higher viscosity of Hyskon makes it easier to maintain uterine distension and lens washing. Low-viscosity liquids require a fairly high flow in the small uterine cavity to wash away blood and debris. The requirement of high flow makes it difficult to achieve satisfactory intrauterine pressure with low-viscosity liquids. In each case the choice of fluid can be individualized, as there is no incompatibility among the liquids, and change from one to the other is easy and useful during surgery, depending on the problem. The fit between hysteroscopic cannula and the cervical canal is important. It is desirable to have a comfortable fit. A tight fit will not permit much liquid to flow out between the cervix and cannula. A loose fit means that even a high-viscosity liquid runs out so fast that the uterine cavity cannot be distended. Control of this factor is managed by careful dilatation or cross clamping a floppy cervix.

Following the surgery, bleeding may continue to be a problem. The use of an intrauterine balloon distended to conform to the cavity and achieve a pressure of 80 to 100 mm Hg is an excellent means of controlling and preventing postoperative bleeding. The balloon pressure can be released several hours later, and if no bleeding occurs it can be removed thereafter. A small ball valve in the stem is designed for easy bedside control, and the stem lies comfortably in the vagina.

PRECISION TECHNIQUES

The key feature of precise surgery is control of the instruments with full knowledge of the surgical field. Hysteroscopy is central to this precision. The operating instruments are also important. The scissors, clamps, laser, electrosurgical instrument, or catheter for injection of Silastic into the tubes must be understood by the surgeon and employed with control and confidence. Safety is important for confidence, and simultaneous laparoscopy is very helpful in many procedures, particularly where cutting or burning are involved.

It is important to know the details such as the length of the cutting blade of scissors, the diameter of the fiberoptic bundle for the YAG laser and the width of the resectoscope loop in order to maintain high precision. The watts of cutting or coagulative effects of the YAG laser are important to know in order to achieve a desired effect and avoid complications. For example, the ablation technique is designed to produce a burn of the endometrium to a depth just below the basal gland layer. In an early proliferative endometrium, this is approximately 4 mm deep. Using the YAG laser, the depth of burn with the fiber tip 1 mm away from the surface produces a 4-mm deep coagulation effect. Touching the tissue will produce carbonization and a deeper burn. In general, therefore, the touch technique will give a more effective destruction of the endometrium. However, it is slightly more risky with respect to producing a deeper myometrial or even a serosal burn of the uterus and damage to surrounding tissues touching the uterus. Such considerations are important to executing the surgery precisely, effectively, and with a minimal risk to the patient.

HYSTEROSCOPIC MYOMECTOMY TECHNIQUE

The principles of hysteroscopic surgery are embodied in the myomectomy technique. The method rests first on accurate diagnosis and presurgical appraisal. The diagnosis is always established by hysteroscopic confirmation, at which time our operative appraisal is also made. If fertility is desired, the operative selection is more rigid. That is, the myoma should not be more than 3 cm across at its junction with the normal myometrium (Fig 21–4). This criterion is based on the need for the raw surface to be re-epithelialized in the postoperative period with little, if any, scar formation. If multiple fibroids are present they should not be on opposite sides of the endometrial cavity. The rationale is the same: to minimize postoperative intrauterine adhesions.

If fertility is not a serious consideration the procedure can be more destructive and indeed may be associated with endometrial ablation. Therefore, a larger intramural diameter of a submucous-intramural fibroid is acceptable, and multiple fibroids around the cavity are not contraindications.

The diagnosis and appraisal can be done in the office or the ambulatory surgical unit and need not be performed at the same time as the surgery. In fact, separate appraisal is helpful as it gives the opportunity to choose those cases to be done hysteroscopically from those best performed abdominally.

The consent for myomectomy always includes laparoscopy, possible laparotomy, and possible hysterec-

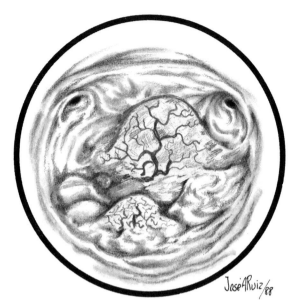

FIG 21–4.
Hysteroscopy is performed to make an accurate diagnosis of submucous myomata. At this examination the size and location of these lesions are ascertained in order to determine whether an operative hysteroscopic approach is possible.

tomy. The patient can be admitted the evening before, or directly to the operating room. We have made it a custom to observe the patient overnight for bleeding or unrecognized injury. Blood is available on call.

The procedure starts with hysteroscopy, using CO_2 gas or Hyskon. With the decision to proceed, laparoscopy is performed, and an insulated probe is placed between the uterus and sigmoid colon. The 8-mm resectoscope is inserted, and 30 W of cutting current is used (Fig 21–5). If an ablation is to be done, it is usually performed first as it produces less blood and debris. Then the myomectomy is performed. Ablation is done preferably when the endometrium is thin, using 30 to 40 W of coagulating current and dragging a resectoscope loop or other insulated electrode across the surface to produce a white coagulation of the endometrial tissues and superficial myometrium. Very little carbonization is seen.

Resection of a submucous fibroid can be performed with the loop of the resectoscope, drawing it in toward the operator (Plate 239). The loop can also be kept at a fixed length from the resectoscope sheath and drawn back, much as a curette, under direct visualization of the hysteroscopic light and optical system. We have found Hyskon uniquely suitable to this type of surgery because of the bleeding, the pressure required for uterine distention, and the washing necessary from a liquid medium.

As the resection procedure progresses, the slices of tissue will float in the endometrial cavity and may lodge over the objective lens. These fragments can be removed by withdrawal of the resectoscope from the sheath to allow them to flow out. Alternatively, they can be removed with an ovum forceps after the whole resectoscope is removed.

The objective is to shave the submucous myoma down to the plane of the endometrial cavity (Plate 240). As the procedure progresses it usually becomes more bloody; therefore, more hysteroscopy skill is necessary later in the procedure, particularly with a large myoma (Fig 21–6; Plates 241 and 242). If the myoma is on a pedicle it can be reduced in size to the point where the ovum forceps can grasp it, twist it off, and extract it. Then the resectoscope is reinserted and inspection carried out to control the bleeding and review the appearance of the endometrial cavity (Plate 243). Clearly, laparoscopic control is critical in these aggressive procedures to warn of perforation or bleeding into the peritoneal cavity or broad ligaments.

Postoperatively hemostasis is important. We have used an intrauterine hemostasis balloon which is inserted with a smooth forceps and partially inflated, after which the forceps is removed. The inflation is then completed until the pressure reaches arterial pressure and the bleeding stops. Postoperatively the balloon is released several hours later, and if there is no bleeding it is removed thereafter. The patients are treated with antibiotics. If ablation is performed, danazol has been used to attempt to suppress endometrial regeneration for two weeks. If future fertility is desired, Premarin, 2.5 mg per day, has been used for 10 days to stimulate endometrial repair to resurface the raw areas left by the resection. The short hospitalization, speed of recovery, and high degree of success in control of bleeding has made this

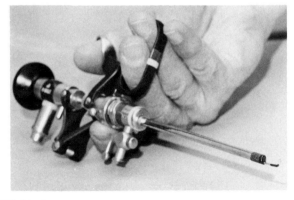

FIG 21–5.
A cystoscopic-resectoscope is used with the loop drawn in toward the operator or kept at a fixed length from the sheath.

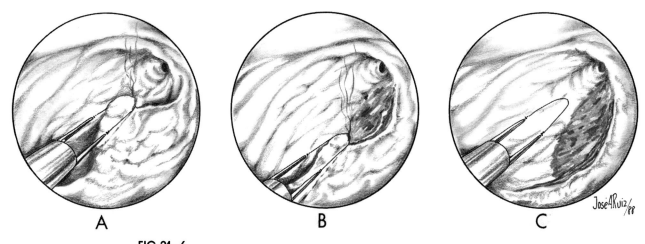

FIG 21–6.
A–C, submucous myoma being shaved down to plane of endometrial cavity.

procedure very promising as an alternative to classic abdominal myomectomy, abdominal hysterectomy, and vaginal hysterectomy.

SUMMARY

With the acceptance of hysteroscopy as a valid, useful diagnostic method, selected surgical techniques have been designed for therapeutic effect. All of these surgical techniques depend on the skill of the hysteroscopist with the equipment, distension media, and hemostasis methods in order to offer the advantages of the hysteroscopy approach to therapy. Once he or she has mastered the equipment and distension techniques, full understanding of the intervention technology such as laser cautery, Silastic rubber, or mechanical instruments will enable the hysteroscopic surgeon to offer safe and effective therapeutic options that avoid the necessity for open abdominal or vaginal surgery.

BIBLIOGRAPHY

DeCherney AH, Cholst I, Naftolin F: The management of intractable uterine bleeding utilizing the cystoscopic resectoscope, in Siegler AM, Lindemann HJ (eds): *Hysteroscopy, Principles and Practice.* Philadelphia, J B Lippincott Co, 1984, part II, chapter 29, p 140.

Lindemann HJ: Transuterine tubal sterilization by CO_2 hysteroscopy, in Sciarra JJ, Butler JC, Speidel JJ (eds): *Hysteroscopic Sterilization.* New York, Intercontinental Medical Book Corp, 1974, p 61.

Neuwirth RS: Some new applications for hysteroscopy. *Contemp Obstet Gynecol* 1987; (special issue) 3:11–28.

Neuwirth RS: Hysteroscopic resection of submucous leiomyoma. *Contemp Obstet Gynecol* 1985; 25:103–123.

Neuwirth RS: Hysteroscopic management of symptomatic submucous fibroids. *Obstet Gynecol* 1983; 62:509.

Neuwirth RS: A new technique for and additional experience with hysteroscopic resection of submucous fibroids. *Am J Obstet Gynecol* 1978; 131:91.

Neuwirth RS, Amin HK: Excision of submucous fibroids with hysteroscopic control. *Am J Obstet Gynecol* 1976; 126:95.

Neuwirth RS, Richart R, Israngkun C, et al: Hysteroscopic sterilization, in *Hysteroscopic Sterilization.* New York, Intercontinental Medical Book Corp, 1974, p 121.

Quinones R, Alvarado A, Aznar R: Tubal electrocoagulation under hysteroscopic control, in *Hysteroscopic Sterilization.* New York, Intercontinental Medical Book Corp, 1974, p 95.

22

Laser Hysteroscopy

Jack M. Lomano, M.D.

Improved hysteroscopic techniques coupled with advances in laser technology have led to an interest in using laser energy to treat intrauterine disease processes. At the present time, the carbon dioxide laser, the Nd-YAG laser, and the argon laser have been used in gynecology to treat extrauterine disease. These lasers have been primarily used to treat pelvic endometriosis, cervical dysplasia, condylomata acuminata, pelvic adhesive disease, and premalignant diseases of the vulva and the vagina.

Laser energy with its advantages of precise tissue destruction, better hemostasis, and rapid tissue healing combined with hysteroscopy and its advantage of accessibility to the uterine cavity with a minimum of discomfort and expense to the patient provides an excellent combination of medical technology. Laser hysteroscopy can be used to treat chronic menorrhagia, myomata, septa and other uterine abnormalities incorporating both convenience and cost effectiveness. Clinicians should become familiar with these techniques as well as their limitations and potential benefits.

WHAT IS A LASER?

When external energy such as electrical current, light, or heat is applied to an atom, the electrons orbiting that atom jump to a higher energy level. This unstable condition lasts for a very short time, and when the electron returns to the ground state, a packet of energy is emitted in the form of a photon (Fig 22–1,A). If the atoms are stimulated in a medium with parallel mirrors at either end, the photon of light will reflect back and forth between the two mirrors. As these generated photons hit other atoms in the unstable state, additional

photons of energy will be emitted from the atom as electrons drop back to their lower energy level. The additional photons will be in phase, i.e. flow in the same direction and frequency as the photon which initially struck the atom (Fig 22–1,B). By continuing to put energy into these atoms, more and more photons will be discharged, thus creating a beam of light which has three distinguishing characteristics that differ from ordinary light. Laser beams are collimated, or parallel, which creates a minimal amount of divergence as the light is transmitted from its source. The laser energy is coherent, that is, all of the waves are in phase. The laser light is monochromatic, or only one color.

When a partially transmitting mirror is placed at one end of the optical chamber, a portion of the laser light can be released from the chamber in a controlled fashion (Fig 22–2,A). Thus, we have *light amplification* by the *stimulated emission* of *radiation*, which has become an acronym, laser.

The carbon dioxide laser has been the primary instrument utilized for gynecologic surgery. The specific absorption of its far infrared output by cell water is independent of tissue color. The CO_2 laser minimizes deep tissue damage because the laser energy is instantly absorbed and there is no scattering into the tissues of the body (Fig 22–2,B). These facts make the CO_2 laser a precise surgical instrument which can be used for vaporizing tissue or cutting tissue with a hands-off technique. The hallmark of the CO_2 laser is its surgical precision. The CO_2 laser energy currently cannot be transmitted through a fiber, thus making it difficult to deliver this into the uterine cavity.

The argon laser was first developed for the treatment of diabetic retinopathy in 1965. This laser produces a visible blue-green light (488 and 515 nm),

186

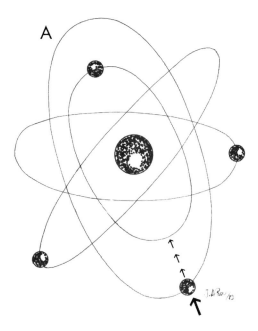

A

B ⟶ photon

Stimulated Emission

FIG 22–1.
A, orbiting electrons are stimulated to a higher energy level (metastable). The atom remains in the unstable state for a very short time since the electron quickly drops to a more stable orbit *(arrows)*. **B,** when a photon is driven into an unstable atom it drives the electron (stimulated) into an inner orbit and liberates two photons traveling in the same direction and with the same frequency as the incoming photon.

which is easily transmitted through clear aqueous tissues. Certain tissue pigments such as melanin and hemoglobin will selectively absorb argon laser light. The interaction of low levels of blue-green light with highly pigmented tissue results in coagulation of these pigmented tissues. The argon laser can be transmitted to tissue sites by way of fine quartz fibers and can efficiently be conducted through liquid media. It is a highly effective system for endoscopic delivery.

The Nd-YAG laser is a solid crystal made up of yttrium, aluminum, and garnet with surrounding neodym-

ium. The Nd-YAG light emits in the near infrared region with a wavelength of 1,064 nm. The beam is transmitted through clear liquids, which allows its optimal use in water-filled cavities such as the eye, the bladder, or the uterus. Its absorption is not highly color specific like the argon laser; however, the beam is more efficiently absorbed by dark pigment. The Nd-YAG laser has a characteristic physical property of front scatter and penetrates deeply, resulting in a homogenous zone of thermal coagulation which may extend from 1 to 4 mm beyond the site of impact. The Nd-YAG laser is an ex-

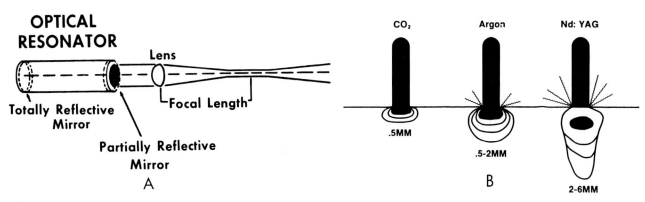

OPTICAL RESONATOR

Lens

Focal Length

Totally Reflective Mirror

Partially Reflective Mirror

A

TISSUE REACTION

CO₂   Argon   Nd: YAG

.5MM

.5-2MM

2-6MM

B

FIG 22–2.
A, schema of laser tube. The laser beam leaves the tube by way of partially reflective mirror. **B,** three surgical lasers utilized in gynecology. Note the levels of tissue coagulation for each laser.

cellent tool for tissue coagulation, and like the argon laser, can be delivered through fiberoptic systems. By applying a sapphire tip to the Nd-YAG laser fiber, one can focus the laser to a fine point which will allow it to perform as a cutting tool with precision similar to the CO_2 laser.

A relatively new laser is based on the frequency doubled YAG laser which utilizes a KTP (potassium triphosphate) crystal to double the wavelength of the YAG laser, thus resulting in a 532-nm beam. This wavelength is in the green range similar to that of the argon laser. Its tissue effects are virtually identical to those of the argon laser (Plate 244).

TISSUE EFFECTS OF LASERS

When laser light strikes an object including cellular tissue, it may be reflected, transmitted, scattered, absorbed, or a combination of these (Fig 22–3). Since lasers are a special form of light, they obey all of the physical principles of light energy. Whatever occurs when a laser beam strikes tissue, depends on the wavelength, intensity, duration of the irradiation, and the type of tissue impacted (Fig 22–4).

CO_2, argon, and Nd-YAG lasers can be used in a continuous mode, that is, allowing a noninterrupted stream of light energy to flow from the laser tube. This energy can then be focused or defocused by a lens system, thus altering the spot size. A larger spot size will diffuse the energy over a greater surface of the target tissue, thus allowing for less penetration. A focused laser beam, on the other hand, will concentrate the laser energy onto a very small area of the tissue, permitting deeper penetration. A deeper tissue effect can also be obtained by increasing the amount of laser light passing through the partially transmitting mirror. Thus, the term *power density* best describes the quantity of laser energy absorbed per unit of tissue (Fig 22–5). One can increase the power density by decreasing the spot size or increasing the power that is transmitted from the laser. Tissue penetration is also controlled by length of exposure. If the laser is allowed to strike the tissue for a long time, the beam will penetrate deeper.

DELIVERY SYSTEMS

The carbon dioxide laser can be utilized via the hysteroscope, but the beam must be directed through a system of reflecting mirrors and focused, with difficulty down the length of the hysteroscope's operating channel. The inability of the CO_2 laser to transmit via a

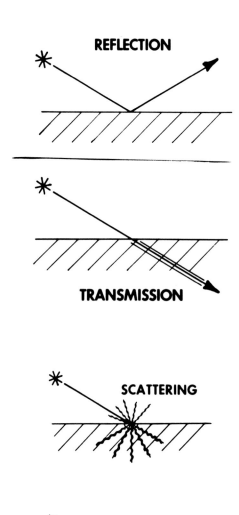

FIG 22–3.
Laser light may be reflected, transmitted, scattered, or absorbed.

quartz fiber makes this system very difficult to utilize for intrauterine surgery.

The Nd-YAG, argon and KTP 532 lasers can be passed through a flexible fiberoptic guide (Fig 22–6). All of these lasers have been used laparoscopically as well as hysteroscopically. The flexible tip of the fiber may be passed through the hysteroscope and will allow the operator to reach remote areas of the uterine cavity. The fibers can be directed with an Albarren's bridge similar to those used for cystoscopic work (Fig 22–7). A sapphire crystal can be attached to the laser fiber which then concentrates the energy, and thus increases the capacity of these lasers to actually cut through intrauterine structures.

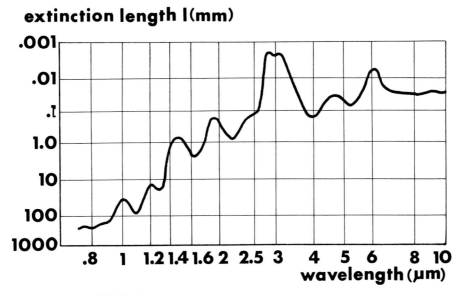

FIG 22–4.
The action of a given laser on tissue is a function of its wavelength. Penetration is greater for the short wave lengths and diminishes at the long end of the electromagnetic spectrum.

ENDOMETRIAL ABLATION

Hysterectomy is the most frequent performed major genital operation in the United States (570,000 to 735,000 per year). One fourth to one half of these patients will develop some type of morbidity. Although many infections are treated very easily with modern an-

tibiotics, 600 women die as a result of complications secondary to the operation in any given year, and $1.7 billion in health care funding is spent each year to perform this operation. If one estimates that 30% of hysterectomies are done for some type of abnormal bleeding, there would be considerable savings in morbidity, mortality, and health care dollars if there were a conserva-

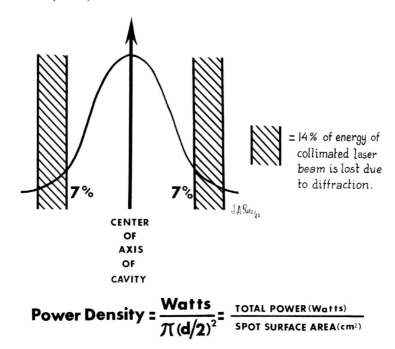

$$\text{Power Density} = \frac{\text{Watts}}{\pi (d/2)^2} = \frac{\text{TOTAL POWER (Watts)}}{\text{SPOT SURFACE AREA (cm}^2)}$$

FIG 22–5.
The quantity (watts) of laser energy interacting per square unit of tissue area *(cm²)* is referred to as the power density. The CO_2 laser is most efficiently absorbed. The Nd-YAG laser penetrates deeply and creates the greatest area of coagulation.

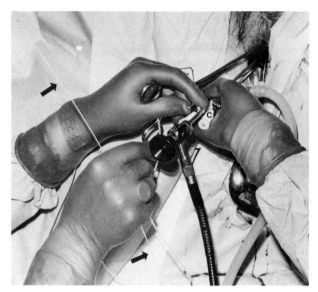

FIG 22–6.
The laser fiber *(arrows)* delivers coherent light to the intrauterine target by way of the hysteroscope operating channel *(c)*.

tive method of treating chronic menorrhagia. Past investigators have attempted various physical and chemical means to damage the endometrial cavity in order to create an Asherman's syndrome. Most of these methods have failed, because of (1) inadequate destruction of the endometrial lining, or (2) complications related to the physical or chemical material introduced into the uterine cavity. In 1981, Goldrath et al. described the first cases of ablation of the endometrium utilizing the Nd-YAG laser to create an Asherman's syndrome. This work was also repeated by Lomano when patients refractory

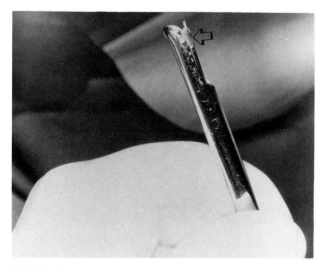

FIG 22–7.
The fiber can be directed by way of an Albarren's bridge *(arrow)*.

to both hormonal therapy and diagnostic curettage and faced with the prospect of hysterectomy were given an alternative of endometrial ablation for the treatment of chronic uterine bleeding.

Patients with a history of heavy menstrual flow failing to respond to surgical and medical management were treated with the YAG laser at a power setting of 40 to 60 W. The YAG laser energy was introduced through the hysteroscope using a 0.6-mm quartz fiber. Five percent dextrose in normal saline (D_5S) was used as the distending medium and the photocoagulation process was carried out from the corpus of the uterus down to the internal cervical os (Fig 22–8).

The goals of endometrial ablation were to decrease menorrhagia sufficiently to obviate the need for hysterectomy and to hopefully attain complete amenorrhea. All patients were sterilized or willing to be sterilized since the outcome of a pregnancy following this procedure has not been established. Ablation of the endometrium using the Nd-YAG laser was removed from FDA protocol in March 1986 (Fig 22–9).

The procedure is accomplished on an outpatient basis and takes from 20 to 45 minutes of operative time. A general anesthetic is used and the patients are discharged on the day of the surgery. They resume normal activities two to three days following the procedure.

A multicenter study was established to determine the effectiveness of YAG laser ablation on the endometrium. This study was carried out at four units across the United States and included 61 patients who ranged in age from 27 to 55 years. Sixty-two percent of the patients reported flows greater than 7 days in duration. Eighty-nine percent of the patients needed to wear more than 20 pads per menstrual period. Following the ablation procedure, 77% of the patients flowed less than 6 days and 23% became totally amenorrheic. All 61 patients used fewer than 20 pads per menstrual period following ablation of the endometrium with the Nd-YAG laser.

Over 300 patients have undergone this procedure and, with few exceptions, most have been able to avoid hysterectomy. Complications have been infrequent. In one patient pulmonary edema developed which was treated with intravenous diuretics. A second patient had a uterine perforation secondary to introduction of the hysteroscope. A third patient who was on high doses of warfarin (Coumadin) required a hysterectomy because of recurrent menorrhagia several weeks following the procedure. Endometrial ablation has been established to be a reasonably safe, effective, and convenient alternative to hysterectomy for selected cases of chronic menorrhagia. The operation can be accomplished on an outpatient basis with an anticipated rapid return to normal activity, adding to the procedure's cost effectiveness.

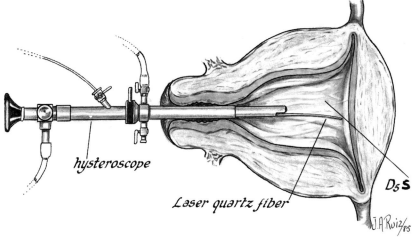

FIG 22–8.
The Nd-YAG fiber can be seen within the uterine cavity. The uterus is distended with D_5S.

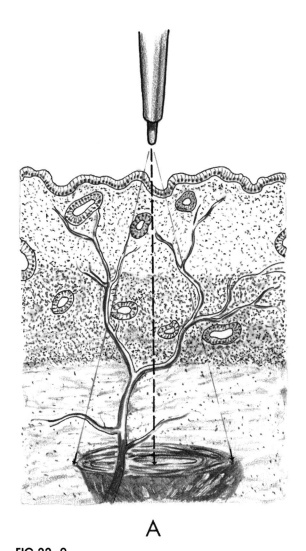

A

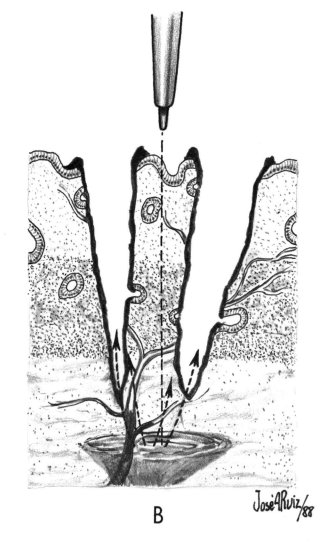

B

FIG 22–9.
A and **B,** as the Nd-YAG beam contacts the target, it continues to penetrate deeply (front scatter). The tissue is destroyed and the beam reflects back toward the surface (backscatter) and disrupts the surface cells (popcorn action).

SPECIFIC TECHNIQUES FOR THE PROCEDURE OF ENDOMETRIAL ABLATION

Patients who are candidates for endometrial ablation are seen on the night before the scheduled surgery. Most patients elect to have a general anesthetic since it is often difficult for them to remain perfectly still for the 20- to 45-minute duration of the operation. After a general anesthetic is administered, the vagina and vulva are prepped in the usual fashion. A urologic collection system is then placed under the perineum in order to collect all irrigating fluids that emerge from the patient. A weighted posterior speculum is inserted into the vagina and a double-tooth tenaculum is applied to the anterior cervix. The cervix is dilated so that the hysteroscope can be easily directed through the internal cervical os. We generally overdilate the cervix so that the flow of the fluid from the endometrial cavity is around the hysteroscope, rather than through the egress channel from the hysteroscope itself. A thorough hysteroscopic evaluation is done to evaluate the cornual ostia, the thickness of the endometrial lining, and the demarcation of the internal cervical os. A 0.6-mm fiberoptic fiber is used to deliver the YAG laser energy to the endometrium. This easily fits through the operating channel of the hysteroscope.

There are generally two techniques that have been employed for endometrial ablation. The first is the so-called "dragging technique," which involves placing the fiberoptic fiber in direct contact with the endometrium and then slowly dragging the fiber through the endometrium until there is superficial vaporization of the endometrial lining (Fig 22–10). At a power setting of 30 to 50 W, this technique will eventually result in a coagulation defect that extends 4 to 6 mm into the uterine wall. This amount of coagulation defect destroys all of the endometrial glands, especially in those patients with adenomyosis. As the laser beam traverses the veins of the endometrium, there is damage to some of these veins, which results in two technical problems. First, the patient may have bleeding back into the distending media, making visualization more difficult. Secondly, infusion of the distending fluid from the endometrial cavity into the veins of the patient can result in a fluid overload, especially in patients with a compromised cardiovascular function.

A second technique, called the "blanching technique," employs the same 0.6-mm fiberoptic fiber and powers in the range of 50 to 60 W (Fig 22–11). Using this technique, the fiber is placed 1 to 5 mm away from the endometrium and the laser energy is applied. The fiber is slowly moved across the endometrial surface un-

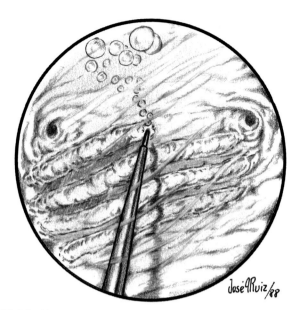

FIG 22–10.
The "touch technique" allows the fiber to contact the endometrium, creating furrows in the tissue.

til there is a blanching from the normal pink endometrium to that of a coagulated white endometrium. Using this technique, the superficial endometrium is coagulated. The "blanching technique" may be safer in that much less fluid is absorbed by the patient and the distending medium remains clear (Plate 245,A and B); however, it does not penetrate as deeply as the touch technique.

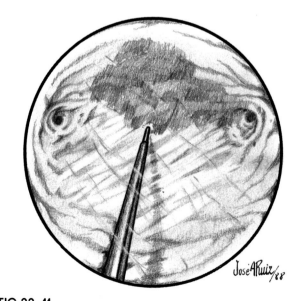

FIG 22–11.
The "blanch technique" allows the fiber to dwell above the surface, creating a whitening of the otherwise pink mucosa.

EXCISIONAL PROCEDURES WITH THE LASER HYSTEROSCOPE

Vaporization of uterine septa, precise removal of submucous fibroids, and lysis of the intrauterine adhesions can all be accomplished via laser hysteroscopy. The carbon dioxide laser must be used in a gas distending medium and must be used in a focused mode in order to allow precise tissue removal. The fiberoptic lasers (Nd-YAG, argon, and frequency-doubled YAG) may be used with a crystal focusing tip or with the bare fiber (Fig 22–12). All of the lasers capable of fiberoptic conduction are used with fluid distending media. Excisional procedures performed by laser hysteroscopy differ little from conventional techniques, which are described elsewhere in this book. The tissue to be removed, whether it be uterine muscle, uterine fibroid, uterine adhesions, or uterine polyp, is simply excised or incised using laser energy rather than the mechanical energy of a hysteroscopic scissor, biopsy forceps, or urologic wire loop cautery. The laser techniques offer the distinct advantage of precise removal with minimal damage to surrounding normal uterine structures. The laser techniques can be accomplished with less bleeding and no increased risk of perforating the uterus and damaging adjacent pelvic structures. A fluid distending medium will allow for cooling of the laser tip as well as removal of debris in order to facilitate visualization during the hysteroscopic excisional procedure. Smaller lesions can be vaporized by placing the bare fiber tip directly on the tissue to be removed. Fiberoptic lasers used with a focusing sapphire crystal must be limited to less than 20 W of power in order to avoid fracture of the crystalloid material. The surgical technique with the contact probes is very similar to that of a knife dissection in that the probe must be brought in direct contact with the base

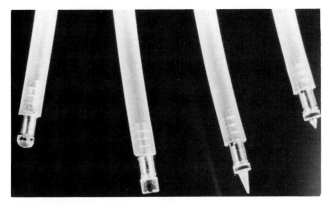

FIG 22–12.
Sapphire tips are mounted at the end of Nd-YAG laser fibers. The sapphire crystal allows the beam to be focused.

of the structure to be excised. The laser is then activated and the tissue is precisely excised.

PHOTODYNAMIC THERAPY

Dougherty et al. have described the use of hematoporphyrin derivative for the treatment of cancer. Patients with malignant tumors will selectively take up hematoporphyrin derivative when this drug is injected intravenously. Normal cells will excrete this material after a lapse of 72 hours. When laser light emitting at 630 nm is applied to cells containing hematoporphyrin derivative, singlet oxygen forms, resulting in cell death (Plate 246).

Photodynamic therapy for neoplasms previously sensitized with hematoporphyrin derivative provides a new modality of treatment. The first case of hysteroscopic photodynamic therapy was reported by McCaughan in 1985. Patients were given 2.3 to 3 mg of hematoporphyrin derivative per kilogram of body weight 2 to 6 days prior to photodynamic therapy. A tunable dye laser system using 20 W of argon power coupled with a rhodamine B tunable dye laser was used to provide a 630-nm light source. Malignant lesions involving the uterine cavity can be treated with this system, so long as it is realized that there is a limitation on the penetration of the 630-nm light (1.5 to 2.0 cm into the tissue).

SAFETY CONSIDERATIONS

Hysteroscopic laser surgery presents certain risks which may not be considered with conventional hysteroscopic surgery. The YAG, frequency-doubled Nd-YAG, and argon lasers carry a risk for the doctor as well as the patient. Eye injury from backscatter following tissue impact is a danger for the surgeon. Use of special safety filters with the hysteroscope therefore is mandatory. For the patient, the principal risk is occult damage to pelvic contents if the beam penetrates through the uterine wall. If the surgeon follows the principles of power density that have been outlined in this chapter, this risk should be kept to a minimum. The extremely thick muscular wall of the uterus provides a significant safety factor for the gynecologist when compared to other laser surgeons using similar laser energy in the bladder, bowel, or stomach. Although the safety record of hysteroscopic laser surgery has to date been good, more widespread use by inexperienced persons will cause the misadventure rate to rise. It is mandatory that all surgeons be trained by attending specific hands-on courses in addition to thorough didactic instruction. It is important that surgeons read the manufacturer's manual and instructions prior to using the laser. Finally, prospective hysteroscopic laser surgeons should attend preceptorship programs sponsored by experienced surgeons who are competent with hysteroscopic laser techniques.

SUMMARY

Recent technical advances in laser surgery combined with improved hysteroscopic techniques have provided a basis for a new horizon in hysteroscopic laser surgery. The carbon dioxide, Nd-YAG, argon, KTP 532, and tunable dye lasers have been used effectively in treating intrauterine disease via the hysteroscope. Ablation of the endometrium for chronic menorrhagia has proved to be an effective alternative to hysterectomy for patients with chronic menorrhagia refractory to medical and surgical therapy. Hysteroscopic excision with lasers can be accomplished with substantial hemostatic benefits. Tunable dye laser therapy incorporating hemtoporphyrin derivative has been shown to be effective in treating some forms of malignant disease. The future of laser hysteroscopy will be determined by the advances in laser biophysics as they are coupled to the needs of the practicing physician. The approach of laser hysteroscopy offers the advantages of simplicity and decreased costs. Physicians must become familiar with both the difficulties and the potential benefits of this new and rapidly developing technology.

BIBLIOGRAPHY

Asherman JG: Amenorrhea traumatica (atretica). *J Obstet Gynecol Br Emp* 1948; 55:23.

Daniell JF: Pesonal communication, Use of KTP crystal laser and argon laser in excision of uterine septa, 1986.

Dougherty TJ, Kaufman JE, Goldfarb A, et al: Photoradiation therapy for the treatment of malignant tumors. *Can Res* 1978; 38:2628–2635.

Droegemueller W, Greet BE, David JR, et al: Cryocoagulation of the endometrium at the uterine cornua. *Am J Obstet Gynecol* 1978; 131:1.

Droegemueller W, Greet B, Makowski E: Cryosurgery in patients with dysfunctional uterine bleeding. *Obstet Gynecol* 1971; 38:256.

Goldrath M, Fuller T, Segal S: Laser photovaporization of endometrium for the treatment of menorrhagia. *Am J Obstet Gynecol* 1981; 140:14.

Keye WR, Maston GA, Dixon J: The use of the argon laser in the treatment of experimental endometriosis. *Fertil Steril* 1983; 39:1.

Lomano JM: Ablation of the endometrium with the neodymium:YAG laser: A multi-center study. *Colpos Gynecol Laser Surg* 1986; 4:203.

Lomano JM: Photocoagulation of the endometrium with the Nd-Yag laser for the treatment of menorrhagia: A report of 10 cases. *J Reprod Med* 1986; 31:26.

Lomano JM: Photocoagulation of early pelvic endometriosis with the Nd-YAG laser through the laparoscope. *J Reprod Med* 1985; 30:2.

McCaughan JS, Schellhas HF, Lomano J, et al: Photodynamic therapy of gynecologic neoplasms after presensitization with hematoporphyrin derivative. *Lasers Surg Med* 1985; 5:491–498.

Oelsner G, David A, Insler V, et al: Outcome of pregnancy after treatment of intrauterine adhesions. *Obstet Gynecol* 1974; 44:341.

Tadir Y, Raif J, Dagan J, et al: Hysteroscope for CO_2 laser application. *Lasers Surg Med* 1984; 4:153.

23

Hysteroscopic Sterilization

Rafael F. Valle, M.D.

Sterilization of women was greatly enhanced and simplified with the introduction of laparoscopy which, since the late 1960s, has become one of the most common methods for tubal sterilization of women in the non-puerperal state. Nonetheless, the method, although highly effective, in the majority of cases is performed under general anesthesia. The risks associated with laparoscopy are also associated with tubal sterilization. For these reasons, new, simpler methods of tubal sterilization that are well-tolerated by patients, effective, and perhaps eventually reversible are still being sought.

Modern hysteroscopy was introduced in the early 1970s as a method of visualizing the uterine cavity and uterotubal junctions, and the idea of occluding this area by hysteroscopy was revived with great interest. In 1878 Kocks attempted to occlude the uterotubal junctions blindly by a transcervically inserted electrode; despite numerous other attempts to improve this rudimentary technique by guiding an electrode with fluoroscopy, this method did not produce significant clinical success. It was associated with unacceptable failures and serious complications. Although the idea of utilizing hysteroscopy as a guide to tubal occlusion goes back to the 1920s and indeed was explored in clinical trials in the 1950s, particularly by Japanese investigators, these preliminary attempts again did not produce significant acceptable results. It was not until the early 1970s that serious and well-designed clinical trials were initiated in several centers, utilizing electrodes delivered directly under hysteroscopic guidance at the proximal segment of the intramural portion of the fallopian tubes. These clinical trials were performed particularly in West Germany by Lindeman, in Japan by Sugimoto, in Mexico by Quinones, and in the United States by Neuwirth. Once hysteroscopy was seen as a practical technique to deliver thin electrodes to the uterotubal junctions, other methods of tubal occlusion began to be explored.

The various hysteroscopic techniques to attempt occlusion of the intramural portion of the fallopian tubes are the following:

1. Electrocoagulation and cryocoagulation
2. Injection of chemicals either for permanent closure, such as quinacrine; gelatin, resorcinol, and formaldehyde (GRF); and methyl cyanoacrylate (MCA).
3. Nondestructive occlusion by plastic formed-in-place plugs.
4. Mechanical devices or tubal plugs that are placed at the proximal portion of the interstitial oviduct.
5. Intratubal devices.

ELECTROCOAGULATION AND CRYOCOAGULATION

Electrocoagulation

Electrocoagulation of the intramural portion of the fallopian tubes by hysteroscopy was the main hysteroscopic method of investigation in the early 1970s. Nonetheless, although the technique itself was fairly standard, the coagulation of this tubal area varied among investigators, particularly in the wattage and time of delivery; nonetheless, the preliminary results seemed comparable with 75% to 80% bilateral initial closure with one application and about 85% to 90% closure with a second application. Nonetheless, the complications and specific failures were not uniform.

Because of reports of pregnancies and major complications associated with this technique, a hysteroscopic sterilization registry was established at Columbia University in 1975. Ten collaborators from the United States, Thailand, West Germany, India, and Singapore were enrolled in the study, and a total of 587 cases were analyzed with 333 (57%) found to have bilateral tubal closure at subsequent testing. There were 229 women (39%) who had one or both fallopian tubes open at subsequent testing or who had become pregnant despite tubal closure at patency test. What was most distressing in the analysis of these 587 cases were the major complications, which included tubal and cornual ectopic pregnancies, uterine perforations, bowel damage, peritonitis, acute endometritis, excessive uterine bleeding, and one death as the result of bowel perforation and peritonitis. The overall rate of major complications was 4.3%. When this study was completed in 1977, hysteroscopic sterilization by electrocoagulation was just beginning to peak and expand to several centers. Nonetheless, in view of the failure rate and complications, most clinical trials were stopped altogether, and further investigation did not seem warranted.

Although multiple factors seemed to be related to the failures and complications, it was evident that the most important factor seemed to be lack of standardization and control of the current utilized and the time of its delivery. This was impossible to monitor, particularly thermal injury to this anatomic area, which is thinner than the uterus (Plates 247–250; Fig 23–1).

Cryocoagulation

Cryocoagulation of the endometrium and uterotubal junctions has also been investigated as a method to occlude the fallopian tubes for permanent sterilization. The tissue effects of cryosurgery are coagulation necrosis, due to biochemical and biophysical changes, with cellular and nuclear damage produced by the subfreezing temperatures. The final result is avascular necrosis of tissues. Because of the rapid regeneration of the endometrium when cryosurgery has been applied, collagen plus 2-mm in diameter and 8-mm long have been placed at the cornual junctions following freeze-thaw cycles and abrasion. The initial experiments have been performed in animals and in selected human volunteers prior to hysterectomy; nonetheless, although no extended clinical trials have been performed to determine the permanent damage to the tissue and the results of tubal occlusion and subsequent recanalizations, the initial results appear promising.

HYSTEROSCOPIC INJECTION OF CHEMICALS

Utilizing hysteroscopy as a platform to deliver chemicals into the fallopian tube to produce tubal occlusion has constituted another attempt at tubal steriliza-

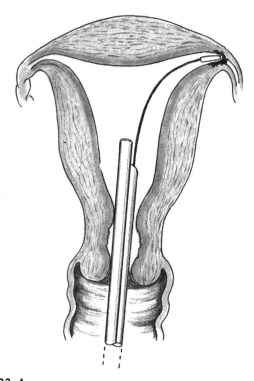

FIG 23–1.
A (see Plate 250), blanching of tissue produced by transmission of the electric current as electrode (shown in Plates 248 and 249) is activated. **B** (above), schematic view of the events shown in Plates 247 through 250.

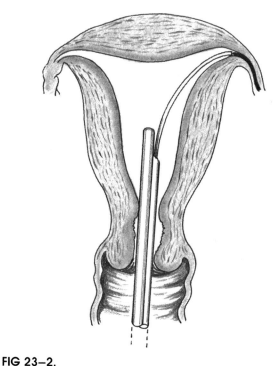

FIG 23–2.
Various sclerosing materials have been injected into the oviduct by a catheter delivered through the hysteroscope.

tion, either permanent or temporary. Of the various sclerosing substances utilized to produce permanent occlusion of the fallopian tubes, the most relevant have been quinacrine, GRF, and MCA (Fig 23–2).

Quinacrine

Zipper studied the effects of quinacrine in the fallopian tubes by transcervical injection in 1970. A 50% bilateral occlusion was obtained with one injection of quinacrine in 1,000 patients; when the instillation rate was increased to three at 1-month intervals, the closure rate rose to 80%. In 1976, Alvarado et al. described the preliminary results with the hysteroscopic instillation of quinacrine to attain tubal occlusion in 60 patients, and only six out of 16 cases under hysterosalpingographic control showed bilateral obstruction. After 3 months of application, of 16 of 30 patients, bilateral obstruction was achieved in 6 cases, unilateral obstruction in 6, and bilateral patency in 4. No further clinical trials were performed, and quinacrine delivered under hysteroscopy was not deemed feasible for tubal closure.

Gelatin, Resorcinol, and Formaldehyde

Of the tissue adhesives studied in an attempt to occlude the fallopian tubes, a combination of gelatin, resorcinol, and formaldehyde was investigated in 1964 by the Battelle Laboratories. This adhesive substance permitted ingrowth and, being biodegradable, could be used safely in these investigations. Although GRF has never been used in human clinical trials, some preliminary studies in animals show its potential for tubal blockage. Nonetheless, although theoretically the substance could be delivered through hysteroscopy, perhaps difficulty in confining the substance to the fallopian tubes and/or avoiding reflux have halted any further attempts to study this approach.

Methyl Cyanoacrylate

Another tissue adhesive evaluated for occlusion of the fallopian tubes is MCA (Crazy Glue), which—injected as a fluid—polymerizes rapidly upon hydration. One of the problems in using MCA for surgical application has been its localized effect on surrounding tissues, which developed necrosis, inflammation, and fibrosis. Although the application of MCA to the fallopian tubes has been tried by means of a balloon catheter to prevent reflux, hysteroscopy was also attempted by Lindemann with fair success.

The utilization of MCA has been facilitated by a device called FEMCEPT for its delivery. The FEMCEPT sys-

tem requires transcervical introduction of a cannula with a distal balloon. Insufflation places the tip of the device with lateral openings, facilitating delivery of substances directly into the fallopian tubes without reflux. The device has been designed so as to deliver a volume of 0.06 ml (0.2 in tubes) of MCA per instillation (Fig 23–3). Bilateral tubal closure rate has been achieved in these preliminary trials in 72% of tubes with a single application, and in 96% with two applications 1 month apart (Table 23–1).

HYSTEROSCOPIC TUBAL OCCLUSION WITH SILICONE RUBBER PLUGS

In 1975, Erb proposed the use of silicone rubber plugs directly formed in place to block the oviducts as a

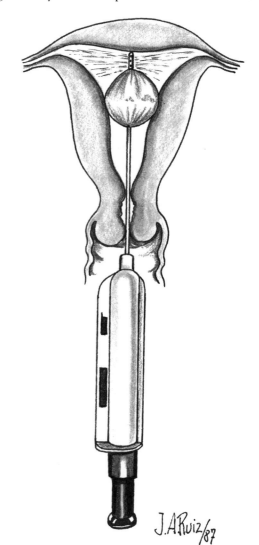

FIG 23–3.
Distal balloon of FEMCEPT device inflated in the uterine cavity.

TABLE 23–1.

Electrocoagulation, Cryosurgery, Sclerosing Chemicals, and Tissue Adhesives*

Procedure	Animal Studies	Clinical Trials	Efficacy (% Tubal Occlusion)	Present Status
Electrocoagulation				
(Darabi/Roy, Richart)	None	587 women (registry)	57	Discontinued
(Quinones et al.)	None	1,284 women	80 (1 procedure)	Follow-up
(Lindemann, Mohr)	None	360 women (high frequency of coagulation)	89 (9 pregnancies)	
		260 women (microcoagulator)	89.4 (7 pregnancies)	
		48 women (NTC thermoprobe)†	56 (2 pregnancies) (variable depending on temperature)	
Cryosurgery				
(Droegemueller et al.)	Baboon	Preliminary		Research
Quinacrine	Various species, various responses			
(Alvarado et al.)	None	60 women		Abandoned
GRF	Rabbit	None		No recent studies
MCA				
(Lindemann/Mohr)	None	50 women (only 16 had follow-up at 8 wk)	81.2	Discontinued
FEMCEPT-MCA (Bolduc/Neuwirth/Richart)	Effective if delivered directly; no hysteroscopic studies reported			

*Adapted and modified from Sciarra JJ: Hysteroscopic approaches for tubal closure, in Zatuchni GI, Labbok MH, Sciarra JJ (eds): *Research Frontiers in Fertility Regulation.* Hagerstown, Md, Harper & Row, 1980, chapter 26, p 283.
†NTC = negative temperature coefficient.

method of tubal occlusion, utilizing a cornual salpingo-guide guided directly under fluoroscopy. With direct visualization of the uterotubal junctions through the hysteroscope, this approach was logical for the direct placement of the liquid silicone in the oviducts. The viscous liquid is injected through a specially designed dispenser with a special catalyzer that produces the cure of the formed plug. The silicone does not adhere to or invade tissue; therefore, destruction of the epithelium is minimal. The silicone is injected by means of two concentric polysulphone catheters inserted through the operating channel of the hysteroscope. The obturator tip is custom-molded from a composition of silicone rubber, spherical silver powder, radiopaque, and stannous octoate.

Although the original design of this plug with a retrieval loop was intended for possible reversible sterilization, experience has shown that the method cannot be offered as such but as a permanent method of contraception.

Because the rubber silicone accommodates itself to the convolutions of the intramural portion of the fallopian tubes and its total length, it is easily introduced and acts as a perfect tubal plug. Clinical studies were initiated in 1980 and expanded to several centers, giving an overall occlusion rate of 80% at the first instillation which, in the best conditions, rose to 90% with two or three applications (Fig 23–4).

The method is applicable as an outpatient method of sterilization, requiring only local anesthesia and avoiding surgical incisions. With the tubal occlusion rate and time consumed in the procedure, however, as well as need for a careful follow-up of these patients to assure tubal occlusion with a subsequent hysterosalpingogram, the technique requires additional refinements to be applicable to most patients requesting it. Furthermore, the expense to these patients as compared with an outpatient technique available today does not favor its use as the most simple method of sterilization. Important considerations are the selection of patients, the instrumentation needed, and the skill of the operator. Nonetheless, of the methods studied at present, it seems to offer the most reliable and safe hysteroscopic method of occluding the oviducts at present. Although the plugs are not approved by the U.S. Food and Drug Administration at present, in the near future, they will undoubtedly be available to patients under the trademark of Ovabloc.

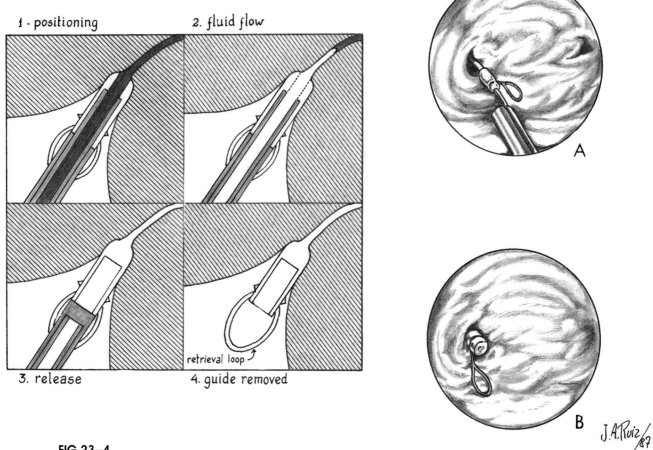

FIG 23–4.
Sequences (*1* to *4*) in the formation of silicone-elastic plugs. Hysteroscope and guide *(a)*; silicone plug in situ *(b)*.

MECHANICAL OCCLUSIVE DEVICES OR TUBAL PLUGS

Another promising approach to tubal sterilization by hysteroscopy has been in the use of mechanical occlusive devices made of solid inert materials to occlude the proximal intramural portion of the fallopian tubes. Several problems have been encountered, nonetheless, in the development of these plugs, and also their proper insertion and retention. The objective of using these devices is not only to achieve tubal occlusion but also to permit potential reversal of sterilization; therefore, long-term follow-up clinical studies are of utmost importance.

Although there have been many designs of such intratubal plugs, few have entered the clinical human trials. Of these, the most promising ones are the uterotubal junction devices proposed by Hosseinian and the hydrogel tubal plugging device or P-block as proposed by Brundin.

UTEROTUBAL JUNCTION BLOCKING DEVICES

These devices are made of silicone rubber with four anchoring spines made of elgiloy which serve to fix and keep the device in place by penetrating the adjacent myometrium. There is an assembly screw of stainless steel which attaches the anchoring spines to the plug and provides a grasping base for the device carrier. The plug itself, made of silicone, is cone-shaped and measures 1 mm or less at the tip and increases to about 2 mm at the base. The length of the device varies from 7 to 9 mm.

The original studies made in primates were 100% successful in 21 baboons, for a minimum of eight breedings. The reversibility potential of this technique after removal was studied in 15 baboons, and eight of these animals became pregnant, achieving a total of 12 pregnancies (Plate 251 and Fig 23–5). Encouraged by these results, investigators began clinical trials in two phases:

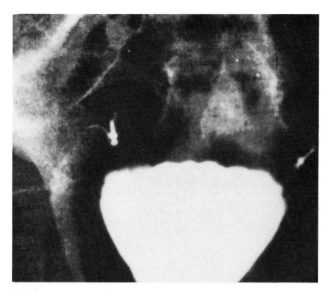

FIG 23–5.
Hysterogram of the baboon's uterus with radiopaque plugs seen.
(Courtesy of Dr. A. Hosseinian.)

first, to evaluate the capability of these plugs to occlude the uterotubal junctions and, second, to determine the extent of tissue reaction and reestablishment of tubal patency after the device was removed. This was carried out in three volunteers who were scheduled for hysterectomy for a variety of gynecologic conditions. The efficacy of closure was achieved in 91% of the tubes, and one pregnancy occurred. Only minimal to moderate tissue reaction around the anchoring spines was observed at the removal and some widening of the tubal lumen and flattening of the endosalpingeal cells where the plug had been. In 20 women, 90% of the tubes regained their patency after the device was removed. In Phase II, 11 volunteers underwent device implantation under local anesthesia. Five of these women developed an intrauterine pregnancy, and no further clinical trials were performed until this unacceptable failure rate could be solved. Perhaps modifications in the plug itself, and in its delivery, and improved instrumentation to view the tubal opening and direct the plug properly could result in lower failures (Fig 23–6,*1* and *2*).

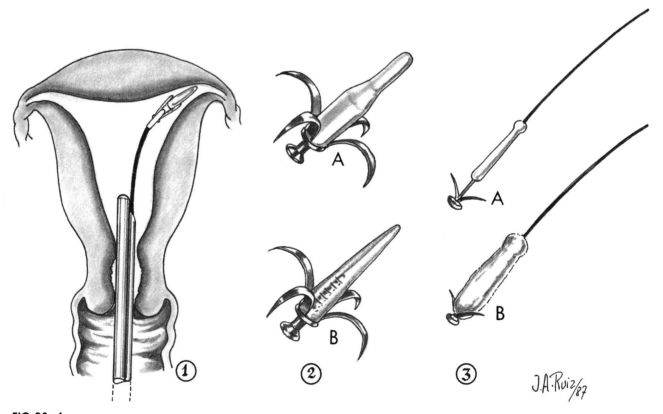

FIG 23–6.
Tubal plugs for hysteroscopic placement: *1,* hysteroscopic delivery of a tubal plug. *2,* Hosseinian blocking device with anchoring spines: *(a)* polyethylene device, *(b)* silicone device. *3,* the Brundin P-block; *(a)* in dry state, *(b)* after hydration.

TABLE 23–2.

Mechanical Occlusive Devices*

Procedure	Animal Studies	Clinical Trials	Efficacy (% Tubal Occlusion)	Present Status
Silastic oviductal plug (Reed/Erb)	Rabbit and rhesus monkey	350 women	78.8	Pending FDA approval
(Houck/Cooper/ Rigberg (Loffer)		415 women 206 women	80 (1st attempt) 90 (2nd attempt) 80.6 (1st attempt 91.3 (several attempts)	Pending FDA approval Pending FDA approval
UTDJ (Hosseinian et al.	Baboon	Phase I 33 women (Prior to hysterectomy) Phase II 11 women	91 (1 pregnancy) 72.2 (5 pregnancies)	Ongoing research Ongoing research
P-Block (Brundin)	None	35 women	48.5 (4 pregnancies)	Ongoing research
ITCD (Sugimoto)	None	32 women	Spontaneous expulsion (1 side in 3 women)	Ongoing research
Rigid plastic plug (Lindemann)	Not specified	12 uteri	Insertion problems (5 perforations)	Ongoing research
Intratubal devices (Hamou)	None	157 women	95 successful insertion (5 pregnancies)	Ongoing research

*Adapted and modified from Sciarra, JJ: Hysteroscopic approaches for tubal closure in, Zatuchni, GI, Labbok, MH, Sciarra, JJ. (eds.) *Research Frontiers in Fertility Regulation.* Hagerstown, Md, Harper & Row, 1980. Chapter 26, p. 284.
†90% patency following plug removal from 30 patients

HYDROGEL TUBAL BLOCKING DEVICES

The P-block tubal plug is made of a hydrogel body 4 mm long and 1.2 mm wide which is fixed on a nylon skeleton in its dry state and has 2-mm wide nylon wings at the top to prevent expulsions from the tube before hydratization. Swelling of the plug with moisture takes about 30 minutes. Hydrogel is a polymeric compound of polyvinylpyrrolidone, a hydrophilic substance; methylacrylate; and hydrophobic material. This plug has undergone considerable modifications. When tested in 35 women volunteers under paracervical block, it was found to be easy to insert and well tolerated. Nonetheless, bilateral occlusion was achieved in the first attempt in only 15 of the 35 women, and in two other women, a second procedure was necessary to produce successful occlusion on both tubes. The long-term results, nonetheless, in these 15 women show four subsequent pregnancies, all due to faulty placement or expulsion of the device. Furthermore, in 15 patients insertion was not possible. This problem, plus the high failure rate after

bilateral occlusion, has prompted plans to design the plug to better suit the tubal anatomy (Fig 23–6,3).

Other tubal plugs have been designed to occlude the uterotubal junctions by hysteroscopy; nonetheless, no clinical trials have been performed and the design of the plugs is still under investigation (Table 23–2).

INTRATUBAL DEVICES

Jacques Hamou in Paris has proposed a new approach for tubal sterilization by hysteroscopy. The Hamou device is simply a nylon thread 1 mm in diameter and 23 mm in length, which is placed by microhysteroscopy, without anesthesia, in the interstitial portion of the fallopian tubes. At the distal end of the device, there is an open loop of the nylon, which prevents migration of the device into the uterine cavity. At the proximal end, another loop attached to the nylon allows for retrieval. Because the intratubal device is flexible, it may be introduced safely into the interstitial portion of the

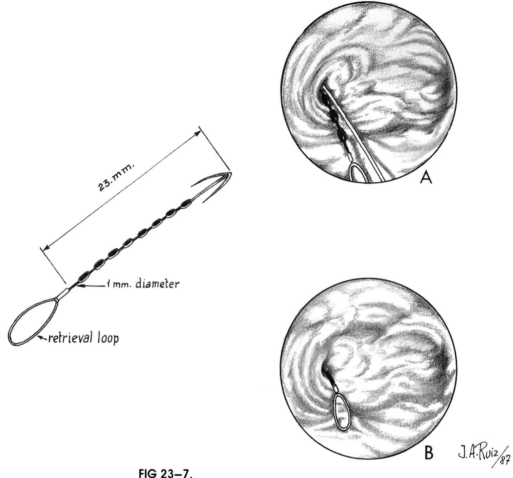

FIG 23–7.
Nylon intratubal device: *(a)* hysteroscopic placement of the intratubal device, *(b)* the intratubal device in place. The distal open loop protrudes into the uterine cavity.

fallopian tube. The device is placed by microhysteroscopy under 20 + magnification, and the patient may require local or no anesthesia. The intratubal device is inserted 1 to 1½ cm in the fallopian tube, utilizing a 6.5-mm operative sheath of the microhysteroscope. The distending medium is CO_2 gas under low intrauterine pressures of 60 mm Hg and a flow of 30 to 40 ml/min (Fig 23–7).

This device does not appear to produce total tubal occlusion, as has been demonstrated by hysterosalpingography. At present, it is under investigation, and although 140 patients have undergone the procedure, follow-up periods have been short (Plate 252). Successful insertion of this device has been achieved in about 95% of the patients, but five pregnancies have occurred. Nonetheless, because this technique is in its developmental stages, further follow-up study is necessary before definite conclusions can be drawn. Tubal reaction and possible damage appear to be minimal, so the po-

tential for reversibility is great. Nonetheless, this benefit must be balanced against the achievement of an acceptable failure rate. It is possible that this device could be used also as a vehicle of pharmacologic spermicidal and/or gametocidal substances enhancing the mechanical effect of the intratubal device.

Although no hysteroscopic method of tubal occlusion can be accepted as practical at present, it seems reasonable to expect that the hysteroscopic approach remains promising. Electrocoagulation offers little promise for the future, but new designs in tubal plugs may offer efficient occlusion and simplicity of insertion and warrant further investigation; intratubal devices used also as therapeutic vehicles may serve as a simple and effective method of tubal sterilization by hysteroscopy. There are, nonetheless, major issues that must be solved before these methods can be offered as practical and effective sterilization alternatives for women. These include efficacy, tissue destruction and subsequent sequelae, intrauterine and/or ectopic pregnancies, and potential reversibility.

BIBLIOGRAPHY

Alvarado A, Quinones R, Aznar R: Tubal instillation of quinacrine under hysteroscopic control, in Sciarra JJ, Butler JC, Speidel SJ (eds): *Hysteroscopic Sterilization.* New York, Intercontinental Medical Book Corp, 1974, pp 85–94.

Bolduc LR, Neuwirth RS, Richart RM: Design objectives for the FEMCEPT device, in Zatuchni GI, Shelton JD, Goldsmith A, et al (eds): *Female Transcervical Sterilization.* Hagerstown, Md, Harper & Row, 1983, pp 192–195.

Brundin J: Hydrogel tubal blocking device: P-Block, in Zatuchni GI, Shelton JD, Goldsmith A, et al (eds): Female Transcervical Sterilization. Hagerstown, Md, Harper & Row, 1983, pp 212-218.

Darabi K, Richart RM: Collaborative study on hysteroscopic sterilization procedures: Preliminary report. *Obstet Gynecol* 1977; 49:48–54.

Darabi KF, Roy K, Richart RM: Collaborative studies on hysteroscopic sterilization procedures: Final report, in Sciarra JJ, Zatuchni GI, Speidel JJ (eds): *Risks, Benefits, and Controversies in Fertility Control,* Hagerstown, Md, Harper & Row, 1978, pp 81–101.

Droegemueller W, Greet BE, Davis JR, et al: Cryocoagulation of the endometrium at the uterine cornua. *Am J Obstet Gynecol* 1978; 131:1–9.

Erb RA: Silastic: A retrievable custom-molded oviductal plug, in Sciarra JJ, Droegemueller W, Speidel JJ (eds): *Advances in Female Sterilization Techniques.* Hagerstown, Md, Harper & Row, 1976, pp 259–271.

Falb RD, Lower BR, Crowley JP, et al: Transcervical fallopian tube blockage with gelatin-resorcinol-formaldehyde (GRF), in Sciarra JJ, Droegemueller W, Speidel JJ (eds): *Advances in Female Sterilization Techniques.* Hagerstown, Md, Harper & Row, 1976, pp 208–215.

Greer BE, Droegemueller W, Binham PE, et al: Uterine cryosurgery in baboons, in Sciarra JJ, Droegemueller W, Speidel JJ (eds): *Advances in Female Sterilization Techniques.* Hagerstown, Md, Harper & Row, 1976, pp 231–258.

Hamou J: Personal communication, 1986.

Hamou J, Sabat-Baroux J, Uzan H: Intratubal devices for contraception. Presented at the Annual Meeting of the American Association of Gynecologic Laparoscopists, San Diego, Calif, November 10–14, 1982.

Hayashi M: Tubal sterilization by cornual coagulation under hysteroscopy. *Hum Sterilization Med* 1981; 26:375–382.

Hosseinian AH, Lucero S, Kim MH: Hysteroscopic implantation of uterotubal junction blocking devices, in Sciarra JJ, Droegemueller W, Speidel JJ (eds): *Advances in Female Sterilization Techniques.* Hagerstown, Md, Harper & Row, 1976, pp 169–175.

Hosseinian AH, Morales WA: Clinical application of hysteroscopic sterilization using uterotubal junction blocking devices, in Zatuchni GI, Shelton JD, Goldsmith A, et al (eds): *Female Transcervical Sterilization.* Hagerstown, Md, Harper & Row, 1983, pp 234–239.

Houk RM, Cooper JM, Rigberg HS: Hysteroscopic tubal occlusion with formed-in-place silicone plugs: A clinical review. *Obstet Gynecol* 1983; 62:587–591.

Kocks J: Eine neue Methode der Sterilisation der Frauen. *Centralblatt Gynaekol* 1878; 2:617–619.

Lindemann HJ: Transuterine tubal sterilization by CO$_2$ hysteroscopy, in Sciarra JJ, Butler JC, Speidel JJ (eds): *Hysteroscopic Sterilization.* New York, Intercontinental Medical Book Corp, 1974, pp 61–73.

Lindemann HJ, Mohr J: Review of clinical experience with hysteroscopic sterilization, in Sciarra JJ, Droegemueller W, Speidel JJ (eds): *Advances in Female Sterilization Techniques.* Hagerstown, Md, Harper & Row, 1976, pp 153–161.

Loffer FD: Hysteroscopic sterilization with the use of formed-in-place silicone plugs. *Am J Obstet Gynecol* 1984; 149:261–270.

Neuwirth RS, Levine RU, Richart RM: Hysteroscopic tubal sterilization: I. A preliminary report. *Am J Obstet Gynecol* 1973; 116:82–85.

Quinones-Guerrero R, Aznar-Ramos R, Duran HA: Tubal electrocauterization under hysteroscopic control. *Contraception* 1973; 7:195–201.

Reed TP, Erb R: Hysteroscopic tubal occlusion with silicone rubber. *Obstet Gynecol* 1983; 61:388–392.

Richart RM, Neuwirth RS, Nilsen RS, et al: The effectiveness of the FEMCEPT method and preliminary experience with radiopaque MCA to enhance clinical acceptability, in Zatuchni GI, Shelton JD, Goldsmith A, et al (eds): *Female Transcervical Sterilization.* Hagerstown, Md, Harper & Row, 1983, pp 212–218.

Sciarra JJ: Hysteroscopic approaches for tubal closure, in Zatuchni GI, Labbok MH, Sciarra JJ (eds): *Research Frontiers in Fertility Regulation.* Hagerstown, Md, Harper & Row, 1980, pp 270–286.

Sugimoto O: *Diagnostic and Therapeutic Hysteroscopy.* Tokyo, Igaku-Shoin, 1978, pp 208–210.

Sugimoto O: Hysteroscopic sterilization by electrocoagulation, in Sciarra JJ, Butler JC, Speidel JJ (eds): *Hysteroscopic Sterilization.* New York, Intercontinental Medical Book Corp, 1974, pp 107–120.

Yasui S: Sterilization of the female by electrocoagulation of the uterine cornu. *Japan Med J* 1952; No. 1475.

Zipper J, Stachetti E, Medel M: Human fertility control by trans-vaginal application of quinocrine on the fallopian tubes. *Fertil Steril* 1970; 21:581–589.

24

Hysteroscopic Sterilization With Formed-in-Place Silicone Rubber Plugs

Theodore P. Reed III, M.D.

Neuwirth, in his text on hysteroscopy, first stated that the ideal sterilization procedure for women would be one that would have minimal surgical intervention, together with cosmetic appeal, a high rate of effectiveness, low cost, a low rate of complications, and potential reversibility.

These desirous features seem to be applicable to hysteroscopic insertion of intraluminal tubal devices for the purpose of sterilization. Although many attempts at this have been made, only two procedures have met with any degree of success in a significant number of patients. The failure of most devices seems to be the fact that although they fit into the tubal lumen and are anchored there by various means, the expulsion rate for practically all of these devices has been too high to be acceptable.

The first of the two methods that have met with success has been electrocauterization of the cornual ostium of the tube, which was developed and carried out primarily by Quinones, who did several hundred of these procedures. If he performed a repeat procedure in those for whom the first procedure had failed—as observed by patency with hysterosalpingogram—his success rate was in the area of 90%. He used unipolar cautery and did not report any serious complications. However, when others tried this, there were a few serious complications in the nature of perforation, bowel injury, and death. The procedure was abandoned outside of Quinones' work.

The other procedure that has met with reasonable success is the use of formed-in-place silicone rubber plugs developed by Erb. Erb developed the instruments to apply this, did the original studies in animals, and had instruments patented while working at the Franklin Research Institute in Philadelphia. These patents were sub-sequently purchased by Ovabloc Corporation, which now owns them. Ovabloc instigated extensive clinical trials and supported them in an effort to get clinical studies to be approved by the U.S. Food and Drug Administration (FDA). These clinical studies were performed from 1978 through 1985. During this time 20 investigators, both in the United States and abroad, entered 2,501 women into the study.

EARLY EXPERIMENTAL TRIALS

Silicone was believed to be an ideal material with which to form plugs because during other uses in the body it appeared to be non–tissue damaging and non-invasive. The animal studies of the substance were conducted by Erb on rabbits and monkeys (Plate 253). Pathologic examination of the removed organs after being instilled with silicone for up to 284 days showed no invasiveness of the material into the tissues and no tissue damage other than some flattening of the tubal cilia. Standard pathologic investigation techniques were used in these studies as well as electron microscopy evaluation of these organs (Plate 254).

Erb got his ideas from suggestions from Corfman and Taylor and also from Hefnawi et al., who in animal studies found silicone to be 100% effective when the material was retained in the isthmus of the tube. The first applications to humans were made by Rakshit, who had a very simple technique. He used a low-viscosity solution of silicone which he injected through the cervical canal by means of a large, cone-shaped syringe to fill the uterine cavity and the fallopian tubes. He had a 50% success rate with this technique and reported no pregnancies in a period of 11 to 24 months in 22 patients who had bilateral occlusion. The excess rubbery solution from the uterine cavity was simply wiped out.

Erb reasoned that if there could be a direct application of the silicone to the tubal ostia at the cornual end, a higher success rate of filling the tubal lumen could be obtained. He also felt that if the material was made more viscous, it would not flow into the abdominal cavity or the uterine cavity as it did so readily with Rakshit's technique. He therefore added a catalyst (stannous octuate) to the mix, which made it cure more rapidly and become more viscous in its liquid form.

Erb and colleagues worked originally with rabbits. Through hysterotomy, they applied the material with a catheter directly into the cornual opening of the fallopian tubes. Afterward, the does were exposed to bucks for up to 280 days, and none of them became pregnant. Following this Erb attempted to apply the procedure in women fluoroscopically with a cannula to the cornual opening of the tube; but as they could not find a proper fitting, they abandoned this approach and began looking at hysteroscopy as a means of visualizing and cannulating the tube.

PLUG AND INSTRUMENT DESIGN

To make this a successful procedure Erb then developed the guide assembly (Plates 255 and 256), the obturator tip (Plate 257), a mixer-dispenser (Plate 258), and the fluid flow actuator (Plate 259). These instruments were developed for the hysteroscopic application of the silicone to the fallopian tubes. The obturator tip (see Plate 257) is a hollow, premolded silicone rubber tip which measures in its original form 2×5 mm. This is placed on the end of the guide assembly, which is 75 cm long and 1 mm in diameter (Plate 260). It is made of polysulfone tubing that has over approximately two thirds of its length a second polysulfone tubing measuring 2 mm in diameter which butts up against the base of the obturator tip (Fig 24–1; Plate 261). The silicone flows through the inner guide, then through the hollow tip; the flowing silicone cross-links to this tip, making the tip a part of the final "formed-in-place" plug (Fig 24–2; Plate 262). With proper viscosity and timing, the viscous liquid silicone will flow through the obturator tip into the fallopian tube to the ampullar section (Fig 24–3; Plates 263 and 264). When it cures, which takes about 5 minutes, the plug has a so called "dumbbell" shape, which is larger on either end than in the middle of the isthmus portion. This is what is believed to be the basic success of the silicone plug over other types of intralumenal devices. The tip, because of the design of

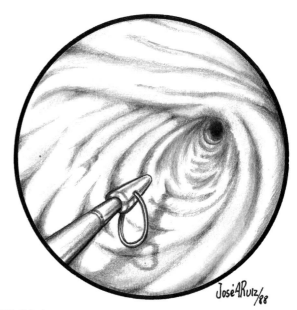

FIG 24–1.
A (see Plate 260) the guide assembly (cannula) approaches the ostium. A test dose of methylene blue is squirted through the assembly. **B** (above), drawing of same.

the guide assembly, can be separated from the attached cured silicone in the remainder of the guide assembly, thus leaving the cured plug (Plate 265) with its tip attached in the tube from the cornu through the isthmus into the ampullar section (Plate 266,A and B; Figs 24–4 and 24–5).

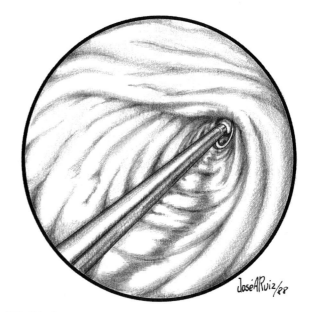

FIG 24–2.
A (see Plate 261) liquid silicone is injected and the operator watches for an air bubble in the cannula. **B** (above), drawing of same.

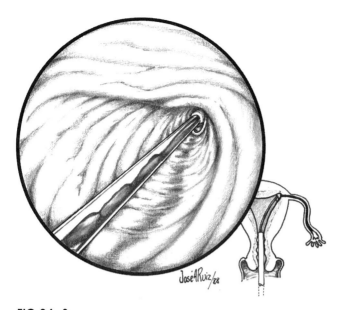

FIG 24–3.
A (see Plate 262), white liquid silicone now flows into the tube.
B (above), drawing of same.

METHODOLOGY OF INSERTION

Hyskon or CO_2 may be used as distending medium. In the author's experience, Hyskon is a little more satisfactory because it will suppress minor bleeding problems that often develop during the relatively long hysteroscopic procedure, but some investigators have preferred CO_2.

The guide assembly, prior to instilling silicone, is

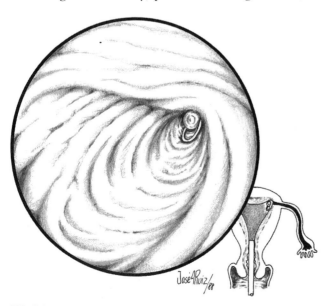

FIG 24–4.
A (see Plate 266), the plug is correctly in place. **B** (above), drawing of same.

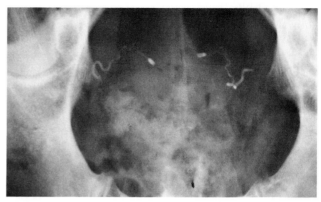

FIG 24–5.
Post operative radiograph reveals correctly placed plugs with cross-linked obturator tip giving it the "dumbbell" shape.

filled with a dilute solution of methylene blue so that after the assembly is placed through the hysteroscope and threaded into the lumen of the tube (see Plate 260), patency and continuity can be tested before the silicone is injected.

The procedure is almost always done under local or paracervical block anesthesia in the physician's office, with about 25% of the patients requiring some mild sedation. In the author's experience in a series of over 600 cases, he only had two or three patients who required general anesthesia for completion of the procedure.

No significant recovery period is required. Most of the patients are able to get up from the operating table immediately upon completion of the procedure and are able to leave the office within a few minutes without any adverse effects.

In regards to complications, minor bleeding problems occurred in fewer than 10% of patients. Two patients had moderately heavy bleeding shortly after the procedure, and this was controlled by medical therapy.

In the author's experience and series of cases, there were three major complications other than pregnancy. One patient had a history of pelvic inflammatory disease, but on preoperative testing with standard hysterosalpingography the fallopian tubes appeared to be open and normal, and there was no reaction to the hysterosalpingogram. However, following the instillation of the silicone plugs the patient developed an acute febrile reaction and required hospitalization with triple antibiotic therapy intravenously. The patient recovered, removal of the plugs was not necessary, and the patient used them for contraception following her recovery. Two patients required laparotomy to remove the silicone because of chronic low-grade pain due to foreign body reaction. In both cases, symptoms were relieved by removal of the material.

Technically, the procedure has some difficulties, and improved instrumentation would be of help in this regard. The only significant change in the instrumentation since the original investigations has been introduction of a wide-angled hysteroscope developed by De-Maeyer and the Wolf Corporation which, according to DeMaeyer, allows him to cannulate tubes more readily. He reports a 95% success rate in cannulization and proper plug formation with the use of this hysteroscope. This is well above the 82% average reported to date.

At the present time further clinical application is awaiting completion and approval of animal studies required by the FDA.

RESULTS

Present statistics show that 2,501 patients were entered in the original FDA clinical study and were considered for the procedure. Of these, 2,054 (82%) had a successful bilateral procedure. At the last follow-up report available, 1,858 (74.3%) of these women still had bilateral normal plugs. The reasons for this decline in status from the original report on the bilateral procedure are as follows: There was migration or expulsion of the plug in 2.9% of the patients, defective plugs developed in 2.9% (there was breakage or change in appearance), plugs were removed in 1.9%, or the patient had intervening surgery that disrupted or caused removal of the plugs in 1%.

As to the reproductive efficacy, 28 patients became pregnant who were felt to have proper plugs and were not using any other method of contraception. Two of these were ectopic pregnancies. This translates into an annual pregnancy rate of approximately 0.77%. In other words, if 10,000 women relied on the Ovabloc device for 1 year, approximately 77 of these women would become pregnant.

There has been very little work done or reported on the possibility of reversal of this procedure. In the author's series, 16 patients underwent reversal. Of these, only two became pregnant after removal of the plugs. Two or three of the patients were followed up with hysterosalpingograms in an effort to see if the tubes were patent, and bilateral blockage was found. One of the patients was referred to a reproductive endocrinologist for definite surgery. At laparotomy, intense fibrosis of the tubes was found.

In summary, it should be stated that this hysteroscopic sterilization procedure can be done in the office on an outpatient basis with the patient under local anesthesia. The pregnancy rate with bilateral plug formation is an acceptable rate. The ectopic pregnancy rate is not excessive. There were practically no serious complications other than pregnancy.

The general experience in achieving proper plug formation in patients who seem suitable for the procedure is somewhere around 85%. The author feels that with improved instruments this success rate in patients who have normal fallopian tubes can be achieved in the low 90% range.

There is very little evidence for the ability to reverse this procedure, but what little evidence there is makes it seem unlikely that reversal would meet with a high frequency of success.

BIBLIOGRAPHY

Corfman PA, Taylor HC: An instrument for transcervical treatment of the oviduct and uterine cornua. *Obstet Gynecol* 1966; 27:880.

Erb RA: Method and apparatus of nonsurgical reversible sterilization of females, U.S. Patent 2,805,767 (23 April 1974); reissue 29, 345 (9 August 1977).

Erb RA, David RH, Kyriazis GA, et al: System and technique for blocking the fallopian tubes. *Adv Planned Parenthood* 1974; 9:42.

Erb RA, Reed TP: Hysteroscopic oviductal blocking with formed-in-place silicone rubber plugs: I. Method and apparatus. *J Reprod Med* 1979; 23:65.

Hefnawi F, Fuchs A, Lawrence KA: Control of fertility by temporary occlusion of the oviduct. *Am J Obstet Gynecol* 1967; 99:421.

Neuwirth R: *Hysteroscopy.* Philadelphia, WB Saunders, 1975.

Quinones R, Alvarada A, Ley E: Hysteroscopic sterilization: Follow-up of 800 cases, in Sciarra JJ, Droegemueller W, Speidel JJ (eds): *Advances in Female Sterilization Techniques.* Hagerstown, Md, Harper & Row, 1976.

Rakshit B: The scope of liquid plastics and other chemicals for blocking the fallopian tube, in Richart RM (ed): *Human Sterilization.* Springfield, Ill, Charles C Thomas, 1972, p 213.

Rakshit B: Attempts at chemical blocking of the fallopian tube for female sterilization. *J Obstet Gynecol India* 1970; 20:618.

Rakshit B: Intratubal blocking device for sterilization without laparotomy. *Calcutta Med J* 1968; 65:90.

Reed TP, Erb RA: Hysteroscopic tubal occlusion with silicone rubber. *Obstet Gynecol* 1983; 61:388.

Reed TP, Erb RA: Tubal occlusion with silicone rubber: An update. *J Reprod Med* 1980; 25:25.

25

Endoscopy During Pregnancy

Michael S. Baggish, M.D.

Jacques Barbot, M.D.

Few endoscopic techniques are either safe or advisable during pregnancy. However, in this regard the contact hysteroscope is a unique instrument since it requires no distending medium to be placed within the pregnancy environment, it provides vision even in the presence of mucus or other body fluids, it allows light contact with the epithelium or structure to be viewed, and it delivers true cold light. If examination is carried out in a careful, systematic manner, complications are minimal. Because the endoscope enters the uterus under direct vision, the risk of perforation is low. No perforations of the uterus have occurred in over 200 examinations during pregnancy to date. The only side effect reported after examination during early or late pregnancy has been light bleeding. No pregnancy to date has been inadvertently terminated following endoscopic examination. Similarly, no patient developed an intrauterine infection as a result of contact endoscopy. Finally unintentional rupture of the membranes secondary to contact endoscopy is rarely encountered.

EMBRYOSCOPY

Examination of intrauterine pregnancies between 4 and 10 weeks of gestation heretofore has not been possible without invading the gestational sac. By means of the contact hysteroscope, the examiner may now view the living embryo without disrupting its environment (Fig 25–1; Plate 267).

The technique of embryoscopy diverges from the routine of general contact endoscopy only after the hysteroscope has entered the uterine cavity. First, the gestational sac is located. This structure protrudes like a ball into the uterine cavity, and as the endoscope makes contact, it pushes off to the side. Light blue patches of chorion stud the otherwise white decidua capsularis (Plate 268). Once the gestational sac is identified, the surface is gently scanned seeking an amniotic window. The latter can be seen in 70% to 80% of cases. The hysteroscope is placed onto this space; then, with a gentle side-to-side motion the window can be enlarged to accommodate the full 6- to 8-mm diameter of the endoscope (Plate 269). If the observer's movement is too rough, bleeding will be initiated and vision will be difficult; in virtually every case this problem can be avoided. The embryo appears stark white as it comes into view against the dark background of the amniotic fluid. Since the chorioamnionic sac is intact and the light is absolutely cold, the natural activities of the embryo can be accurately assessed.

Hysteroscopic examination at early phases of development indicates that the embryo is actively moving. Precise observations of anatomic development and differentiation have been recorded. Gentle pressure of the endoscope on the amniotic window frequently can initiate movement. Since the embryo is so small and because visualization occurs from the contact point to a distance of 5 mm, the view in this circumstance is magnified and panoramic.

At 4 weeks of development, bulbous eminences dominate the head of the conceptus. Initially, these structures were considered to be pathologic cysts, but are now recognized as normal landmarks (Plate 270). Fusion of these structures starts at 5 to 6 weeks of development and is evidenced by the presence of "cranial ridges," which subsequently leads to formation of the skull (Plate 271). These ridges are well developed by 7 weeks. At the 4 to 5 week's stage, the first brachial cleft is another prominent visual structure (Plate 272). By 7

During this embryonic period, the intestine naturally prolapses into the proximal cord, but does not represent an omphalocele (Plate 275). Interestingly, bright-red blood can be seen spiraling through the umbilical arteries. The upper extremities appear initially as paddlelike structures, but, by 7 to 8 weeks, differentiate into unwebbed hands with distinct finger pads and nail beds (Plate 276). In contrast, the inferior extremities lag behind the upper limbs by 2 weeks and remain flipperlike appendages at 8 weeks. At 8 weeks the external genitalia are indifferent, and the most prominent feature seen is the phallus. The labioscrotal folds may be observed beneath the phallus in various states of fusion (Plate 277,A and B).

The technique of embryoscopy does allow complete scanning of the embryo and can be a valuable tool for genetic counseling. Barbot in France has followed four women to term after performing embryoscopic examination to rule out structural abnormalities in the conceptus. Out of 110 examinations done at Mt. Sinai Hospital, Hartford, Conn., two patients have had delayed termination of pregnancy at 2 and 3 weeks after endoscopic study. Neither woman showed signs of threatened abortion in the interval between the endoscopic study and the eventual abortion. Although most of these examinations have been performed in women undergoing pregnancy termination, it has been consistently observed that the cervix promptly closes after withdrawal of the endoscope.

INCOMPLETE ABORTION

Contact hysteroscopy is a feasible and safe method by which to examine the intrauterine milieu in the presence of products of conception, blood, and fluid. Because the cavity is not distended by the endoscope, the hazard of pushing infected debris into the tubes or peritoneal cavity is eliminated. However, the differential diagnosis between incomplete abortion and other causes of uterine bleeding may be difficult; considerations should include threatened abortion, ectopic pregnancy, dysfunctional bleeding, and uterine neoplasia. The question about when and if to perform curettage must be answered. Although dilatation and curettage is the most frequently performed operation in obstetrics and gynecology, it should not be construed to be free of complications. In particular those problems related to future fertility (e.g., uterine synechiae, incompetent cervix, and perforation) are especially worrisome. Contact endoscopy gives a precise diagnosis in suspected cases of incomplete abortion.

Contact hysteroscopy may be carried out in an

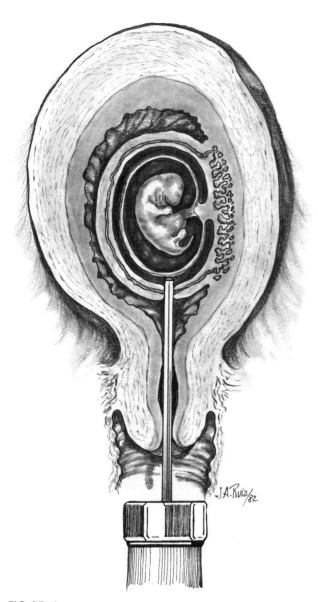

FIG 25–1.
A (above), the hysteroscope makes contact with the embryonic sac. A window in the chorion is located, and direct contact with the amnion is made. **B** (see Plate 267), panoramic view of gestational sac.

to 8 weeks this closes to form the ear. Because no eyelids are present, the blue-black eyes are clearly visible and a retinal-type reflex may be seen in photographs but rarely during direct examination (Plate 273).

Because the integument is very thin and virtually transparent, it has been possible to observe the pumping heart at approximately 4 weeks. The heart during this stage of development occupies most of the chest cavity and appears cherry red. The thorax virtually fuses with the abdomen where the umbilicus enters the latter (Plate 274).

emergency room or private office utilizing a 6-mm hysteroscope without the need of cervical dilatation. The appearance of fresh conceptual products is diagnostic: chorion is slate blue; decidua is white but sprinkled with large, scarlet vessels; the placenta is deep reddish-brown (Plate 278). No intact gestational sac (as in embryoscopy) is seen. In circumstances of ectopic pregnancy, the blue chorionic tissue is absent. Placental polyps lose their reddish hue and degenerate to a whitish color; the blue chorionic tissue also turns green. The polypoid structure of the tissue and the color changes described permit accurate diagnosis and direct the operator to the site of pathologic consideration. Barbot et al. in France avoid curettage unless bleeding is heavy. Weekly contact hysteroscopy is performed on an ambulatory basis.

Barbot discovered that within 1 week of fetal death, 25% of all uteri were spontaneously emptied; at the end of 2 weeks, 50% of the cavities were empty; and at the end of 1 month, 80% were empty. None of these women had a curettage. These investigators were able to differentiate necrotic decidua from placental fragments and observed normal endometrium regenerating at the same time as the necrotic decidua was sloughing (Plate 279). No complications were encountered as a result of the hysteroscopic examinations. By the 6th week, 94% of all cavities were empty. As a result of this study, curettage is no longer a routine procedure in incomplete abortions unless heavy bleeding occurs; patients return once at 6 weeks following abortion for an endoscopic examination; only 5% of the women show real placental retention (Plate 280).

INDUCED ABORTION

Although the number of unsuccessful pregnancy evacuations by vacuum or sharp curettage is less than 1%, the consequences of incomplete removal may be serious for both the patient and her physician. If the pregnancy continues and recognition is delayed, more hazardous second-trimester methodology may be required for successful termination. Should the pregnancy continue beyond the legal time permitted for termination, the possibility of delivering a deformed infant will subject the mother to great anguish and the physician to a malpractice lawsuit. Failure to interrupt a pregnancy is possible when the length of gestation is early, when a uterine septum is present, and when a twin gestation is not diagnosed. For the preceding reasons we have performed contact endoscopy prior to and after pregnancy termination in 155 cases. Once the gestational sac is lo-

cated, the operator can direct the vacuum curette to that specific area. Postcurettage inspection ensures that all the products of conception have been removed. As a result of our study, three instances of retained pregnancy were immediately observed. Repeat evacuation removed the residual products of conception. None of these patients had bleeding beyond 10 days following evacuation. When a septum was noted, the site of gestation was located, avoiding unnecessary trauma to the nonpregnant portion of the uterus (Plate 281).

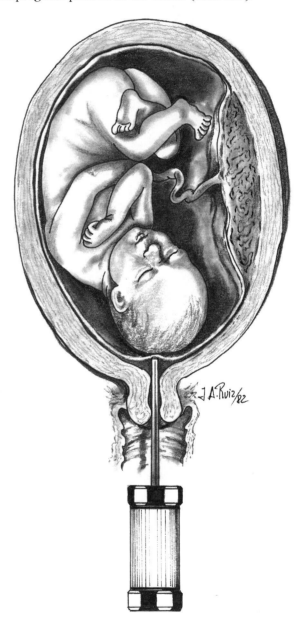

FIG 25–2.
The contact hysteroscope is carefully guided through the cervix, and gentle contact is made with the intact amnion. These examinations may be performed atraumatically between 28 weeks and term.

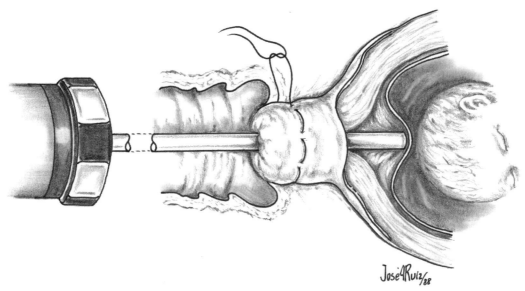

FIG 25–3.
The contact endoscope pushes the amnion upward during placement of cervical suture.

POSTPARTUM HEMORRHAGE

Extensive bleeding may follow term delivery because of the retention of small placental or membrane fragments. Unfortunately, gross inspection of the placenta postpartum frequently fails to locate the missing entity: that is, it usually appears intact. Initial procedures carried out in the face of immediate postpartum hemorrhage consist of uterine massage, inspection for lacerations of the cervix or vaginal fornices, uterine exploration, and administration of oxytocin. When these measures fail, the obstetrician usually resorts to blind use of instrumentation within the cavity in an attempt to stop bleeding. These blind techniques (e.g., sponge stick exploration and/or sharp curettage) carry a significant risk of perforation and myometrial disruption. It would seem preferable to utilize the 8-mm contact hysteroscope to explore the uterus under direct vision, even in the face of major bleeding.

In 10 out of 14 cases of postpartum hemorrhage, membrane fragments were seen in the cornual areas of the uterus; 7 of the 10 were found in the left cornua (Plate 282). Once localization had been achieved, di-

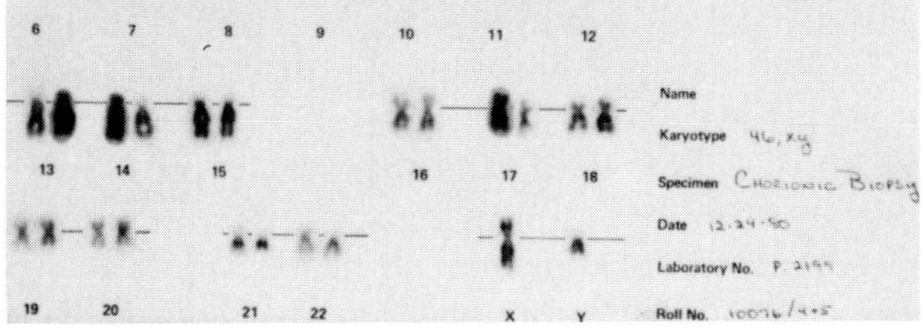

FIG 25–4.
Chromosome spread obtained from chorionic biopsy showing 46 X,Y karyotype.

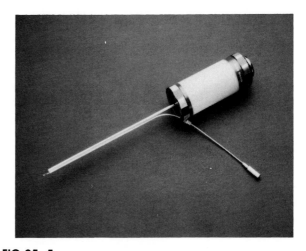

FIG 25–5.
Special 4-mm contact hysteroscope with a channel built in to obtain chorion villus sample.

rected curettage was performed, with prompt cessation of bleeding. None of the women developed postpartum infection, and no perforations occurred.

AMNIOSCOPY

Saling popularized the transcervical approach to observe both the amniotic sac and the color of amniotic fluid as a method of assessing fetal risk. He utilized a cone amnioscope, which unfortunately restricted the use of this technique to late pregnancy and labor (i.e., when the cervix was 2 to 3 cm dilated).

Although the presence of meconium-stained fluid may indicate fetal distress prior to the onset of labor, its significance continues to be debatable. Meconium discoloration postterm is recognized to portend a high-risk status for the fetus and to provide an additional indication for prompt delivery. Another risk attributed to the antepartum passage of meconium is the hazard of meconium aspiration, which results in significant morbidity and mortality during the neonatal period.

The contact endoscope is well suited for amnioscopy because the small diameter of the instruments allows easy passage through the endocervix and atraumatic contact with the amnion (Fig 25–2). The technique for performing contact amnioscopy is also very simple. No tenaculum is required. The cervix can be palpated by digital examination, and the endoscope can then be introduced through the external os. The examining room light is directed onto the light-collecting chamber of the endoscope, and the amniotic sac is located under direct vision. Gentle contact between the distal extremity of the endoscope and the amnion is made, and the color of the fluid is noted. Frequently, vernix may be seen floating in the fluid (Plate 283). Meconium staining can visually range from mild to severe. Additionally, the presentation of the fetus can be conveniently diagnosed, since scalp hair can be seen in vertex presentations. Two recent studies have described the value and ease of performing contact amnioscopy in 610 women. The incidences of meconium staining in general were 5% and 6%, respectively, however, among 25 women who were examined because of prolonged gestation (more than 42 weeks); 20% showed meconium in the amniotic fluid. Three out of five women had fetal distress during induced labor and were delivered by cesarean section. Both studies confirmed the accuracy of the amnioscopy by sampling fluid obtained during amniocentesis. Agreement of diagnosis was found in 100% of the cases tested. Antenatal diagnosis of meconium staining will alert the obstetrician to the risk of meconium aspiration and allow for earlier rupture of mem-

branes, intubation, and suction at delivery. Neither study was associated with any morbidity for mother or infant.

Another alternative use of amnioscopy is as an adjunctive measure to diagnose premature rupture of the membranes. Subtle leakage can be diagnosed even when unaided observation may be questionable. Similarly, spontaneous sealing-off of the membranes after disruption may be confirmed. Additionally, this instrument has proved helpful during the treatment of incompetent cervix. The 6-mm endoscope may be inserted through the internal os and used to elevate the membranes while the purse-string suture is tightened. This maneuver diminishes the risk of inadvertent rupture of the membranes during the operation (Fig 25–3). In the Mt. Sinai study, only 13% of the women demonstrated slight bleeding or spotting after endoscopy. No patient developed infection or inadvertent rupture of the amnion.

HYDATIDIFORM MOLE

Although the diagnosis of hydatidiform mole may be made by ultrasound, occasionally the scan may be equivocal. A definite diagnosis may be made by direct observation of molar vesicles. Since no amnion forms in molar pregnancy, direct entry into the uterus is very easy. Inspection of the uterine cavity following molar evacuation is vitally important to ensure that all the tissue has been removed.

The hysteroscopic view of a molar gestation presents a magnified view similar to what would be seen on gross examination of an evacuated mole (Plate 284,A). The vesicles are bleb-like, and show the characteristic blue color of chorion. Trophoblast, like placenta, is deep red, and the surrounding decidua is shining white (Plate 284,B and C).

CHORIONIC BIOPSY

Several publications have described the advantages of early prenatal chromosomal diagnosis by obtaining first-trimester chorionic biopsies. In this manner, pregnancy termination, if indicated, may be carried out early in the pregnancy. A report from Russia described an experience of 165 cases in which chorionic biopsies were carried out in the first trimester by hysteroscopic guidance. In 26 patients, biopsy was performed for genetic reasons—and when the gestation was continued, no spontaneous abortions were recorded, and the pregnancies finished with delivery of full-term healthy infants. At Mt. Sinai Hospital six chorionic biopsies were per-

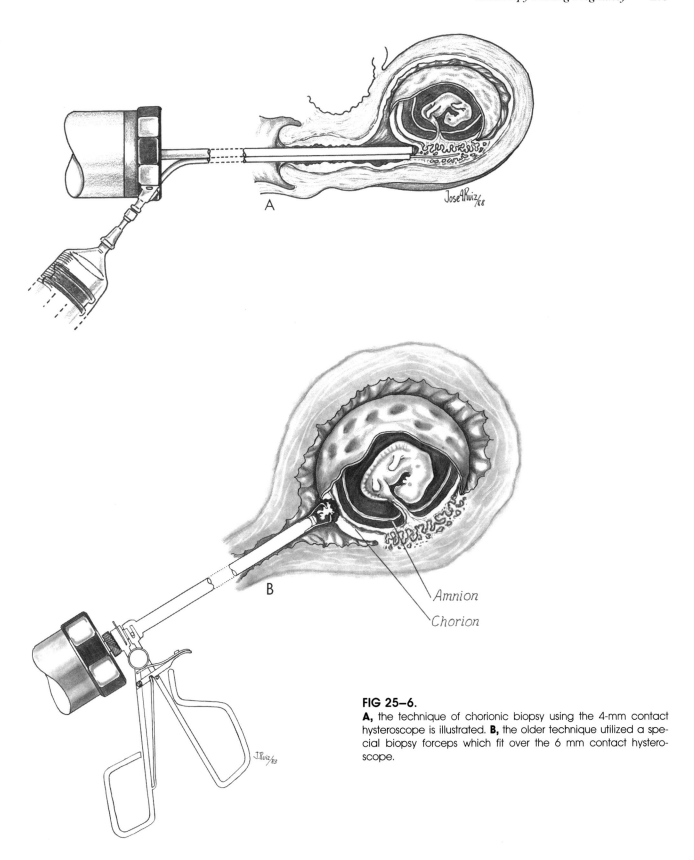

FIG 25–6.
A, the technique of chorionic biopsy using the 4-mm contact hysteroscope is illustrated. **B,** the older technique utilized a special biopsy forceps which fit over the 6 mm contact hysteroscope.

formed with a specially designed biopsy forceps, which was used in conjunction with the 6-mm contact hysteroscope (see Fig 25–6,B). The technique for obtaining biopsy material was very similar to that of embryoscopy; however, in this circumstance the amniotic window was not sought. A peripheral piece of chorionic tissue, measuring 1×1 mm underwent biopsy under direct vision and was immediately placed in thioglycollate broth. The specimen was transported to the cytogenetics laboratory for karyotyping. Successful spreads were obtained without great difficulty (Fig 25–4). It can be anticipated that the use of this technique will increase as more experience is gained with contact embryoscopy. Recently, a 4-mm contact hysteroscope with a channel for a sampling catheter was specifically designed for chorion biopsy procedures (Figs 25–5 and 25–6,B).

BIBLIOGRAPHY

Baggish MS: in Spirt BA, Gordon LP, Oliphant M (eds): *Prenatal Ultrasound* New York, Churchill Livingstone, 1987, pp 13, 21, 26, 37, 44, 47.

Baggish MS: Embryoscopy, in Filkins K, Russo JF (eds): *Human Prenatal Diagnosis.* New York, Marcel Dekker, 1985, p 311–323.

Baggish MS, Barbot J: Contact hysteroscopy. *Clin Obstet Gynecol* 1983; 26:219.

Baggish MS, Barbot J: Contact hysteroscopy for easier diagnosis. *Contemp Obstet Gynecol* 1980; 16:3.

Daker M: Chorionic tissue biopsy in the first trimester of pregnancy, commentary. *Br J Obstet Gynecol* 1983; 90:193.

Hahnemann N: Early prenatal diagnosis. A study of biopsy techniques and cells culturing from extraembryonic membranes. *Clin Genet* 1974; 6:294.

Hahnemann N, Mohr J: Genetic diagnosis in the embryo by means of biopsy from extraembryonic membranes. *Bull Eur Soc Hum Genet* 1968; 2:23.

Kazy Z, Rozovsky IS, Barkarev VA: Chorion biopsy in early pregnancy. A method of early prenatal diagnosis for inherited disorders. *Prenat Diagn* 1982; 2:39.

Ward KHT, Modell B, Petrou M, et al: Method of sampling chorionic villi in first trimester of pregnancy under guidance of realtime ultrasound. *Br Med J* 1983; 286:1542.

26

Hysteroscopic Photography

John L. Marlow, M.D.

The recording of images obtained through the hysteroscope has become an important and integral part of this surgical procedure. Modern instrumentation has simplified the means of obtaining an image record and has also improved its quality. The truism that "a picture is worth a thousand words" is significant in an era of expanding medical records. Long verbal operative reports can be distilled to a few simple photographs. Spatial relationships such as the proximity and orientation of disease to the internal uterine landmarks can be expressed better by pictures than by words. Photographs are useful for communications between surgeon and patient, her family, referring physician, and consultant. It is an essential tool in teaching hysteroscopy. Common anatomy and rare disease alike can be demonstrated to student surgeons and others learning the operative technique. Finally, for medicolegal purposes, the picture is yet another supporting record of the procedure. Some of the uses of hysteroscopic photography are listed in Table 26–1.

HISTORY

The initial image records of hysteroscopy were those of freehand drawings, usually done by the surgeon. The only tools necessary to record these images were a pen and paper, and the only limitation was the surgeon's ability to draw. Later hysteroscopy publications included sketches and paintings by artist illustrators. Subsequently, photography provided a simpler and more accurate tool to record the images of hysteroscopy. A review of the history of photography and the development of this and other techniques for hysteroscopy image documentation is helpful in understanding its present use.

In 1725, Johanne Schulze proved that light caused silver nitrate mixed with chalk to become dark. Later, in 1826, Joseph Nicephore Niepce produced what is considered to be the first photograph. It consisted of the roof line visible from his workshop in France and required 8 hours of bright sunlight to produce a fuzzy permanent image. In 1835 Louis Daguerre, using a pewter plate coated with a light-sensitive varnish of asphalt (Bitumen of Judea) and using oils as a fixing agent, improved the process and made it reproducible using silver copper plates coated with iodine vapor. Later in 1839, Sir John Herschel coined the word "photography." George Eastman selected the word "Kodak" for his camera: "A name that could be pronounced anywhere in the world." He sold his hand camera for twenty-five dollars. After taking the pictures the owner returned the camera to the factory, where for ten dollars, 100 mounted prints were provided, and the camera was reloaded and returned. The single lens reflex camera, the mechanism still in use today, was patented in 1888 by McKellen. It has become the most useful tool for endoscopic photography.

The early lighting available for illumination of the uterine chamber through the hysteroscope was very poor. Candles and sunlight directed to the endoscope by means of lenses and mirrors provided the first light for early endoscopists. The endoscope of Bozzini, the first endoscopist, provided a very weak light and poor visibility. Kerosene and alcohol flame were used by Desormeaux, the surgeon credited with performing the first hysteroscopy procedure, but this light also proved unsatisfactory as well as being hazardous to patient and surgeon alike. A heated platinum wire was used to illuminate the oral cavity, but it also produced significant heat and required use of circulating ice water within the uterine chamber to prevent burns.

TABLE 26–1.

Uses of Hysteroscopic Photography

Records of operative findings
Patient education
Surgeon and health care personnel
    education
Referral reports
Comparisons of before and after surgery
Lecture and educational conferences
Development of research techniques
Historical record of findings for future use
Record of rare and unusual findings
Medico-legal record of surgery
Consultation, including teleconferences

TABLE 26–2.

Color Temperatures of
Common Light Sources

Light Source	°K
Candle	1,000
Tungsten lamp	2,000
Electronic flash	5,000
Bright sunlight	6,000

In the late 1880s, modern lighting techniques for photography began with Thomas Alva Edison, who developed the incandescent bulb. This source of light was adapted to the distal cystoscope by Nitze and improved the quality and intensity of the light available to the endoscopist. The improved light, coupled with advances in cameras, became the basis of hysteroscopic photography. Exacta produced the first commercially available single-lens camera in 1937. Kodachrome, the first three-color subtractive color film, was produced in 1935 for cinematography and in the next year for 35-mm cameras. Also in 1935 came the development of the electronic flash, which provides the optimum light today for 35-mm endoscopic photographs. In 1948, the Polaroid Corporation was able to provide a black-and-white image in 60 seconds. The "instant" color prints became available in 1963.

A major milestone in the development of endoscopy was the development of fiberoptic lighting, which provided the so-called "cold light." For the first time, it provided intense light which was relatively free of the danger of thermal injury. Fiberoptics became available to hysteroscopy in the mid-1960s.

LIGHT

To obtain optimum photographs through the hysteroscope, an understanding of the principles of lighting is necessary. Visible light is generated when energy is added to atoms and subsequently lost in the form of photons. The color of radiation in visible light will vary according to the source of light. In photography, the mixture in a particular light is described in terms of the color temperature, which is expressed in degrees Kelvin (equivalent to Celsius degrees plus 273). In Table 26–2,

the color temperatures of common light sources are listed in degrees Kelvin.

Tungsten provides an inexpensive source of light, but at 2,000°K, the temperature of molten steel, it emphasizes the red tones and may result in color distortions. Another disadvantage is that when the bulb is attached to the distal end of the hysteroscope, its heat production can cause tissue injury. Halogen light is more reliable and intense, as are mercury and xenon high-pressure arc lights. Electronic flash provides the highest intensity, and because of its very brief duration, prevents blurring caused by tissue movements such as vessel pulsations. Flash color simulates daylight and, with the appropriate film, results in the accurate reproductions of the tissue color. The flash strobe light is produced when electrical energy stored in a capacitor is released in a sudden burst of power. This burst is converted to light in the flash tube. The intense light is usually 1/1,000 of a second or shorter in duration.

EQUIPMENT

The essential equipment for hysteroscopic photography consists of the following:

- Light source
- Light cable
- Hysteroscope
- Camera and lens adaptor
- Film or recording media
- Accessory equipment.

Light Source

Electronic flash has been traditionally the optimum light source. For endoscopy, early flash instruments were used intra-abdominally. The tip of the endoscope contained a small strobe light. This provided very adequate light for the abdominal chamber but had the disadvantage of occasionally stimulating muscle contraction

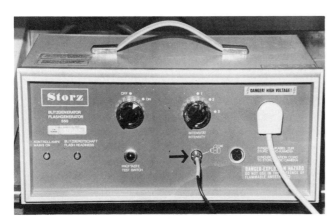

FIG 26–1.
Endoscopic remote electronic flash unit. The intensity of the light may be adjusted. A synchronization cable may be plugged into the unit *(arrow)*.

with the high voltage produced. Another concern was the safety of delivering such high voltage inside the body. This system is no longer in use. Hysteroscopy photography has a working distance usually less than 1 inch and requires less light. On the other hand, the hysteroscope is smaller, so that less light can be transmitted through the instrument. Electronic flash can be delivered attached directly to the hysteroscope or at the remote light source through the light-transmitting cable. Dedicated light sources with interactive light systems which are automatically controlled by the camera for accurate-exposure, through-the-lens computers are also available (Fig 26–1). Flash durations of 1/100 to 1/1,000 of a second are automatically provided according to distance, color, reflectivity, and other factors (Fig 26–2). High-intensity metal halide arc and automatic xenon light sources up to 300 W can also be used for examination, television, still photographs, and cinematogra-

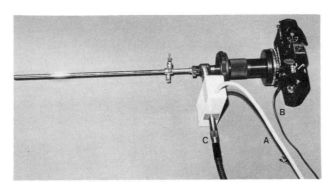

FIG 26–2.
A 35-mm camera attached by a cable to flash unit *(A)*. The synchronization cable plugs into the camera *(B)*. A fiberoptic cable connects to the flash unit cable by a special fitting *(C)*.

phy. These high-intensity lights produce a light in the 6,000°K range. They also produce thermal heat as an additional undesirable byproduct that must be dissipated. This heat can also be transmitted into the light cable and result in tissue burning or ignition of flammable drapes.

Light Cable

Fiberoptic cables became available in the 1960s. Their development was aided by the use of optical fibers for communication, imaging, diagnostics, therapeutics, and lasers in medicine. Light-transmitting optical fibers are a non-order array of fibers that are coupled to a light source. The bundle transmits light and illuminates the uterine chamber. The optical fiber is a special glass which may be 10 to 125 μm in diameter, about the same thickness as a human hair. Electromagnetic waves that constitute light tend to travel through regions that have a high refractive index. The center of the glass strand has such an index and is referred to as the "core." To keep the light inside the core it is covered with material with a lower index of refraction called the "cladding." Light travels with very little loss within the fiber. However, when the fiber is coupled with other instruments, light may be lost.

Light loss sites are:

- The interface of the light source and fiber optical cable, owing to reflections.
- The cable-hysteroscope interface, as a result of fibers that do not align precisely.
- Within the cable at broken fiberoptical fiber sites.
- Within the cable (minor losses) owing to length of the fibers.

Fiber cables are referred to as incoherent and coherent. Incoherent light cables have a random non-order arrangement of the fibers. These are less expensive to construct. Coherent bundles on the other hand have a precise ordered arrangement of the fibers so that any image entering one will be reproduced on the other end. This is used in flexible fiberoptic teaching devices and flexible endoscopes. Another innovation in light-conducting cables has been the fluid light cable. Instead of fiberglass threads, the light is transmitted through a fluid medium illustration. The cable is less flexible and cannot be bent in a short radius but is capable of transmitting more light and a more desirable color temperature.

Fiberoptic systems are also used in the transmission of specialized light such as laser light. Nd-YAG, KTP, and argon lasers are examples of the use of fiberoptics therapeutically. The fibers are also capable of diagnostic uses in systems composed of sensors in which light emitted or reflected is dependent on a chemical or physical quality that can be measured.

Hysteroscope

The hysteroscope is composed of a series of lenses, fiberoptic bundles, and instrument channels. The early hysteroscopes contained an eyepiece, followed by a series of small lenses and a distal lens which directed the viewing angle and field of vision. In the late 1950s, Professor H.H. Hopkins of the University of Reading, England, succeeded in producing a rod lens optical system using glass rods instead of small lenses. This hysteroscope produced a brighter image by means of more light being transmitted, a better resolution and contrast, and a wider viewing angle.

The optimum hysteroscope for photography is one without instrument channels, which allows a large rod lens and fiberoptic light bundle. Hysteroscopes with integrated fiber light-transmitting cables that are continuous from the light source to the tip of the hysteroscope provide maximum light; however, this is not impractical, because with the deterioration of the cable, the hysteroscope must be replaced. Some hysteroscopes are now available with focusing and contact views that can magnify to ×80 and ×150. To photograph at this high magnification, the surgeon must use a high-intensity light flash or very light sensitive film or television cameras.

The distal lens of the hysteroscope can become blurred with blood or mucus, resulting in a poor photograph. The liquid distending media such as D_5W or dextran are more effective in clearing the lens from blood. On the other hand, CO_2 provides the optimum light transmission.

Camera

The 35-mm single lens reflex camera has become the most useful photographic tool for hysteroscopic photography. Excellent photographs can be obtained without difficulty. Adapters between the camera and the hysteroscope adjust for precise focus (Fig 26–3,A and B).

Lens

The purpose of the camera lens is to bend the light to a focal point on the recording media or film surface. The focal length of the lens is the distance from the center of the lens to the point at which parallel rays entering the lens converge. Long-focus lenses see more narrow angles of view, and the image recorded is filled with a small area of the scene. Lenses with focal lengths from 15 to 50 mm can be used for hysteroscopic photography. The focal length of the lens will determine the amount of the 35-mm frame tht is exposed; the longer the focal length, the larger the film image exposed and also the more light that is necessary. The major factors affecting the amount of light reaching the film are the duration of exposure and diameter of the aperture. The aperture is calibrated in F-numbers or stops. Hysteroscopy lenses with F values of 1.2 or 1.4 or less provide the optimum amount of light for exposure (Fig 26–4).

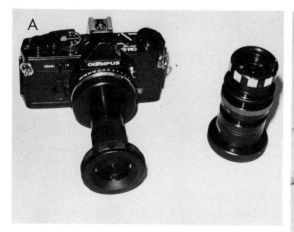
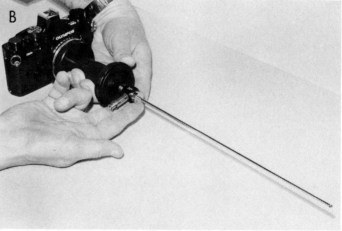

FIG 26–3.
A, Olympus OM-2 35-mm single lens reflex camera with special endoscopic lens attached. **B,** same camera attached to the eyepiece of the hysteroscope.

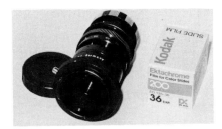

FIG 26–4.
The endoscopic lens is detached from the camera and hysteroscope. Caps provided by the manufacturer protect the lens during storage.

Film

Most hysteroscopy photography today uses color film balanced for electronic flash. This is designated as "daylight film" and emphasizes the blue light spectrum. Film should be stored at 55°F or lower and should be removed from the refrigerator 1 hour before use. The degree of sensitivity of the film to light is designated by the ASA number originated by the American Standards Association. DIN, a German equivalent system, is a similar standard. More recently, light sensitivity has been expressed in a comparable ISO system. Hysteroscopic

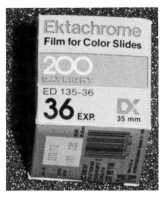

FIG 26–5.
Daylight film with ASA of 200 is used for hysteroscopic photography and consistently obtains excellent pictures.

photography requires film speeds inversely proportional to the light available. Loading film into the camera should be done in low light and in areas free of dust. Glove powder, which may be present during surgery, should be avoided. Compressed air or brushes may be helpful in removing such dust. Care should be made to handle the film on the edges and not on the emulsion side of the film. The four enemies of film are heat, hu-

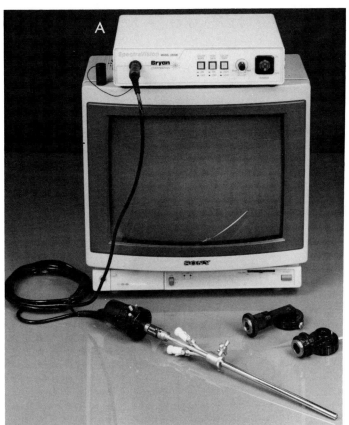

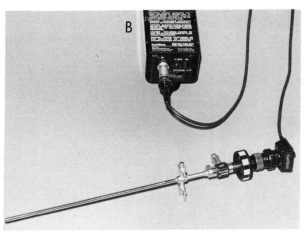

FIG 26–6.
A, endoscopic television camera attached to the eyepiece of the telescope. This-high resolution camera is lightweight and capable of being sterilized by soaking in Cidex. **B,** another chip camera with its control unit, which couples to the television recorder and monitor.

TABLE 26–3.

Uses of Television in Hysteroscopy

Reduces muscle strain and fatigue of surgeon
Coordination of the surgical team
Consultation during surgery
Education of surgeons and health care professionals
Provides accurate tissue color during laser surgery
Provides magnetic and optical disc filing, for easier
  storage and retrieval
Provides immediate hard-copy photographs (Fig
  28–8)

midity, dust, and light. The chances of obtaining good photographs is improved by taking large numbers of pictures. This being the case, it may be necessary to have an assistant in the operating room who is familiar with the camera and able to reload it. Large-volume filmpacks can also be used in some cameras (Fig 26–5).

Accessory Equipment

Television

Television systems have revolutionized endoscopic documentation (Table 26–3; Fig 26–6,A and B). Small (0.5-in.) CCD (charge couple device) chip cameras with combined weights of 6 to 8 ounces provide images with resolutions of over 300 lines per inch and low light photography with minimum illuminations of 1 foot candle (10 lux). Magnetic and optical storage devices and instant thermal printers can be coupled to the television and will become the visual documentation system of the future (Figs 26–7 and 26–8).

Photographic Accessories

Photographic accessories are as important as the primary equipment in obtaining good photographs. Accessories that aid hysteroscopic photography are listed in Table 26–4. There are motor drives for single or multiple exposure. The motor drive frees the surgeon photographer from mechanically advancing the film. Data back recording imprints on the film preselected information including date, patient sequence or number, or combinations of information. Clear viewing screens specifically for endoscopy provide a superior view through the hysteroscope, especially in low-light situations. This allows for more precise focus and composition. The Olympus No. 1–12 screen is one such screen (Fig 26–9). The usual ground-glass viewing screens do not provide a clear enough view for most hysteroscopic photography. An optical articulated arm made by Karl Storz is useful in taking photographs. It is lightweight and

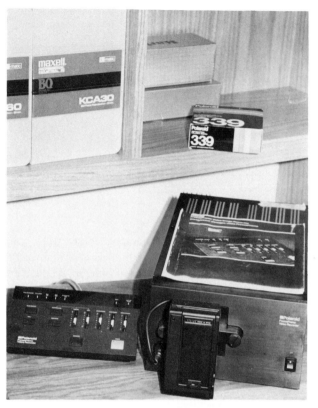

FIG 26–7.
Freeze-frame video image recorder allows still photography directly from the television monitor. Color adjustment is possible. Either 35-mm or Polaroid hard-copy photographs may be optionally taken.

provides for optimal movement with no interference to the surgeon. It consists of two to four joints with a beamsplitter from 50% to 50% or 10% to 90% sharing the image between the examiner and camera. The camera can thus be attached to the arm some distance from the operative field, which allows the hysteroscopist optimum working conditions during photography.

INSTRUMENT MAINTENANCE

Proper care of the hysteroscopy photography equipment is essential. The fiber light-transmitting cables should be checked periodically for broken fibers. This can be done by directing one end of the cable toward a light source and inspecting the opposite end. Broken fibers will appear as dark spots in the cable. This can be quantified by measuring on a light meter the light transmitted from a known constant light source with a fixed cable distance. Light cables with a light loss of over 30% should be replaced. Bending the cable to an acute angle

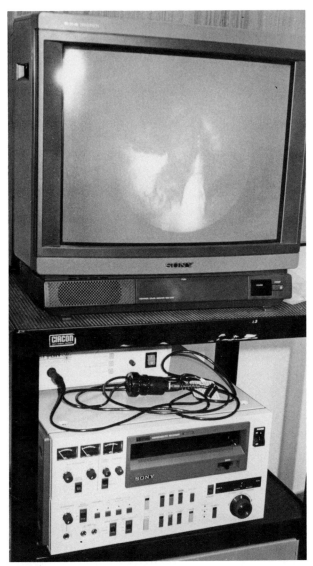

TABLE 26–4.

Hysteroscopic Photography
Accessories

Motor drive
Record data back
Clear viewing screen for endoscopy
Articulated optical arm

storage will decrease instrument damage. Another common time for instrument damage is when the hysteroscope is placed in a tray or basin with a weighted speculum or other heavy instruments that can bend or damage the instrument.

IMAGE IDENTIFICATION AND STORAGE

An efficient system for identification and storage of the image is essential. Data recording back systems, which imprint a data or code on the photograph, are most convenient (Fig 26–10). Television, including prints, can be electronically imprinted with similar data. Log books or computer files are also available for large-volume records and can be filed according to patient

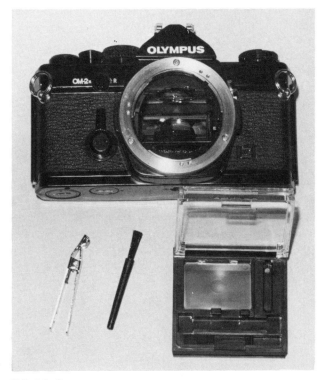

FIG 26–9.
The best hysteroscopic photographs are obtained with a clear viewing screen. The ground-glass screen is replaced with a screen from the kit pictured here.

FIG 26–8.
View of stop action on a high-resolution monitor. Simply pressing the exposure button on the system in Fig 26–7 produces hard copy for record-keeping purposes.

will break the fibers and result in light loss. Bending can be minimized through wall support storage systems for the fiberoptic cable plus careful handling. Boiling water or autoclave heating, followed by rapid cooling, may jeopardize the seals at the ends of the hysteroscope. Gas autoclaving avoids this temperature extreme but is not practical in a busy operative theater.

Instrument warmers raise the temperature of the hysteroscope to body temperature; however, the fogging problem encountered in laparoscopy is not experienced in hysteroscopy.

Instrument damage can occur during the storage of the hysteroscope. Foam rubber or similar protective

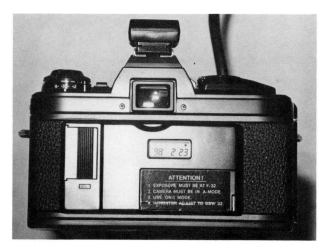

FIG 26–10.
A recording back provides a convenient mechanism for recording identification data directly on the 35-mm film.

name, number, date of surgery, type of surgery, or findings. Computer filing has the advantage of ease of cross-referencing. A simple method of identifying the patient, should these sophisticated systems not be available, is to photograph the patient's chart, including her stamped information identification plate. Photographs should be stored in protective envelopes or trays. Important or unusual photographs should be protected beneath glass or plastic and duplicate slides made.

THE FUTURE

Improvements in recording images promise to make this one of the most dynamic areas of medical records. Available at this writing are optical disc systems which can record over 25,000 visual images, any one of which can be retrieved in less than 0.10 sec. All this is in an 8-inch optical disc. Improved resolution television, which promises to provide 1,000-line resolution or more and which can be immediately printed, will challenge today's photograph. The digitalization of images and the capacity to transmit them by way of telephone lines promises to significantly benefit hysteroscopic visual image recording.

BIBLIOGRAPHY

Busselle M: *Creative Photography.* Mitchell Beazley Publishers, 1977.

Cohen MR: Photograph, in Phillips J (ed): *Laparoscopy.* Baltimore, Williams & Wilkins, 1977, p 300.

Cohen MR: Routine endoscopic photography simplified, in Phillips J (ed): *Gynecological Laparoscopy: Principles and Techniques.* Miami, Symposia Specialists, 1974, p 199.

Croy OR: *Camera Close Up.* New York, Am Photo, 1961, p 14.

Electronic Flash. The Kodak Workshop. Rochester, NY, Eastman Kodak Publication, 1981.

Hansell P: *A Guide to Medical Photography.* Baltimore, Md, University Park Press, 1979.

Hulka J: *Textbook of Laparoscopy.* New York, Grune & Stratton, 1985.

Eastman Kodak Technical Publication: *Clinical Photography* N-3, 1972; *Kodak Filters* B-3, 1970; *Photomacrography* N-12B, 1974; *Medical Infra-red Photography* N-1, 1973; *Photography Through the Microscope* P-2, 1974; *Basic Scientific Photography* N-9, 1970; *Kodak Color Films* E-77; *Professional Photoguide,* 1975. Rochester, NY, Eastman Kodak publications.

Editors of Eastman Kodak Co: *The Joy of Photography.* Reading, Mass, Addison-Wesley, 1979.

Kott DF: Photography, cinematography and television in endoscopy, in Phillips J (ed): *Endoscopy in Gynecology.* Downey, Calif, AAGL, 1978, p 481.

Korff H: *Colour Photography for the Medical Photographer.* New York, American Elsevier, 1973.

Lyons AS, Petrucelli RJ: *Medicine: An Illustrated History.* New York, Harry N. Abrams, 1978.

Marlow J: History of laparoscopy, optics, fiberoptics and instrumentation. *Clin Obstet Gynecol* 1976: 19:261.

Nelson PK: Photography in laparoscopy, in Phillips J (ed): *Endoscopy in Gynecology.* Downey, Calif, AAGL, 1978, p 90.

Semm K: *Operative Manual for Endoscopic Abdominal Surgery,* Friedrich E (trans). Chicago, Year Book Medical Publishers, 1987.

Sugimoto O: *Diagnostic and Therapeutic Hysteroscopy.* New York, Igaku-Shoin, 1978.

27

Establishment of a Hysteroscopy Program

Michael S. Baggish, M.D.

A modicum of thoughtful planning is recommended prior to initiating a hysteroscopy program. Organization beforehand will minimize frequently costly and always aggravating mistakes. The endeavor should be reduced to component parts, which are best transmitted by the written word. Diagrams, photographs, and equipment brochures should be kept in a file entitled, for example, "Hysteroscopy Project." Importantly, an accurate budget should be constructed based on available funds and should be matched line for line with *quoted* costs. Again, word of mouth is a poor substitute for written documentation.

LOCATION FOR PERFORMANCE OF HYSTEROSCOPY

Several sites may be used for this procedure. In the previous chapters mention has been made of the office, surgicenter, and operating room as the most likely locations for the performance of hysteroscopy. Nevertheless, one might also consider that examinations could conceivably be done in the clinic, emergency room, labor and delivery unit, or in-patient treatment room. Fixed or at least stable locations for the more fragile and heavier equipment should be established in areas where the largest number of cases are anticipated. Portable equipment setups should be prepared for use in less likely sites.

For office endoscopy, select the most spacious examining room available and make certain it is adequately wired with three-prong electrical outlet receptacles. An electrically controlled examining table is a necessity because raising and lowering the patient is an anticipated routine during hysteroscopy. A high-intensity, multipositional examining light, preferably wall mounted, is paramount if one anticipates doing contact hysteroscopy. Space should be allocated for a double- or triple-tiered mobile table where prep solutions, swabs, and accessory instruments are placed in addition to the light generator and CO_2 insufflator. Adequate counter, cupboard, and shelf space will pay dividends, as will a sink with running water.

Surgicenter and operating suite locations already have the requisite accoutrements necessary for the performance of diagnostic and operative hysteroscopy. However, dedicated storage space for the concentration of equipment must not be taken for granted. A special shelf, cabinet, or cart should be procured to keep all the hysteroscopy equipment in one place, otherwise things tend to get lost or damaged. Even with the best intentions, new and less experienced nursing assistants will from time to time be called upon to help with hysteroscopy procedures. If the location of everything that is needed to do the operation is known, the sequence of events will progress smoothly rather than helter skelter. Again a shelved, mobile cart is a handy place in which to locate light sources, insufflators, endoscopes, accessories, and supporting packs. When hysteroscopy is ready to begin, the cart is simply wheeled up to the operating table; the fiberoptic cable and CO_2 line are plugged in; the surgeon is ready to go.

PERSONNEL

Under most circumstances another person will be present and will be expected to help with some phase of hysteroscopy. This may range from cleaning the instruments after the procedure is finished to actively assisting with the endoscopy. Nevertheless, rewards will be reaped if these people are at the least given a detailed explanation of what hysteroscopy is about and at the best trained to handle all the equipment properly. If office and operating room personnel know what is going on, they can effectively explain details to the patient and answer questions she poses. Characteristically most patients question nurses, technicians, and secretaries more often than they do their physicians. Both the life of the hysteroscopy equipment and the coronary arteries of the gynecologist will be preserved if the assistant is well versed about sterilizing, cleaning, boxing, and storage of fragile endoscopes. The axiom seems to hold that if everything is properly at hand and in enviable readiness, the whole hysteroscopic procedure goes well from start to finish. The corollary equally follows that, when one has to scramble for needed items and make do with improper instruments, the procedure disintegrates into a fiasco.

The availability of printed and illustrated material answering basic questions in lay terms will not only be very much appreciated by patients, but will substantially reduce the number of time-consuming telephone calls to the physician. Such questions can include (1) What is hysteroscopy? (2) Why is it done? (3) How is it carried out? (4) What will be learned? (5) What will be treated? (6) What risks or side effects are entailed? (7) How long will the procedure take? and (8) How much will it hurt?

EQUIPMENT

Data regarding hysteroscopes, illumination sources, and supporting accessories have been adequately conveyed in preceding chapters. However, a few additional words on this subject should not be considered a wasteful overstatement of details.

One should not be considered dilatory by carefully selecting instrumentation which might serve more than one purpose. In other words, why purchase a particular telescope for office diagnostic use only when another device could be applied to an operative sheath in the surgicenter and with equal facility be inserted into a diagnostic sheath when used in the office. The money saved could be applied to the purchase of an extra accessory.

Common sense would lead the prospective purchaser of precision optics to realize that prices vary in a narrow range between competitive manufacturers. Nevertheless, Americans continue to pursue the relentless quest of obtaining "something for nothing," the driving philosophy of every bargain hunter. Invariably this "bargain" purchase subsequently turns out to be in reality inferior goods and a financial liability. Another peculiar logic construes that the choice between two items matched and faithfully equal in every aspect of excellence must be made in favor of the more expensive product. This decision is steeped in a long-held tradition that greater cost always translates to mean superior quality. The smart shopper will endeavor to learn as much about the material to be acquired, then personally examine and compare instrumentation. Clearly, the best place to view and handle hysteroscopy instruments is at a dedicated course, at the annual congress of the American College of Obstetricians and Gynecologists, or at a subspecialty meeting, for example, the Gynecologic Laser Society or American Fertility Society. Once the decision to purchase a specific number and type of instruments has been made, manufacturer's representatives may be approached to obtain the most favorable value for the money.

Equipment stored out of sight tends to be underutilized. Also, a certain degree of uncertainty and inertia must be overcome when embarking on a new procedure or technique. Frequent use breeds familiarity and vice versa. We recommend having everything needed for hysteroscopy conveniently within reach. Additionally, a simple reminder protocol should be posted within a close viewing distance of the operating field. Similarly, a plan for quickly cleaning, sterilizing, and rinsing instruments should be at hand. The latter means that Cidex, soaking containers, sterile water, and sterile towels must be acquired and have predetermined and functional locations.

No single instrument will fulfill every need or clinical circumstance. Therefore, the pursuit and acquisition of skills utilizing a variety of hysteroscopes is commendable. For example, although panoramic endoscopy permits one to view the endocervical canal, contact hysteroscopy provides a better comprehension of detail and hence a more accurate diagnosis.

Finally, only trained persons should use shared hysteroscopy equipment. Damage inflicted as the result of ignorance and carelessness infuriates the experienced practitioner who quickly learns to depend on this equipment for his/her daily practice of gynecology. Categorically, there is no excuse for infliction of injury secondary to a lack of familiarity with instrumentation.

CREDENTIALING

As with any manipulative or operative procedure, the ability to perform hysteroscopy skillfully and safely requires documentation. The "see one, do one, teach one" mentality is based on inappropriate reasoning in light of contemporary practice standards.

What constitutes adequate knowledge of hysteroscopy, and how does one qualify for hysteroscopy privileges?

First, proof must be established that bona fide training has been obtained. This may take the form of a certificate of participation in a hysteroscopy course, preferably with "hands-on" sessions. A letter from the director of a residency training program attesting to the fact that hysteroscopy skills were taught to and adequate "hands-on" experience was acquired by the candidate as an integral part of his/her residency training will equally suffice.

Second, a detailed explanation and demonstration concerning the proper use and care of the instruments should be arranged with the manufacturer's representative. It is most convenient to have nurses and assistants present at the demonstration in order to ensure that the entire team is synchronized insofar as instrumentation details are concerned. At this time, it is convenient also to catalogue the equipment, mark it with identifying tape or etchings, and have all questions answered.

Third, initial learning should follow the plan presented in the chapter titled "How to Learn Hysteroscopy."

Fourth, the learning curve for both diagnostic and operative hysteroscopy may be substantially shortened by attending a preceptorship program with an experienced endoscopic surgeon. There is no substitute for scrubbing in and handling the hysteroscope during an actual operation, but only under the watchful eyes of an expert. Fine nuances can render any procedure easier to perform, particularly if they are seen and learned in supervised settings.

Fifth, repetition with the same assisting team leads to steady improvement in performance from all aspects. Constantly changing personnel and techniques make things difficult and retard attainment of confidence.

Sixth, complications should be tracked from the standpoint of quality assurance. Surgeons who have a record of excessive complications and unsuccessful procedures should repeat the early instructional steps and definitely attend a preceptorship.

Continuous review of the credentialing process is imperative in updating endoscopists in new techniques such as laser hysteroscopy. When additional equipment is obtained, further in-service training should be required for everyone prior to usage. Similar standards with practical but equivalent strategies should be promulgated for office hysteroscopy programs as well.

28

Future of Hysteroscopy

Michael S. Baggish, M.D.

Rafael F. Valle, M.D.

Hysteroscopy, as a bona fide technique, has received accelerated acceptance during the 1980s and will reach its acme during the 1990s to the extent that it will be a required skill for residency training programs. Without exception, any center dedicated to women's health care will have hysteroscopy performed by the majority of gynecologists. This rapid expansion will prompt manufacturers to introduce innovations in instrumentation for both diagnostic and operative hysteroscopy, resulting in diverse instruments with superior optics and better lighting, which will in like fashion lead to creative surgical accessories and techniques.

PRESENT STATUS OF HYSTEROSCOPY

In previous chapters the numerous indications for hysteroscopy have been presented in detail. Intrauterine visualization for the evaluation of patients with abnormal uterine bleeding represents the "gold standard" today. The ability to observe the entire endometrium provides accuracy and precision in sampling, allowing truly directed biopsies for abnormal lesions that are focal or located in the uterotubal cones. The probability of missing structural abnormalities (e.g., submucous leiomyomas, endometrial polyps, and septae) is virtually nullified.

As pointed out, hysteroscopy can confirm or correct an abnormal hysterosalpingogram, rectifying the false positive readings secondary to distortion of the uterine cavity, blood clots, mucus, debris, or air bubbles. Additionally, with the ability of performing direct biopsies under visual control, hysteroscopy brings the accuracy of the diagnosis to a level comparable to colposcopy. The three areas in which hysteroscopy helps in the eval-uation of the abnormal hysterosalpingogram for its confirmation or rectification are infertility, intrauterine adhesions, and pregnancy wastage. An abnormal hysterogram is the main indication for hysteroscopy in infertile patients. The false positive filling defects may be confirmed or rectified, and lesions suggesting neoplasia can undergo biopsy and sometimes be removed transcervically under visual control. Polyps, submucous leiomyomas, intrauterine adhesions, and uterine septa may be diagnosed and treated by hysteroscopy. Blind division of intrauterine adhesions by curettage should be relegated to the past in the same vein as high forceps operations. The facility of direct vision has now resulted in precision dissection and division of adhesions with minimal trauma to the surrounding normal endometrium. Contemporary hysteroscopy is the accepted method for the evaluation and treatment of intrauterine adhesions. Statistically, the visual approach to these adhesions has improved the pregnancy rate while simultaneously diminishing the risk of uterine damage.

In the evaluation of patients with pregnancy wastage, hysteroscopy is combined with the hysterosalpingography in providing visualization of the endocervical canal and the internal cervical os. The observation of this anatomic area, as well as visual evaluation of the extension of uterine anomalies and the distortion of the uterine architecture, has led to their direct treatment through hysteroscopy. Hysteroscopy, however, as used today, does not exclude the hysterosalpingogram; rather, it complements its findings and adds to its accuracy. The hysterosalpingogram offers more areas of examination than hysteroscopy: for example, it permits appraisal of the fallopian tubes and their architecture, intratubal defects, possible intratubal adhesions, the presence of tubal diverticuli, and tubal patency.

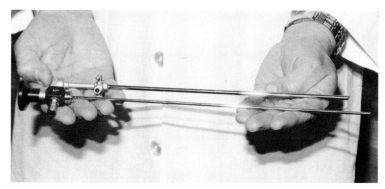

FIG 28–1.
A 3-mm telescope and accompanying 4-mm (O.D.) sheath. The wide-angle optics of this small-caliber instrument provide an excellent view of the uterus and it is ideal for office hysteroscopy using CO_2 as the distending medium.

A common problem until recently was misplacement and/or embedment of intrauterine devices. Although the majority of the misplaced devices predominantly lie in the uterine cavity, blind transcervical manipulations with curettes, forceps, catheters, or hooks are rather barbaric and invariably traumatize normal tissue during extractions. Persistence with such blind techniques may eventuate in uterine perforation and the danger of bleeding or infection. The comfort of visualizing the uterine cavity directly permits detection of embedment or fragmentation of the device and adds enormously to the safe evaluation of these patients, offering not only the ability to diagnose directly whether the foreign body is in the uterine cavity or not, but also the possiblity of immediate direct transcervical removal.

Use of hysteroscopy for this purpose has obviously decreased with the current removal from the market of most IUDs. Predictably, IUDs will make a future comeback, similar difficulties may accrue, and again the most efficient atraumatic method for removal will be hysteroscopy.

The clinical applications of hysteroscopy continue to proliferate in direct proportion to the proficiency and acumen of gynecologic surgeons. Modifications and refinements in instrumentation specifically designed for intrauterine viewing have occurred. Because more therapeutic applications are performed and will undoubtedly increase with time, new technology will be required by more skilled endoscopists performing an increasing variety of therapeutic procedures by means of hysteroscopy. Although hysteroscopy at present is a practical method of examination and treatment for sundry intrauterine conditions, three major areas hold promise for simplification and expansion of the technique as a diagnostic method, and predictably will open new avenues for therapeutic applications: (1) the refinement of instrumentation and introduction of new techniques; (2) the expansion of clinical applications, both diagnostic and therapeutic; and (3) introduction of the hysteroscope to new reproductive technologies.

NEW INSTRUMENTATION AND TECHNIQUES

The introduction of small-caliber telescopes (less than 4 mm OD) in the early 1980s permitted the use of hysteroscopy as an office procedure without the need for cervical dilatation and therefore avoided trauma to the endocervical canal. This not only facilitated the procedure but also reduced the need for anesthesia. Cervical endoscopy has become a standard procedure to be used in conjunction with colposcopy. This technique will supersede blind endocervical curettage as the method of choice to evaluate the endocervix in cases of intraepithelial neoplasia. Currently, office hysteroscopy can be carried out expeditiously, safely, and without discomfort for the patient. Because of the small caliber of

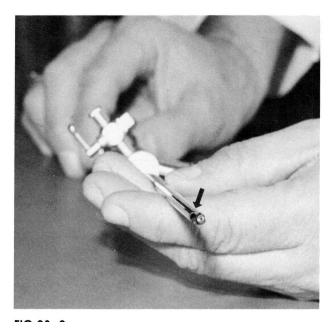

FIG 28–2.
This special operating (single-channel) hysteroscope measures 5.5 mm and permits operative procedures to be performed with minimal cervical dilatation.

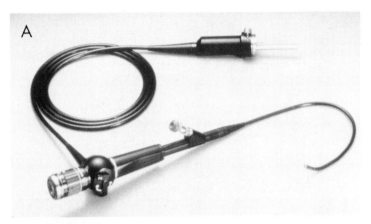

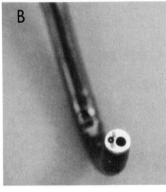

FIG 28–3.
A, small size steerable fiberoptic hysteroscope offers the advantage of entering hard-to-reach spaces within the uterus and likewise provides excellent operative access to all areas of the uterus. **B,** close-up view of steerable hysteroscope and operating channel.

the endoscope, the only practical medium for uterine distension is the CO_2 gas, which can be delivered safely by machines specifically designed for hysteroscopy. These permit electronic control of the flow of the gas and the intrauterine pressure (Figs 28–1 and 28–2).

New instruments are currently under evaluation for visualizing the uterine cavity. Flexible systems, which can be steered to observe the lateral portions of the uterus, particularly the uterotubal cones, can also deliver flexible instruments, catheters, or fibers, and be deflected by an operator-controlled positioning mechanism. These instruments are available in different sizes: the smaller instruments with a 4-mm OD for diagnostic purposes, and the larger instruments of 5-mm diameter with an operating channel. The distal tip can be deflected upward or downward at 160° to 130°. The operating channel varies from 2 to 2½ mm in diameter (Fig 28–3).

The flexibility and the steerability of the distal end allow introduction of the instrument atraumatically into uteri that are markedly anteflexed or retroflexed, and permit inspection of the cornual areas of the uterus, particularly the uterotubal junctions in those patients with acutely angulated uterotubal cones. Further, miniaturized equipment offers an alternative to direct view of the tubal openings for possible occlusion and/or inspection. Potentially, because of its extended flexibility, the small-diameter endoscope permits insertion of fibers that can help in the delivery of laser systems to areas that are difficult to reach with rigid instruments. This is particularly helpful for ablation of the endometrium or to treat laterally located lesions such as intrauterine adhesions, which are difficult to reach using rigid ancillary instruments with the present hysteroscopes. The role of these flexible endoscopes in hysteroscopy is not yet clear; nonetheless, they offer promise, particularly for the delivery of flexible fibers conducting lasers, and perhaps eventually for tubal occlusion, which was the main reason for their original introduction in gynecology.

Another innovative approach to visualization of the uterine cavity, particularly the first portion of the intramural fallopian tubes, is the use of small, flexible optical catheters from 1 to 3 mm in outer diameter, which can be inserted atraumatically and without cervical dilatation and can be illuminated with portable battery-operated units (microvasive catheters). The portable lightweight battery pack includes a focusing device and can be sterilized. Furthermore, the catheters could be used as a miniendoscope to be delivered through the standard hysteroscope. This technology is under evaluation at present (Fig 28–4,A and B). Even smaller (less than 1

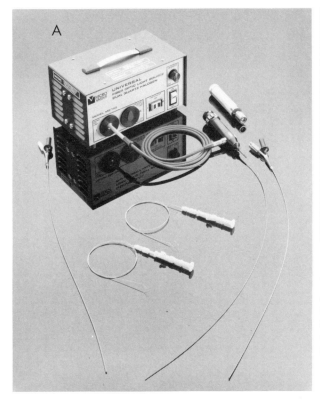

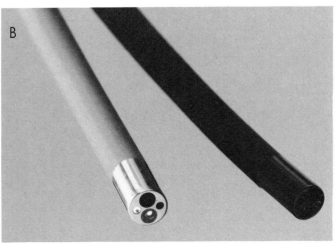

FIG 28–4.
A, flexible operating hysteroscope with a variety of endoscopic catheters and operating accessories. **B,** distal tip of endoscope seen in **A.** The optics and operating channels measure less than 4 mm in diameter. The accessory channels measure 0.9 and 0.4 mm in diameter.

mm) flexible endoscopes are being investigated in entering and exploring the oviduct. Such tiny viewing devices combined with fine laser fibers will allow intratubal surgery (Figs 28–5 through 28–7).

Video telescopes that permanently incorporate a chip-type endoscopic video camera into the construction of a high-resolution, wide-angle, 4-mm hysteroscopic telescope have several advantages over current separate-component systems. The video images produced with the new equipment, particularly when coupled to monitors with fewer than 400 resolution lines will result in pictures of substantially better quality. Since hysteroscopic surgery, particularly laser surgery will increasingly be performed by viewing the operative field through a high-resolution video monitor, the quest for improved television pictures will be unending. The video hysteroscope offers tremendous advantages insofar as sterilization is concerned. Since this is a single, completely sealed system, it can be soaked or gas sterilized with equal facility. Additionally, compared with current technology, the videoscope's camera housing will be miniaturized to a greater degree than instrumentation now available, making the overall system lighter. A single illuminating source coupled with an automatic iris and linked to the television governing system will permit single-cord operation. Farther down the road, we will witness further reduction in size of the chips that have so greatly influenced the development of videohysteroscopy. When these tiny chips are commercially available they will be placed at the terminus of flexible

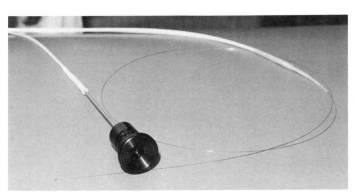

FIG 28–5.
World's smallest endoscope couples illumination and optics in a bundle measuring 400 μm.

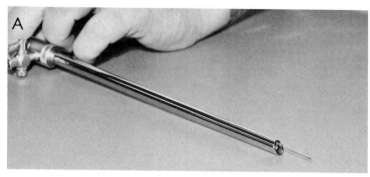

FIG 28–6.
The AIS endoscope is delivered to the ostium of the oviduct through one channel of an operating dual-channel hysteroscope. One microchip video camera is attached to a rigid 4-mm hysteroscope; another microchip camera is attached to the microendoscope's eyepiece.

fiberoptic instruments, which can be bent in a fashion similar to gastroscopes but which will enable a picture quality heretofore delivered to the monitor screen only by means of rigid instrumentation. This may also open the door for stereoscopic television surgery.

Several instruments still in the minds of endoscopists and designers are anticipated to be shown in the near future, particularly items helpful for operative hysteroscopy. As of today, we must rely on biopsy forceps, grasping forceps, miniature scissors, electrodes, probes,

and catheters. Since these manipulative tools are dependent on the sheath diameter, they are necessarily small and operations are tedious and prolonged. We expect to see these drawbacks being solved by technology employing miniature morcellators activated by hydraulic or electric systems that could easily be used for removal of submucous leiomyomas, polyps, and other mass lesions. Variations of existing technology used in other disciplines (e.g., arthroscopic shavers) could also be adapted to hysteroscopy.

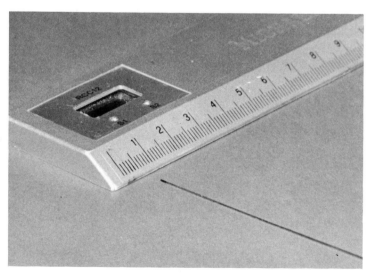

FIG 28–7.
Close-up view of the AIS microendoscope and a reference ruler.

New hysteroscopes have already been developed with multiple channels for surgery, in-flow, and out-flow. These may be particularly useful in allowing simultaneous operation with washing or aspiration, and have already proved of great value in laser applications for the ablation of the endometrium as well as other operative procedures.

The modified urologic resectoscope has been used extensively, and new modifications and adaptations of this valuable instrument are foreseen. For example, redesigning the coagulating loop so as to permit retraction without interference with vision and developing several types of interchangeable loops are expected in the near future. Smaller, safer modifications of this rather old design will enable hysteroscopic surgeons to perform more hemostatic operations and perhaps re-look at coagulative sterilization techniques in the 1990s. These coagulating instruments may be utilized for selective destructive procedures, for example, conservative therapy of uterine diverticulosis (adenomyosis) of the uterus.

NEW CLINICAL APPLICATIONS

Hysteroscopy is now used routinely by most endoscopists for the treatment of intrauterine adhesions, the division of uterine septa, and the removal of some submucous leiomyomas and polyps. In general, hysteroscopic evaluation can rule out morphologic and anatomic defects that distort the symmetry of the uterine cavity. There are, nonetheless, several other applications under evaluation that may prove to be of benefit, particularly those related to evaluation of the endometrium to assess its proper growth maturity or dysmaturity. Use of the panoramic and contact microcolpohysteroscope, facilitated by the use of biological dyes such as methylene blue, may help in the evaluation of tissues at the cellular level, and may be of assistance in predicting the normal proliferation and maturity of the endometrium. Particular interest is now developing toward a quantitative approach to the diagnosis of hormonally related bleeding problems whose extremes are well recognized, for example, anovulatory endometrial patterns and mixed endometrium. The intermediary states of these disorders have defied diagnosis and properly tuned medical therapy. Hysteroscopically directed sampling for receptor assay may provide the information necessary to tailor therapy to the disorder.

Despite sporadic attempts in the 1960s to utilize hysteroscopy for the early detection and staging of endometrial carcinoma, there is less enthusiasm for this indication than for other aspects in gynecology. None-theless, introduction of the small (less than 4 mm OD) caliber endoscopes, particularly because fractional curettage has long been known to carry significant drawbacks in the clinical staging of this disease, has caused hysteroscopy to become a more attractive evaluation method of these neoplasias. Because the prognosis is based on early diagnosis and because screening analogous to cervical Papanicolaou smears has yet to be achieved for endometrial neoplasia, new methodology is urgently required in the face of a predicted upsurge in the proportion of elderly women. The future will see the appearance of 1 to 2 mm disposable viewing devices combined with sampling brushes, which will permit easily performed, direct view sampling of the endometrial cavity.

Perhaps endometrial neoplasias may be treated by the combination of photoactive drugs interacting with laser light delivered to the uterine interior by hysteroscopes. This type of innovative, cheap therapy would only be possible for incipient neoplasia, but would obviously be highly advantageous in realizing a reduction in invasive disease. The technology for such programs is currently in the developmental phase, but research and feasibility studies will not linger far behind the emergence of the required technology. When invasive cancers are diagnosed hysteroscopy will also be useful to map lesions and permit small radiation sources, such as cesium needles, to be implanted directly into the tumor prior to hysterectomy. Clinical staging, particularly of cervical extension will be made more accurate by direct examination of the isthmus and endocervix. Perhaps preoperative plugging of the tubal ostia will be examined to determine whether dissemination of malignant cells during uterine removal can be diminished. If indeed a practical fallopian tube endoscope is produced, high-risk women might undergo regular ovarian observation and cell retrieval techniques to attempt earlier diagnosis of ovarian cancer.

Other therapeutic applications also offer a bright horizon, particularly in the use of small, portable lasers delivered through endoscopes utilizing CO_2 wave guide technology. Those laser delivery systems are currently being employed for operative laparoscopy and have the advantage of controlled penetration without backscattering. They can offer other therapeutic applications besides ablation of the endometrium. The free electron laser, the erbium-YAG laser, and the carbon monoxide laser represent only a few potential systems destined for future endoscopic applications, particularly when very fine cutting is required and thermal injury is to be minimized. Clearly the advantages of fine fiber delivery and the elimination of the thermal actions of the current laser technology will improve our future operative capabilities. Fibers with diameters of less than 300 μm could easily be delivered to the target tissue through 0.5-mm operating channels. If one were to combine these surgical tools with 2.5-mm endoscopes, the entire delivery package could measure less than 4 mm in diameter.

THE HYSTEROSCOPE APPLIED TO NEW REPRODUCTIVE TECHNOLOGIES

Because the hysteroscope offers an excellent platform to deliver instrumentation and/or substances to the fallopian tubes from the uterine side, several techniques of intratubal manipulation have been attempted, including tubal insemination and delayed postcoital testing, with evaluation of the spermatozoa directly removed from the fallopian tubes. The GIFT and/or ZIFT techniques may be modified to transfer the gametes or the zygote into the fallopian tubes from the uterine side rather than the fimbriated end. The feasibility of this approach remains to be proved. Nevertheless, utilizing the hysteroscope as a vehicle to transmit the gametes or zygote to the fallopian tube is promising, particularly because it may simplify the technique of GIFT which has proved to be successful in achieving conception for those couples otherwise unsuccessful in achieving pregnancy. It is possible with experience based on the simplification of the office hysteroscopy equipment that evaluation of the endometrium for in vitro fertilization candidates may become a routine examination to determine beforehand maturity or dysmaturity of the endometrium and predict the probability of successful implantation. Furthermore, it is tempting to believe that the transfer of the early embryo could be accomplished under careful visual control and the fertilized ova placed into the endometrium at chosen sites rather than relying on the rugged blind techniques of today.

Chorionic villus sampling by ultrasound and aspiration catheters is now a routine method of evaluation in prenatal diagnosis because of its simplicity, accuracy, and feasibility during early stages of pregnancy, with relatively quick results from the cytogeneticist. There have been attempts to use endoscopy to improve the relatively blind sampling of the chorionic villus by aspiration and to identify villi appropriate for biopsy that carry the best vascularization. This technique requires dexterity and gentleness but has proven feasible and accurate. Because of the need for and expertise in endoscopy, this technique has not achieved widespread acceptance; however, the concept remains attractive, in that the chorionic villus is selected and a biopsy sample obtained with little or no disturbance of the surrounding tissue,

particularly the amnion. Ultrasound scans by vaginal probes have offered increased advantages to the gynecologist. One could imagine intrauterine ultrasonographic probes directed to various sites by guidance systems. This technique might find important application for studying the embryo or young fetus and allowing early diagnosis of malformations. Additionally, these techniques could be utilized for intrauterine fetal surgery.

The future of hysteroscopy is promising, and we can foresee that the present diagnostic and therapeutic indications will not only consolidate but also expand to replace many other procedures still performed by gynecologists, such as curettage of the uterus, hysterotomies to remove submucous leiomyomas, blind division of intrauterine adhesions, and abdominal metroplasties to treat the septate uterus. The last mentioned procedure will without doubt be relegated to historical reviews as gynecologists gain proficiency and confidence in the utilization of hysteroscopy. Hysteroscopic examinations in the office will encompass all diagnostic procedures, and with the advance in instrumentation and portable units as well as in lasers, many operative procedures will eventually be performed in ambulatory units with the patient under local anesthesia. Most gynecologists now finishing their postgraduate training are being trained to use hysteroscopy in a manner analogous to laparoscopy and it is not overly optimistic to predict in the near future that all gynecologists will be able to perform diagnostic and therapeutic hysteroscopy.

In less than 2 decades, modern hysteroscopy has evolved rapidly to be a practical method for the evaluation of the uterine cavity with well-established indications. As the use of hysteroscopy increases and more practitioners utilize the technique for diagnostic or therapeutic reasons, new instrumentation and operations will evolve, and will simplify not only diagnostic examinations but also difficult and complex surgical interventions. Flexible endoscopes are being tested for possible use in the uterine cavity, and operative hysteroscopes with practical inflow and outflow accessory channels have been introduced. The accessory operative instrumentation has also been expanded and refined, and portable units for office examinations have been developed. The trend in the development of instrumentation is to provide small-diameter hysteroscopes equipped with high-resolution lenses and with wide fields of view, together with adequate accessory channels.

The future of hysteroscopy is assured. The day is not far off when this procedure will occupy the same preeminent position in gynecology as cystoscopy holds in urology.

BIBLIOGRAPHY

Baggish MS: New instruments and techniques for hysteroscopy. *Contemp Obstet Gynecol Technol* 1984; pp 67–83.

Baggish MS, Baltoyannis P, Badawy S, et al: Carbon dioxide laser laparoscopy performed with a flexible fiber in humans. *Am J Obstet Gynecol* 1987; 157:1129.

Bordt J, Belkien L, Vancaillie T, et al: Ergebnisse Diagnostischer Hysteroskopien in einem IVF/ET - Program. *Geburtshilfe Frauenheilkd* 1984; 44:813.

Brueschke EE, Wilbanks GD: A steerable fiberoptic hysteroscope. *Obstet Gynecol* 1974; 44:273.

Chorionic villus sampling. Diagnostic and therapeutic technology assessment (DATTA). A report from 31 physicians' panelists. *JAMA* 1987; 258:3560.

Confino E, Friberg J, Gleicher N: Transcervical balloon tuboplasty. *Fertil Steril* 1986; 46:963.

Cornier E: Interet de la fibroscopie uterine souple. *Contraception-Fertilite-Sexualite* 1984; 12:891.

Cornier E: La fibro-hysteroscopie operatoire souple. Technique, indications, premiers resultats. *Gynecologie* 1984; 35:281.

Daniell JF, Miller W: Hysteroscopic correction of cornual occlusion with resultant term pregnancy. *Fertil Steril* 1987; 48:490.

DeCherney AH: Anything you can do I can do better . . . or differently. *Fertil Steril* 1987; 48:374.

Fayez JA, Muttie G, Schneider PJ: The diagnostic value of hysterosalpingography and hysteroscopy in infertility investigation. *Am J Obstet Gynecol* 1987; 156:558.

Ghirardini G, Camurri L, Gualerzi C, et al: Chorionic villi sampling by means of a new endoscopic device, in Fraccaro M, et al (eds): *First Trimester Fetal Diagnosis,* Berlin, Springer-Verlag, 1985; pp 54–59.

Gustavii B: Direct vision technique for chorionic villi sampling in 100 diagnostic cases, in Fraccaro M, et al (eds): *First Trimester Fetal Diagnosis.* Berlin, Springer-Verlag, 1985, pp 46–50.

Hamou J: Microhysteroscopy. A new procedure and its original applications in gynecology. *J Reprod Med* 1981; 26:375.

Lindemann HJ: *Atlas der Hysteroskopie.* Stuttgart, Gustav Fisher Verlag, 1980, pp 33–35.

Lindemann HJ: Pneumometra fur die Hysteroskopie. *Geburtshilfe Frauenheilkd* 1973; 33:18.

March CM, Israel R, March AD: Hysteroscopic management of intrauterine adhesions. *Am J Obstet Gynecol* 1978; 131:539.

Mencaglia L: Hysteroscopy and gamete transfer: New modalities. Presented at the Third World Congress and Workshop of Hysteroscopy, Miami Beach, Florida, January 15–18, 1987.

Mencaglia L, Perino A, Hamou J: Hysteroscopy in perimenohot6pausal and postmenopausal women with abnormal uterine bleeding. *J Reprod Med* 1987; 32:577.

Mencaglia L, Tantini C, Colafranceschi M, et al: Hysteroscopic evaluation of precancerous endometrial lesions, in van der Pas H, van Herendael B, van Lith D, et al (eds): *Hysteroscopy.* Boston, MTP Press Limited, 1983, pp 129–132.

Menken FC: Endoscopic observations of endocrine processes and hormonal changes, in Albrecht FR, Sanchez JR, Willowitzer H (eds): *Simposio Esteroides Saxuales.* Berlin, Saladruck, 1969, pp 276–281.

Nordenskjold F, Gustatvii B: Direct-vision chorionic villi biopsy for prenatal diagnosis in first trimester. *J Reprod Med* 1984; 29:572.

Parent B, Guedj H, Barbot J, et al: *Panoramic Hysteroscopy.* Paris, Maloine S.A., 1985 (translated edition distributed by Williams & Wilkins, Baltimore, 1987).

Quinones-Guerrero R, Alvarado-Duran A, Aznar-Ramos R: Tubal catheterization: Applications of a new technique. *Am J Obstet Gynecol* 1972; 114:674.

Savino L, Scarselli G, Branconi F, et al: Usefulness of hysteroscopy in endometrial adenocarcinoma staging. *Eur J Gynaecol Oncol* 1982; 3:210.

Schellhas JH, Schnieder DF: Hematoporphyrin derivative photo-radiation therapy applied in gynecology. *Colposcopy Gynecol Laser Surg* 1986; 2:53.

Siegler AM, Kemmann E: Location and removal of misplaced or embedded intra-uterine devices by hysteroscopy. *J Reprod Med* 1976; 16:139.

Sugimoto O: Diagnostic and therapeutic hysteroscopy management of intrauterine adhesions. *Am J Obstet Gynecol* 1978; 131:539.

Sulak PJ, Letterine GS, Hayslip CC, et al: Hysteroscopic cannulation and lavage in the treatment of proximal tubal occlusion. *Fertil Steril* 1987; 48:493.

Taylor PJ, Hamou JE: Hysteroscopy. *J Reprod Med* 1983; 28:359.

Valle RF: Hysteroscopic evaluation of patients with abnormal uterine bleeding. *Surg Gynecol Obstet* 1981; 153:521.

Valle RF: Hysteroscopic removal of intrauterine devices with missing filaments. *Obstet Gynecol* 1977; 49:55.

Valle RF: Hysteroscopy in the evaluation of female infertility. *Am J Obstet Gynecol* 1978; 131:425.

Valle RF, Sciarra JJ: Current status of hyteroscopy in gynecologic practice. *Fertil Steril* 1979; 32:619.

Index